PROLACTIN : PHYSIOLOGY
AND CLINICAL SIGNIFICANCE

PROLACTIN : PHYSIOLOGY
AND CLINICAL SIGNIFICANCE

David F. Horrobin, M.A., D.Phil., B.M., B.Ch.
Reader in Physiology, The Medical School,
University of Newcastle upon Tyne, England.

Springer-Science+Business Media, B.V.

ISBN 978-0-85200-065-6   ISBN 978-94-010-9695-9 (eBook)
DOI 10.1007/978-94-010-9695-9

The Blackburn Times Press

SBN 852 000 65 0

CONTENTS

1. Introduction

SECTION A :
PHYSIOLOGY AND PATHOPHYSIOLOGY OF PROLACTIN

2. Isolation, structure and cells of origin
3. Assay of prolactin
4. Biochemistry and effects on metabolism
5. Effects of metabolic and environmental stimuli on prolactin secretion
6. Control of prolactin secretion
7. Prolactin in male and female reproduction
8. Pregnancy
9. Lactation
10. Prolactin and thyroid function
11. Prolactin and cancer
12. Prolactin and fluid and electrolyte balance and the cardiovascular system
13. Other effects of prolactin

SECTION B :
PROLACTIN AND HUMAN DISEASE

14. Introduction. Hormones and disease
15. Tests of the prolactin secreting system
16. Drugs which alter prolactin secretion
17. Puerperal lactation and galactorrhea
18. Premenstrual syndrome and pregnancy toxemia
19. Disorders of fluid and electrolyte balance
20. Nephrotic syndrome
21. Thyroid disease
22. Adrenal disease

SECTION C :
HYPOTHESIS

PREFACE

I first became interested in prolactin a little over two years ago. I was then
working in Nairobi and I knew nothing about the hormone apart from its role
in lactation. Professor Mohammed Hyder of the Department of Zoology in the
University of Nairobi was interested in the endocrine mechanisms which enable
Tilapia fish to adapt to water with a very high electrolyte content. He invited
me to a seminar given by Professor Howard Bern which was largely concerned
with the role prolactin plays in fluid and electrolyte balance in sub-mammalian
vertebrates. This inspired me to begin a programme of research into the roles
prolactin plays in man and other animals.

Very few physiologists or clinicians seem aware of the multifarious effects of
prolactin in mammals. This book therefore aims to give a comprehensive account
of the mammalian physiology of prolactin and to make suggestions about its
possible role in diseases ranging from cancer to mental illness. The two subjects
which have been previously widely covered, the roles of prolactin in lactation
and in rat mammary cancer, are presented relatively briefly though with a full
list of references. Other subjects are dealt with more extensively and I hope that
many research workers and clinicians may find the book helpful.

The ideas presented have been extensively discussed with my colleagues,
notably Peter Burstyn, Ieuan Lloyd and M.S. Manku, and I should like to
record here my gratitude to them. I should also like to thank my secretary,
Mrs. Pat Haselhurst for working so hard on this book.

David F. Horrobin
Newcastle upon Tyne
May 1973

Chapter 1

INTRODUCTION

Until very recently, interest in mammalian prolactin was confined to those with a specific concern for reproductive physiology. Scientists dealing with non-mammalian vertebrates were aware of a much wider spectrum of action. There is some evidence that phylogenetically a form of prolactin may be the oldest pituitary hormone and in view of this it is not surprising that it has widespread effects on many tissues. It seems to be of particular importance in osmoregulation and is the hormone which permits species like the eel and the salmon to move from sea water to fresh and vice-versa: it regulates salt gland function in birds and helps to control fluid and electrolyte movements in the anuran bladder. In amphibians particularly, it has important effects on maturation, stimulating the growth of larval structures by blocking the effects of TSH on the thyroid gland and of thyroxine on the tissues. In a number of species it shows interactions with other hormones either facilitating or inhibiting their target organ effects. As in mammals, in the non-mammals it is a major reproductive hormone with important actions on reproductive behavior and reproductive physiology, particularly in connection with mechanisms for ensuring adequate nutrition of the young. (Bern, Nicoll, 1968: Meites, Nicoll, 1966: Nicoll, Bryant, 1972: Turkington, 1972d.)

In the past decade there has been an explosion of interest in the effects of mammalian prolactin. The themes have been largely those which might have been predicted from a knowledge of its functions in non-vertebrates. Prolactin has been shown to modify the actions of a large number of mammalian hormones including LH, FSH, insulin, estrogens, cortisol, thyroid hormones, progesterone, aldosterone, ADH, erythropoietin and ACTH. It has been shown to control some aspects of fluid and electrolyte metabolism. It is a hormone of major importance in mammalian reproduction and as well as its well known effects in lactation it may have roles in the estrous and menstrual cycles, in pregnancy and in male reproduction. Two themes which might not have been predicted from its role in the non-mammals are its possible roles in both the initiation and prevention of cancer and in mental disease

Introduction

In the past three years interest in human prolactin has grown rapidly, following the increasingly convincing demonstration that human prolactin is an entity distinct from growth hormone. The development of radioimmunoassays has set the seal on this demonstration and the stage is now set for exploration of its role in human physiology and disease. There are already indications that it may be involved in a wide spectrum of illnesses whose mechanisms have up to now been obscure.

Although several volumes of symposium and conference proceedings and monographs on particular aspects of prolactin biology have been published in recent years there has been no systematic review of its overall physiology and no attempt to relate aspects of this physiology to clinical problems. This book is such an attempt and such is the growth of this area of research that 1973 may well be the last date when a volume like this could be attempted by a single author. The book strictly confines itself to mammalian and human species. It is divided into three very different sections:

A.   *Review of prolactin physiology.* This is a strictly factual account and I have attempted to keep all speculation, personal or otherwise, out of this section. It covers papers which were listed in the Index Medicus under the heading of prolactin up to and including December, 1972. Papers appearing later than this in some journals which carry many reports on prolactin are also included. A list of most of the papers consulted is to be found in the bibliography. This is relatively complete from 1960 onwards and includes selected papers before that date. Papers not listed have for the most part been unobtainable by me and all those which are listed have been personally consulted. The bibliography is in alphabetical order as this seems to be the most generally useful form. This does, however, make a system of numbered references difficult to operate as the addition of a single reference may then require extensive alterations throughout the text. I have therefore decided to quote authors' names in full in the text. This too leads to problems as the text can become difficult to read when long lists of names come between every successive sentence. In order to allow the book to be read smoothly all the references supplying information dealt with in a particular paragraph or section are listed in alphabetical order at the end of that paragraph or section. It is my impression that only a very small proportion of people reading any one paragraph will actually want to identify and look up the references with which the paragraph deals. Since the titles of the papers are given in full in the bibliography, it should be relatively easy for someone who does want to locate a particular reference to do so. The majority who do not want to look up the references will be able to read smoothly and continuously. I am aware that my opinions on this matter may not be shared by other scientists and I would appreciate their comments so that, if necessary, the system may be changed in the next edition. I have made no attempt whatsoever to get involved in priority disputes: since prior publication is no guarantee of prior discovery a reader who is not intimately involved in the matter cannot hope to know the truth.

B. *Application of knowledge of prolactin to human disease.* This section attempts to assess the possible roles of prolactin in human illness. Its aim is to show what we now know and to point out possible future lines of research. It includes speculation by others and by myself and should be of particular interest to the clinician. It discusses the possibilities that prolactin may be involved in many conditions apart from the obvious galactorrhea. These include the pre-menstrual syndrome, cancer of various organs, migraine, asthma, myocardial infarction and other forms of thrombo-embolic disease, and mental illness.

C. *Hypothesis.* This is an attempt to draw together the various concepts of the role of prolactin discussed in sections A and B, and to use them to develop a unifying hypothesis of the role of prolactin in human biology.

Because of a clear understanding on the part of the publishers of the importance of rapid publication of this type of volume, this book will be available within six weeks of delivery of the final typescript. Inevitably this means that some of the normally leisurely proof reading processes will be more hastily carried out and that there may be more minor errors than usual in a printed work. However, we believe that rapid production is more important than the final elimination of relatively insignificant errors. We hope that readers will also agree but either I or the publishers would welcome reactions from readers to this approach.

Section A: Physiology and Pathophysiology of Prolactin

Chapter 2

ISOLATION, STRUCTURE AND
CELLS OF ORIGIN

Ovine prolactin was prepared in a relatively pure form in the 1930's and is now readily available in relatively large quantities. The modern preparations contain very little, if any, growth hormone but freedom from such contamination cannot yet be guaranteed. Almost all studies of the effects of prolactin in mammals have used ovine prolactin preparations. Small amounts of pure prolactin from other sources, notably rats, mice, cattle, monkeys and humans have also been obtained but usually in quantities necessary for the development of radioimmunoassays rather than for studying the effects of exogenously administered hormone. (Bryant, Greenwood, 1968: Cheever, Seavey, Lewis, 1969: Chrambach, Bridson, Turkington, 1971: Friesen, Guyda, Hardy, 1970: Guyda, Friesen, 1971: Lewis, Singh, Seavey, 1972: Meites, Kahn, Nicoll, 1961: Reisfield, Tong, Riches, Brink Steelman, 1961: Schams, Karg, 1970: Sinha, Selby, Lewis, Vanderlaan, 1972: White, 1949.)

Human prolactin and growth hormone

Human pituitary prolactin has proved very elusive and for a time there were serious doubts as to its separate existence. It was suggested that in man its role might be shared between growth hormone and placental lactogen and that most studies of so-called prolactin in man were in fact studies of growth hormone. Since growth hormone has lactogenic activity and prolactin has somatotrophic activity the problem could not be resolved with certainty by bioassay techniques.

It now appears that much of the difficulty arose from the fact that relatively small amounts of prolactin are stored in the human pituitary and much of the prolactin that is there seems to disappear within a short time after death, possibly because of lysosomal destruction. This problem was largely surmounted by the development of techniques for the culture in vitro of monkey and human pituitary glands taken from both fetuses and mature individuals. The human fetal pituitary has been reported to begin prolactin secretion as early as five weeks after conception. (Brauman, Brauman, Pasteels, 1964: Friesen, Guyda, 1971: Friesen, Guyda, Hwang,

1971: Gala, 1971: Hwang, Friesen, Hardy, Wilensky, 1971: Lewis, Singh, Seavey, 1971: Nicoll, Parsons, Fiorindo, Nichols, Sakuma, 1970: Pasteels, 1963: 1972b: Pasteels, Brauman, Brauman, 1963: Siler, Morgenstern, Greenwood, 1972.)

The crucial factor in the proof of a difference between human growth hormone and prolactin was the development of a radioimmunoassay for the former. It rapidly became apparent that in dwarfs lactation could occur in the absence of growth hormone and that in normal lactating individuals there was no parallelism between growth hormone levels measured by RI assay and prolactin levels estimated by bioassay. In patients with acromegaly and in those with galactorrhea there was also often a clear dissociation between plasma lactogenic activity and growth hormone levels measured by radioimmunoassay. Furthermore, while in some types of patients such as some acromegalics, antisera to growth hormone could remove most of the lactogenic activity, in most cases lactogenic activity was completely or partially unaffected. Finally when pituitaries were maintained in culture, growth hormone secretion declined while prolactin secretion increased. (References to previous paragraph plus Forsyth, Myres, 1971: Frantz, Klienberg, 1970: Frantz, Kleinberg, Noel, 1972: Guyda, Hwang, Friesen, 1971: Hwang, Guyda, Friesen, 1972: Nichol, Blair, Nichols, Russell, Taylor, 1972: Nicoll, Parsons, Fiorindo, 1969: Peake, McKeel, Jarrett, Daughaday, 1969: Rimoin, Holzman, Merimee, Rabinowitz, Barnes, Tyson, McKusick, 1968.)

The development of effective radioimmunoassays for human prolactin (discussed in the next chapter) has finally put an end to the idea that human growth hormone and prolactin may be identical.

Prolactin structure

The primary structures of human growth hormone, human placental lactogen and ovine and bovine prolactins have now been published. Although the workers in this field continue to dispute about details, there can be little doubt that these structures are substantially correct. All the hormones contain about 190 amino acid residues and have molecular weights somewhere in the region of 22,000 Approximately 80% of the residues are shared between human growth hormone and placental lactogen whereas the pituitary prolactins share only about 20% of the residues with growth hormone. This emphasises the difference between prolactin and growth hormone. Prolactin seems to be the most potent lactogenic hormone but both growth hormone and placental lactogen also have substantial lactogenic activity. In contrast, placental lactogen is only 10-20% as active as human growth hormone in promoting growth as shown by the rat tibia test: in this same test pituitary prolactin has virtually no activity. It is probable that tertiary structure of the hormones is not required for activity, since both human growth hormone and placental lactogen may be oxidised with performic acid without major loss of biological activity. Partial enzymic digestion of the hormones may also be carried out with retention of biological potency suggesting that the latter may be determined by relatively small parts of the molecule. (Belanger, Shome, Friesen, Myers, 1971: Bewley, Li, 1970, 1971, 1972: Li, 1969, 1972: Li, Dixon, Chung, 1971: Li, Dixon, Liu, 1969: Li, Dixon, Lo, Schmidt, Pankou, 1970: Li, Yamashiro, 1970: Niall, 1971, 1972: Seavey, Lewis, 1971: Sherwood, 1967, 1971: Sherwood, Handwerger, McLaurin, 1972: Sherwood, Handwerger, McLaurin, Lanner, 1971: Sherwood, Handwerger, McLaurin, Pang, 1972: Wallis, 1971.)

Within the prolactin molecule itself there appear to be four main areas of internal homology. This suggests that prolactin may have evolved from a much shorter primitive polypeptide by means of two successive reduplications. Since prolactin-type molecules are found even in the more primitive vertebrates while growth hormone and placental lactogen are later developments, it is possible that the last two molecules evolved from prolactin. (Niall, Hogan, Sauer, Rosenblum, Greenwood, 1971.)

The structure of human prolactin has yet to be determined but the fact that some radioimmunoassay procedures based on ovine prolactin cross react with human prolactin but not significantly with growth hormone suggests that prolactin from humans is closely related to that from the sheep. (Jacobs, Bauman, Daughaday, 1971: L'Hermite, Stauric, Robyn, 1972: L'Hermite, Delvoye, Nokin, Vekemans, Robyn, 1972.)

Cellular origin

Our knowledge of the cellular origin of prolactin derives largely from work done by Belgian scientists. In the rat, guinea pig, monkey and human, specific prolactin secreting cells distinct from growth hormone secreting cells (somatotropes) have been identified by both histological staining and fluorescent antibody techniques. Somatotropes stain with orange G and fluoresce with antibodies to growth hormone while prolactin secreting cells may be identified by Herlant's stain and by their binding of fluorescent anti-prolactin antibodies. (Herbert, Hayashida, 1970:

Herlant, Pasteels, 1967: Pasteels, 1963, 1972: Pasteels, Brauman, Brauman, 1963: Pasteels, Gausset, Danguy, Ectors, 1972: Pasteels, Gausset, Danguy, Ectors, Nicoll, Varavudhi, 1972: Vodian, 1970.)

Prolactin secretion from cultured human fetal pituitaries has been observed as early as five weeks after conception but prolactin secreting cells have not been identified until four months gestation. They then increase progressively until parturition. They may be difficult to identify in children and young males but can be readily seen in women of reproductive age. During pregnancy, hyperplasia and/or hypertrophy begins at about the third month and is very marked at term. Some atrophy seems to occur with age but does not occur in patients who have been ovariectomised without hormone replacement. Hypertrophied pituitary cells have been seen in people dying with hepatic cirrhosis and severe untreated myxedema and in those on estrogen, progestin, or testosterone therapy. Adrenal steroid treatment or adrenalectomy had no obvious effect. The prolactin cells tend to be arranged peripherally and adjacent to the neural lobe. Electron microscopy has shown release of granules in response to suckling and apparent lysosomal destruction and digestion of granules at the termination of lactation or following treatment with ergot alkaloids. Maturation of secretory granules has also been observed in lactating rats. Removal of the litter for twelve hours caused a marked increase in the number of mature granules while return of the litter for 15 minutes led to very marked granule extrusion. (Pasteels, 1972: Pasteels, Gausset, Danguy, Ectors, 1972: Shiino, Williams, Rennels, 1972: Siler, Morgenstern, Greenwood, 1972.)

In spite of all the evidence for separate growth hormone and prolactin secreting cells, there are two reports which suggest that at least some pituitary cells may secrete both hormones. Cytoplasmic secretory granules have been isolated from bovine pituitaries. Acidophilic granules contained only growth hormone and prolactin. Lighter granules with a diameter of 250-300 mμ contained growth hormone almost exclusively while heavier granules (diameter about 450 mμ) seemed to contain a mixture of growth hormone and prolactin Growth hormone seemed to occur only as a monomer while prolactin was found in both monomer and polymer forms. In another species, the rat, a clonal strain of cells derived from a pituitary tumor was found to be capable of secreting both prolactin and growth hormone. Thus while it seems very likely that separate prolactin and growth hormone secreting cells exist, the possibility that there is a population of cells which secretes both cannot be excluded. (La Bella, Krass, Fritz, Vivian, Shin, Queen, 1971: Tashjian, Bancroft, Levine, 1097.)

Effects of cyclic AMP and the ionic environment

Several investigators have studied the actions of the ionic environment and of cyclic AMP in cultured pituitaries. Glands cultured in media similar to Krebs-Ringer bicarbonate buffer and inoculated with ^{3}H-leucine release most of the labelled prolactin into the medium but retain labelled growth hormone in the gland. Replacing the bicarbonate with phosphate causes retention in the gland of prolactin as well as growth hormone. Removal of potassium or calcium ions from the medium greatly reduces synthesis and release of prolactin with the effect on release being apparently greater. Elevation of calcium concentration stimulates synthesis and release of prolactin but not growth hormone while elevation of potassium concentration stimulates growth hormone synthesis and release but has no effect on prolactin. Raising both potassium and calcium concentrations elevates secretion of both hormones. Studies on prolactin in culture may be complicated by the presence of several pools of the hormone within the gland. (MacLeod, Fentham, 1970: MacLeod, Lehmeyer, 1972: Parsons, 1969, 1970: Parsons, Nicoll, 1971: Swearingen, 1971: Wakabayashi, Arimura, Schally, 1972.)

Cyclic AMP causes secretion of prolactin from cultured pituitary glands within a matter of minutes. Theophylline also causes prolactin secretion apparently by a cyclic AMP mediated mechanism. The main action seems to be on release of preformed prolactin rather than on synthesis, and extrusion of secretory granules can be observed. Cyclic AMP stimulates the secretion of growth hormone as well as of prolactin. (Bowers, 1971: Lemay, Labrie, 1972: Nagasawa, Yanai, 1972: Pelletier, Lemay, Beraud, Labrie, 1972.)

Chapter 3

ASSAY OF PROLACTIN

The assay of prolactin has improved rapidly in recent years and reliable forms of both bioassay and radioimmunoassay are now available. There is a tendency to dismiss bioassay because of the greater sensitivity and capacity of RI assay techniques but there will always be a need to control and to check RI assays with reliable bioassays. One form of bioassay for which there is an urgent need and which has not yet been devised for any hormone is an assay of the effectiveness of prolactin in the individual whose body fluids are being sampled. As well as knowing that the concentration of prolactin in a fluid is X ng/ml we want to be able to know what effect X ng/ml will have in that individual. The dramatic variability in individual response to a standard exogenous dose of any hormone indicates that X ng/ml in individual A may have quite different effects from Xng/ml in individual B. What is required is some form of biological activity coefficient by which a hormone concentration could be multiplied in order to give a measure of the biologically active concentration in any one individual.

Bioassay of prolactin in blood

Since both growth hormone and placental lactogen have lactogenic activity and since all bioassays in use employ either the pigeon crop sac or the mammary gland as a target organ, bioassay results can be said to be specific for pituitary prolactin only if the fluid to be tested is previously neutralised with an antiserum to growth hormone and, when appropriate, an antiserum to placental lactogen. Alternatively, growth hormone and placental lactogen levels may be simultaneously measured by radioimmunoassay.

Until recently the pigeon crop sac assay was the standard prolactin assay but it suffered from a lack of sensitivity and a susceptibility to false positive results occurring because of an inflammatory response to the fluid being assayed. The use of steroids minimises inflammation but even so the value of this assay in a modern laboratory is doubtful, even if only because workers using RI assays and other bioassays are likely to disbelieve the results! (Apostolakis, 1968: Berswordt-Wallrabe, Herlyn, Flaskamp, Hellige, 1971: Berswordt-Wallrabe,

Herlyn, Jantzen, 1965: Lyons, Page, 1935: Meites, Nicoll, 1966: Nicoll, 1967, 1969.)

A number of in vivo tests have been used in mammals but are difficult to make specific because of the problem of endogenous hormone production. They include local mammary development after intraductal administration of the test fluid to estrogen or HCG - primed rabbits and the histological examination of mammary glands in estrogen-primed rats after sub-cutaneous injection of the test material (mammotropic index). (Sulman, 1971.)

Because of the difficulties of in vivo testing, recently bioassay technology has concentrated on the development of in vitro tests. Four such assays have gained acceptance as being relatively reliable. Two use histological methods with an assessment of the cellular development and amount of alveolar secretion in portions of mammary gland maintained in culture. One of these uses culture of the mid-pregnant mouse mammary gland and the other the pseudopregnant rabbit gland. (Forsyth, 1970, 1972: Forsyth, Edwards, 1972: Forsyth, Myres, 1971: Frantz, Kleinberg, 1970: Frantz, Kleinberg, Noel, 1972a, 1972b: Kleinberg, Frantz, 1971.)

The other two assays use biochemical endpoints and employ the mid-pregnant mouse mammary gland. One depends on the prolactin-stimulated incorporation of ^{32}P into casein and the other utilises the induction of the activity of the enzyme N-acetyllactosamine synthetase which catalyses the following reaction

N-acetylglucosamine + UDP-galactose $\longrightarrow$ N-acetyllactosamine + UDP

All four of these modern bioassays can detect prolactin activity in pregnancy, in lactating women and in situations such as galactorrhea where prolactin levels are abnormally elevated. They are, however, rather complex to carry out and cannot reliably measure activity in normal males or non-pregnant, non-lactating females. The published versions of the biochemical assays have used male "normal" plasma as a diluent and in view of the demonstration by radio-immunoassay that prolactin levels in male plasma may vary considerably from individual to individual, this procedure will need to be revised. (Loewenstein, Mariz, Peake, Daughaday, 1971: Turkington, 1971a.)

Radioimmunoassay of prolactin in blood

The major difficulty with radioimmunoassay is the preparation of highly purified
hormones for iodination and the raising of antisera. Good materials are now
available for rat and mouse radioimmunoassay and the materials for one form of
the rat assay are available in kit form from the National Institute of Arthritis and
Metabolic Diseases, Bethesda, Maryland, U.S.A. (Cheever, Seavey, Lewis, 1969:
Dilley, 1966: Kwa, Gala, 1972: Kwa, Verhofstad, 1967, Neill, Reichert, 1971:
Sinha, Selby, Lewis, Vanderlaan, 1972.)

The domestic animals are also well catered for. Sheep and goats can apparently
share the same assay, while a separate bovine assay has been developed. (Bryant,
Greenwood, 1968: Bryant, Linzell, Greenwood, 1970: Davis, Reichart, Niswender,
1971: Fell, Beck, Brown, Cumming, Goding, 1972: Hart, 1972: Kann, 1971:
McNeilly, 1971: Schams, Karg, 1970.)

The main problems have arisen with human prolactin because of the lack of
availability of adequate amounts of pure hormone of adult human origin. In an
attempt to get round this prolactins from a number of sources including cultured
fetal pituitaries, monkeys, sheep, and pigs, and a denatured form of placental
lactogen have all been used either for ^{131}I labelling or for raising antisera. The
striking thing is that almost all studies using these different preparations are in
broad agreement as to the situations in which prolactin levels may be elevated
and as to the stimuli and drugs which may change prolactin levels. Unfortunately,
as was dramatically pointed out by Cotes, when the various assays are applied
to the same plasma sample there is appallingly little agreement as to the absolute
levels of hormone present. Estimates ranged from 0 to 171 mamp equiv/ml.
It is therefore safe to conclude that while the present assays may be
internally relatively self consistent and valuable for discovering differences in
prolactin levels between populations and in individuals subjected to changing
conditions, they cannot yet be employed with certainty for the assessment of
absolute levels. A central source of adequate amounts of human prolactin for
both iodination and the raising of antisera is urgently required in order to
allow comparison of results from different laboratories. (Bryant, Greenwood, 1972:
Bryant, Siler, Greenwood, Pasteels, Robyn, Hubinont, 1971: Cotes, 1972:
Frantz, Kleinberg, Noel, 1972b: Friesen, Belanger, Guyda, Hwang, 1972:
Friesen, Hwang, Guyda, Tolis, Tyson, Myers, 1972: Greenwood, 1972: Greenwood,
Siler, Bryant, Morgenstern, 1972: Josimovich, Boccella, Levitt, 1971: L'Hermite,

Stauric, Robyn, 1972: L.Hermite, Delvoye, Nokin, Vekemans, Robyn, 1972: Hwang, Guyda, Friesen, 1971: Jacobs, Mariz, Daughaday, 1972.)

Assay of prolactin in other body fluids

The older bioassays have been employed to measure prolactin in urine but as yet neither the newer bioassays nor the radioimmunoassays have been used for this purpose. There is a tendency to look down upon urinary estimations as a poor man's plasma assay but when a hormone like prolactin is involved which shows large fluctuations in plasma level during a 24-hour cycle and which has a very short half-life, the assay of the amount in a 24-hour specimen of urine may have considerable value. It can supply information which a single plasma sample cannot. Since plasma sampling every 10-15 minutes throughout a 24-hour period is not a practical clinical procedure, a 24-hour urine sample may be the next best simple estimate of prolactin secretion. The value of this approach has already been proved with cortisol and a radioimmunoassay applicable to urine is therefore urgently required. (Dilley, 1966: Fraser, Spicer, Williams, Young, 1961: Fujii, Uruta, 1965: Ivanteeva, 1963: Lyons, 1937: Mitsuda, 1965: Vilar, Alvarez, Davidson, Mancini, 1964.)

Radioimmunoassay techniques have been applied to the measurement of prolactin in human milk and amniotic fluid. (Friesen, Hwang, Guyda, Tolis, Tyson, Myers, 1972: Friesen, 1972c.)

Chapter 4

BIOCHEMISTRY AND
EFFECTS ON METABOLISM

Although prolactin appears to have widespread metabolic actions, the only target
organ which has been extensively studied from a biochemical point of view is
the mammary gland. This chapter will discuss those aspects of mammary prolactin
biochemistry which seem likely to be generally applicable. The specific actions
of prolactin on the mammary gland which are peculiar to that gland will be
discussed in the chapter on lactation.

Prolactin in blood

There is very little evidence about the form in which prolactin is transported in
the plasma but it seems possible that it travels as the free molecule unbound to
anything else. The main evidence for this is that the immunoreactive prolactin
present in sheep plasma fractionates on Sephadex and in sucrose density gradients
as a single peak which appears identical to the peak observed with freshly
dissolved ovine prolactin. (Bryant, Greenwood, 1968.)

There is no evidence as to the precise mechanism of prolactin metabolism
but it does seem to be bound by the liver and it is widely assumed to be inactivated
there. Its inactivation is very rapid. In the human its half-life seems to be in the
region of 15-20 minutes and similar results have been obtained in rabbits and cattle.
In all species studied peaks of prolactin in the plasma are followed by falls which
indicate a short half-life. (Birkinshaw, Falconer, 1972: Friesen, Hwang, Guyda,
Tolis, Tyson, Myers, 1972: Schams, Karg, 1970: Turkington, 1972b.)

Metabolic clearances have been most extensively studied in rats. Two or more
phases have been identified, the half-life of the first major one ranging from 2-12
minutes. When bovine prolactin was administered to untreated adult rats the half-
life for the first phase was 6 minutes. Treatment with a low estrogen dose lowered
this to 3 minutes and with a high estrogen dose to 2 minutes. (Grosvenor, 1967:
Koch, Chow, Meites, 1971: Kwa, Feltkamp, Van der Gugten, Verhofstad, 1970:
Watson, Krulich, McCann, 1971.)

13

Prolactin receptors

The identification of tissues to which prolactin is bound can form a good starting point for a biochemical study. Several groups have labelled prolactin with [125] I and after injection into animals have sought for sites where it is preferentially taken up and bound. Not surprisingly there is no doubt that mammary glands take up the hormone and do so more avidly in the pregnant and lactating states than in non-pregnant individuals. Other organs which seem to have specific prolactin receptors are the ovary, uterus, liver, kidney, cerebral cortex and seminal vesicle. Under the experimental conditions spleen, lung, heart, testis and prostate did not specifically bind prolactin and other tissues do not appear to have been studied as yet. Remarkably, the half-life of the labelled prolactin in rabbit mammary tissue was fifty hours indicating that a single brief pulse of prolactin secretion, detectable in the plasma for only half an hour or so, may have a tissue action persisting for several days. (Birkinshaw, Falconer, 1972: Shani, Givant, Sulman, Eshkol, Lunenfeld, 1972: Turkington, Frantz, 1972.)

Molecular biology of prolactin

The fundamental actions of prolactin on cellular biochemistry using the mammary gland as a model have been worked out in a long series of complex papers by Turkington and co-workers. The initial process is the binding of prolactin to the mammary cell membrane. It seems probable that prolactin does not need to. enter the cell to exert its effects since prolactin bound to Sepharose beads is as biochemically effective as the free hormone. Since the beads are much larger than the cells, prolactin bound to them could not have entered the cell but it is possible that some of the hormone could have become dissociated. (Turkington, 1970: 1972a: Turkington, Frantz, 1972.)

Prolactin is fully effective only on mammary epithelial cells which have been maintained in a culture medium containing insulin and hydrocortisone and which have divided onee. Within the first two hours of addition of prolactin there is a rapid increase inthe rate of histone phosphorylation which is presumably connected in some way with gene expression. Synthesis of nuclear RNA occurs at the same time. This is followed by increase in the activity of RNA polymerase and the synthesis of ribosomal RNA and the appearance of polysomes in the cytoplasm. After about six hours new synthesis of casein begins and after twelve hours lactose synthetase activity develops with the appearance of alpha-lactalbumin and galactosyl transferase. Induction of these last two proteins continues for at least 48 hours. Thus the binding of prolactin to the cell membrane seems capable of initiating all the processes leading to the induction of new enzyme activity. (A long series of papers, all with Turkington as co-author, describes this work.)

Prolactin and cyclic AMP

One of the biochemical success stories of recent years has been the demonstration that many hormones act by becoming bound to a cell membrane and there initiating the manufacture of cyclic AMP, the so-called second messenger, which is the intracellular mediator of the action of the hormone. The cyclic AMP is produced in a reaction catalysed by the enzyme adenyl cyclase. It was therefore natural to investigate the action of prolactin on this system.

One enzyme whose activity was studied was phosphokinase II which catalyses histone phosphorylation and may therefore be involved in the regulation of gene expression. This enzyme can be activated by exogenous cyclic AMP added to the system, and it seemed possible that prolactin might activate the enzyme by a mechanism involving activation of adenyl cyclase and cyclic AMP synthesis. In fact the action of prolactin turned out to be quite different. Instead of activating the adenyl cyclase it caused induction of the phosphokinase II without affecting cyclic AMP levels: half maximal levels of the phosphokinase were found after 30 minutes and maximal levels after four hours. Thus prolactin did interact with the cyclic AMP system, not by altering the concentration of the cyclic AMP itself but by inducing the enzyme which is activated by cyclic AMP. If a similar mechanism is found in other tissues it could help to explain how prolactin is able to interact with so many other hormones. In rat prostate, prolactin has been shown to have a more conventional effect in increasing cyclic AMP production. (Boyns, Cole, Golder, Danut Harper, Brownsey, Cowley, Jones, Griffiths, 1972: Majumder, Turkington, 1971a, 1971b: Turkington, 1972.)

Prolactin and the ovary

The actions of prolactin on steroid secretion by the ovary have been observed in several species. At mid cycle in the sheep hypophysectomy causes a sharp fall in progesterone secretion. In the hypophysectomised or intact animal at this stage both LH and prolactin increase progesterone secretion. FSH inhibits progesterone secretion. In the later part of the cycle none of the hormones has any effect. Negative reports on the effect of prolactin administration on progesterone output in the sheep occur only with observations made either for brief periods after prolactin administration or in the later part of the cycle. About 30 minutes seems required for the effect to become clearly established (Baird, 1969: Cook, Kaltenbach, Niswender, Norton, Nalbandov, 1969: Domanski, Skrzeczkowski, Stupnicka, Fitko, Dobrowolski, 1967: Hixon, Clegg, 1969: Short, McDonald, Rowson, 1963.)

The major progestin secreted by the rabbit ovary seems to be 20α-hydroxypregn-4-en-3-one. LH acts on ovarian interstitial tissue to increase the synthesis and release of the 20α steroid and at the same time depletes cholesterol stores. After a large dose of LH cholesterol stores may be so depleted that hormone synthesis is depressed with a low basal outout and a lack of responsiveness to further LH treatment. Prolactin treatment restores the cholesterol stores and basal 20α secretion to normal and increases the sensitivity of the ovary to LH. Hypophysectomy of rabbits 24 hours after ovulation leads to atrophy of the newly formed corpora lutea and also of the interstitial tissue with depletion of cholesterol stores. Prolactin maintains the interstitial tissue but does not prevent luteal atrophy. Estrogen maintains the luteal tissue but does not prevent interstitial atrophy. Estrogen plus progesterone prevent atrophy of both luteal and interstitial tissues. (Hilliard, Spies, Lucas, Sawyer, 1972: Horrell, Kilpatrick, Major, 1972.)

In vitro experiments have failed to demostrate an effect of prolactin on steroid secretion in the hamster, opossum or human. However, the detailed work on rabbits suggests that what should be tested is the effect of LH given after a dose of prolactin which might be expected to increase the stores of steroid hormone precursors but to have little direct effect by itself. (Cook, Nalbandov, 1968: Rice, Hammerstein, Savard, 1964: Schenkel-Hulliger, Krahenbuhl, 1971.)

The rat ovary secretes both progesterone and its reduced form 20α-hydroxy-pregn-4-en-3-one. Hypophysectomy elevates the synthesis of the 20α steroid and reduces the synthesis of progesterone by corpora lutea maintained in vitro. Prolactin given in a dose of 200 μg twice daily to the hypox animals could reverse the change and caused progesterone secretion to reach levels above those in pseudopregnant controls. Prolactin injected into intact animals elevated serum progesterone and reduced serum 20α. In luteal tissue prolactin increased the rate of incorporation of acetate-1-^{14}C into cholesterol, triglycerides, fatty acids and progestins. In contrast it had no effect on interstitial tissue which is the reverse of the situation in rabbits. (Armstrong, Greep, 1962: Armstrong, Knudsen, Miller, 1970: Armstrong, Miller,

Knudsen, 1969: Macdonald, 1969: Macdonald, Yoshinaga, Greep, 1971: Marsh. Telegdy, Savard, 1966: Mason, Tinsley, Cochrane, 1969.)

Prolactin and the testis

In mice and rat tests prolactin seems able to induce the activity of the hydroxy-steroid dehydrogenase enzymes which are required for testosterone metabolism. It is capable of doing this in dwarf mice which have a hereditary prolactin defieiency. Prolactin may also reduce the activity of 5α reductase which is involved in the metabolism of testosterone. As with the ovary, prolactin seems important in maintaining a pool of hormone precursors on which LH can act to stimulate testosterone manufacture. In hypophysectomised rats testosterone secretion falls virtually to zero. Prolactin alone and LH alone have only small effects on plasma testosterone levels but treatment with both hormones elevates plasma concentrations above those seen in intact controls. (Evans, 1962: Hafiez, Bartke, Lloyd, 1972: Hafiez, Lloyd, Bartke, 1972: Hafiez, Philpott, Bartke, 1971: Musto, Hafiez, Bartke, 1972.)

Although it breaks the rule of dealing only with mammals it seems appropriate here to mention the elegant experiments of Meier on testicular growth in sparrows. In house sparrows testicular growth was stimulated if prolactin was injected 4-8 hours after corticosterone: other patterns of treatment were ineffective. In contrast in white-throated sparrows the same treatment pattern inhibited testicular growth while an injection of prolactin given 12 hours after corticos-terane stimulated testicular growth. These experiments emphasise the complexity of the interactions between prolactin and other hormones and indicate that experiments which report no effect of prolactin must be interpreted very cautiously. (Meier, Martin, MacGregor, 1971.)

Prolactin and the adrenal

The adrenal glands in humans treated with high doses of steroids become resistant to the action of ACTH and exogenous ACTH fails to increase steroid secretion. In one such patients are treated with prolactin, the ability of the adrenal to secrete steroid hormones in response to ACTH was restored, as indicated by urinary excretion of 17 ketogenic steroids. Thus in the adrenal as well prolactin may be involved in the maintenance of a precursor pool. Prolactin has been shown to increase testost-erone secretion by guinea pig and human adrenal tissue in vitro, especially from the zona reticularis. (Ingvarsson, 1969b: Boyns, Cole, Golder, Danutra, Harper, Brownsey, Cowley, Jones, Griffiths, 1972.)

Prolactin and growth

Because of its relationship to growth hormone there has naturally been interest in the actions of prolactin on growth. In reptiles, birds and amphibians prolactin can certainly increase body size. In young hypophysectomised rats prolactin caused significant increase both in total body weight and in the width of the tibial cartilage. Inhibition of prolactin secretion by CB 154 in young rats greatly reduced normal weight gain. It failed, however, to allow normal compensatory hypertrophy to occur after unilateral nephrectomy while growth hormone injections did allow the hypertrophic response. In rats with mammotrophic tumors which secrete prolactin, growth hormone and ACTH, adipose tissue atrophied while all other tissues increased in size. However the situation is so complex that it is impossible to say whether any of the effect is due to prolactin. Prolactin may stimulate growth in man provided that diet is adequate. (Astarabadi, 1963: Boyns, Cole, Golder, Danutra, Harper, Brownsey, Cowley, Jones, Griffiths, 1972: McGarry, Beck, 1972: Milkovic, Garrison, Bates, 1964: Nicoll, Bern, 1972: Thompson, Crean, 1963.)

Prolactin and carbohydrate metabolism

Almost twenty years ago Houssay and co-workers tested the diabetogenic effects of growth hormone, prolactin and ACTH in hypophysectomised dogs and cats which were also partially pancreatectomized to increase their sensitivity to possible diabetogenic agents. All three hormones caused hyperglycemia, glycosuria, polyuria, polydipsia, polyphagia and ketonuria. Growth hormone was the most potent and ACTH the least, with prolactin in the middle. (Houssay, Anderson, Bates, Li, 1955: Houssay, Penhos, 1966.)

In intact dogs, sheep and normal and juvenile diabetic humans prolactin given in moderate doses or for a short period only had no effect on fasting blood glucose concentration. In large doses (1000 IU) in children it produced a slight elevation of blood glucose, as it did in dogs treated for several days with the hormone. In hypophysectomised juvenile-type diabetics it caused a clear elevation of blood glucose concentration. (Elsair, Denine, 1970: McGarry, Beck, 1962: 1972: Manns, Boda, 1965: Rathgeb, Winkler, Steel, Altszuler, 1971.)

In humans treated with prolactin, for the most part hypopituitary dwarfs, prolactin reduced glucose tolerance. Prolactin treatment in dogs allowed the animals to recover from insulin hypoglycemia slightly more rapidly than usual:

unlike the situation in growth hormone treated animals there was no obvious insulin-resistance. Patients with galactorrhea and very high plasma insulin levels may have normal glucose tolerance tests. (Frantz, Kleinberg, Noel, 1972b: McGarry, Beck, 1972: Noel, Suh, Stone, Frantz, 1972: Rathgeb, Winkler, Steele, Altszuler, 1971.)

In dogs, although prolactin had little effect on plasma glucose concentrations it did cause a marked increase in the glucose release by the liver and uptake by other tissues. The two effects approximately cancel out. In mice doses of prolactin below 100 μg caused a reduction in liver glycogen stores while higher doses elevated liver glycogen stores. All doses lowered blood glucose levels, the higher the dose the more dramatic the effect. This may suggest a biphasic effect of prolactin on the liver but a monophasic stimulation of glucose uptake by the tissues. (Elghamry, Said, Elmougy, 1966: Elghamry, Grunert, 1969: Rathgeb, Winkler, Steele, Altszuler, 1971.)

Again it is very clear that the effect of prolactin depends very much on the hormonal environment in the individual into whom it is injected.

Prolactin and lipid metabolism

In fasting children and in sheep, prolactin elevates plasma NEFA levels. It has little effect in juvenile type diabetics before hypophysectomy, but afterwards produces a clear elevation. (Elsair, Denine, 1970: McGarry, Beck, 1972: Manns, Boda, 1965.)

In adipose tissue from mature rats, prolactin stimulates glucose uptake and protein synthesis but increases lipolysis with release of NEFA. In adipose tissue taken from young rats in contrast, NEFA uptake may be stimulated. In rats with carrying ACTH and prolactin-secreting tumors, protein and lipid synthesis may both be depressed in adipose tissue but elevated in the liver. In hypophysectomised rats conversion of glucose to fatty acids is defective: thyroxine, prolactin and growth hormone may have synergistic effects in repairing the defect. In pregnant and lactating animals liver RNA and DNA synthesis is stimulated. Finally, in a fish, a lizard and a pigeon it has been shown that prolactin injected 6 hours after adrenal steroids causes fat depletion while after a 24 hour delay prolactin causes fat accumulation. (Hamid, Rubenstein, Ferguson, Beck, 1965: Kovaleva, Ryshka, Dilman, 1972: Leake, Mayne, Barry, 1968: MacLeod, Bass, Hwang, Smith, 1968:

Meier, Trobec, Joseph, John, 1971: Moore, Ball, 1962: Nejad, Chaikoff, Hill, 1962.)

Conclusions

It is clear that a vast amount of work needs to be done on the biochemical effects of prolactin. It is also clear that good experiments will not be easy to design since a recurring theme seems to be that prolactin has little effect by itself but modulates the actions of other hormones, often by controlling percursor pools. The levels of many other hormones and the temporal relationships of hormone treatments will need to be carefully considered.

Chapter 5

EFFECTS OF METABOLIC AND ENVIRONMENTAL STIMULI ON PROLACTIN SECRETION

The most extensive experience of plasma prolactin estimations has been obtained by Friesen's laboratory. In their original publications on "normal" prolactin levels, hospitalised patients with no disease obviously associated with an abnormality of prolactin secretion were used as controls. The mean plasma level was 10 ng/ml in adult males, 10 ng/ml in adult females in the follicular phase of the menstrual cycle and 11 ng/ml in the luteal phase. In children the mean level was 11 ng/ml. However it is now known that a number of situations, including hospitalisation itself, may elevate prolactin levels and in a new series of samples taken from normal healthy volunteers, the mean in adult males was 5.0 ng/ml (range 0-28), in adult females 8.1 ng/ml (range 0-28) and in children 10.8 ng/ml (range 7-17). Levels in females in various phases of reproductive life will be discussed later.

24 hour secretion pattern

In rats the activity of the Golgi apparatus in the manufacture of prolactin secretory granules seems to be at a peak about mid-day. Pituitary prolactin content reaches a peak at about 4.00 p.m. Plasma levels appear highest in the evening. During pregnancy and pseudopregnancy the evening surge seems to occur somewhat earlier and there is an additional peak in the late night-very early morning period. In lactating cattle there tends to be a peak in the late afternoon with low levels in the early morning. (Butcher, Fugo, Collins, 1972: Clark, Baker, 1964: Dunn, Arimura, Scheving, 1972: Freeman, Neill, 1972: Gomez, Dumm, Echave Lanos, 1970: Koprowski, 1972: Schams, Bohms, Karg, 1971.)

In human studies plasma levels are lowest in the afternoon. They begin to rise clearly 60-90 minutes after going to sleep, and increase in a series of peaks and troughs to maximal levels between 05.00 and 07.00 hours, just before waking. They fall rapidly in the first hour after waking. There is no clear sex difference. Growth hormone levels in contrast rise rapidly at the onset of sleep but after 2—4 hours fall to low levels. There is no consistent relationship between release of prolactin and growth hormone. (Nokin, Vekemans, L'Hermite, Robyn, 1972: Sassin, Frantz, Weitzman, Kapen, 1972)

Effects of feeding and fasting

In cattle and goats feeding caused an elevation of prolactin plasma levels with in cattle a peak about six hours after the meal. Fasting for 24 or 48 hours caused prolactin concentrations to fall to very low levels. The changes were roughly in phase with, but much more pronounced than, changes in blood glucose level.
In humans no obvious effect of feeding on prolactin levels was noted. (Joke, 1970: McAtee, Trenkle, 1971: Sassin, Frantz, Weitzman, Kapen, 1972: Schams, Karg, 1970.)

It is possible that the long term effect of starvation and malnutrition in humans and animals may be an elevation of prolactin levels. Starvation in rats elevates prolactin synthesis and release. Widespread gynecomastia and occasional galactorrhea were reported to occur in starved prisoners of war during the refeeding period and one case has been reported of a malnourished patient with elevated prolactin levels. Obviously much more work is needed in this area. (Akikusa, 1971: Hibbs, 1947: Jacobs, 1948: Turkington, 1972c.)

Effects of glucose and insulin

There is no agreement as to the effects of glucose tolerance tests on plasma prolactin levels. Friesen et al reported no obvious effect. Forsyth et al reported that in patients with galactorrhea, oral glucose had no effect on prolactin levels in patients with pituitary tumours but suppressed them in four patients with a normal pituitary fossa. Bryant and Greenwood reported no change of prolactin in two subjects, a sharp fall in one, and a sharp rise in a fourth who, however, showed obvious signs of stress. Glucose infusions in fasting cattle with very low plasma prolactin did not elevate prolactin levels but infusions in goats did. (Bryant, Greenwood, 1972: Bryant, Linzell, Greenwood, 1970: Forsyth, Besser, Edwards, Francis, Myres, 1971: Friesen, Belanger, Guyda, Hwang, 1972: McAtee, Trenkle, 1971.)

There was equal uncertainty about the response to insulin until Wilson et al demonstrated that a consistent elevation of plasma prolactin occurred after insulin injection, but only if blood glucose levels fell below 15-20 mg/100 ml. Levels higher than this failed to stimulate prolactin secretion consistently. (Frantz, Kleinberg, Noel, 1972: Friesen, L'Hermite, Delavoye, Nokin, Vekemans, Robyn, 1972: Noel, Suh, Frantz, 1971: Wilson, Percy-Robb, Singhal, Forrest, Cole, Boyns, Griffiths, 1972.)

Effects of amino acids

Intravenous arginine infusions (0.5 g/kg) produced striking elevations of plasma prolactin levels in cows and sheep over a period of a few minutes. Arginine, leucine and phenylalanine given by intra-carotid infusion all elevated plasma prolactin levels in sheep. In most humans intravenous arginine produced some elevation of plasma prolactin but only in a small proportion of individuals was a very clear cut response seen. During the first thirty weeks of pregnancy arginine had no consistent effect on plasma prolactin levels, but in the last ten weeks it tended to produce consistent prolactin elevation at a time when the response of growth hormone was blunted. (Davis, 1972: Friesen, Webster, Hwang, Guyda, Munro, Read, 1972: McAtee, Trenkle, 1971, Tyson, Hwang, Guyda, Friesen, 1972.)

Effects of stressful stimuli

Nicoll et al first suggested that a wide variety of non-specific stresses might initiate prolactin secretion. In estrogen primed rats they demonstrated that animals exposed to abnormal cold, light or heat, those which were starved or restrained and those injected subcutaneously with formaldehyde all showed evidence of lactation. Specific plasma assays have now confirmed that in the experience of most but not all workers, bleeding, restraint and starvation in rats cause elevation of prolactin levels. (Akikusa, 1971: Dunn, Arimura, Scheving, 1972: Grosvenor, 1965: Grosvenor, McCann, Nallar, 1965: Meites, 1972: Nagy, Kurcz, Kiss, Baranyai, Mosonyi, Halmy, 1970: Nicoll, Talwalker. Meites, 1960: Neill, 1970, 1972.)

Similar results have been obtained in sheep and cattle. Venepuncture, restraint, water deprivation and separation from companion animals have all been reported to stimulate prolactin secretion. (Bryant, Linzell, Greenwood, 1970: Davis, 1972: Joke, 1970: Raud, Kiddy, Odell, 1971.)

Results in humans confirm this general picture. Patients admitted to hospital and especially surgical patients before operation have elevated prolactin levels. Minor medical investigations such as gastroscopy and even proctoscopy stimulated prolactin secretion. Sudden exercise (running up stairs) approximately doubled prolactin levels. (Frantz, Kleinberg, Noel, 1972: Noel, Suh, Frantz, 1971: Noel, Suh, Stone, Frantz, 1972.)

Effects of anesthesia and surgery

In rats ether anesthesia and laparotomy produced a rapid elevation of plasma prolactin level within two minutes of induction. Levels reached were two-three times above the baseline. Intraperitoneal phenobarbital also clearly elevated prolactin secretion while control injections had only minimal effects: this rise in prolactin secretion was associated with depletion of hypothalamic PIF. The rise was followed by a prolonged depression and it was observed that sodium pentobarbital added to pituitary culture in vitro could block prolactin release directly. Nembutal could prevent stress induced elevations of prolactin secretion and also the elevation which occurs at proestrus. (Ajika, Kalra, Fawcett, Krulich, McCann, 1972: Blake, Sawyer, 1972: Kalra, Ajika, Krulich, Fawcett, Quijada, McCann, 1971: Neill, 1970: Terkel, Blake, Sawyer, 1972: Wakabayashi, Arimura, Schally, 1971: Wuttke, Gelato, Meites, 1971: Wuttke, Meites, 1970: Yokoyama, 1971.)

Similar results have been obtained in humans. Surgery and anesthesia produced sharp 5-10 fold elevations of plasma prolactin levels at the beginning of the operation. Levels then tended to decline in spite of continuation of the operation. (Frantz, Kleinberg, Noel, 1972: Friesen, Hwang, Guyda, Tolis, Tyson, Myers, 1972: Noel, Suh, Stone, Frantz, 1972.)

Chapter 6

CONTROL OF PROLACTIN SECRETION

It is now firmly established that unlike most of the other pituitary hormones, but like MSH, the predominant influence of the hypothalamus on prolactin secretion is inhibitory. A prolactin inhibiting factor (PIF) is chronically released into the pituitary portal vessels. The main lines of evidence for this well established conclusion are as follows:

1.   Transplantation of the pituitary to another site, normally the renal capsule, leads to an elevation and not a depression of prolactin secretion. (Chen, Amenomori, Lu, Voogt, Meites, 1970: Everett, 1954: Welsch, Negro-Vilar, Meites, 1968.)

2.   When anterior pituitaries are cultured in vitro, prolactin secretion is maintained for many weeks while secretion of other hormones declines rapidly in the first few days. (Pasteels, Brauman, 1963.)

3.   Lesions in the median eminence region which depress secretion of other pituitary hormones elevate prolactin secretion. (De Voe, Ramirez, McCann, 1966: Kanematsu, Hilliard, Sawyer, 1963: Meites, 1972a.)

4.   Section of the pituitary stalk in rats, rabbits, guinea pigs and humans has led to elevated prolactin secretion. Negative results obtained in guinea pigs and sheep may have been due to infarction of the pituitary following the operation or to regrowth of pituitary portal vessels. (Aron, Marescaux, 1962: Bryant, Greenwood, Kann, Martinet, Denamur, 1971: Donovan, van der Werff ten Bosch, 1957: Ehni, Eckles, 1959: Illingworth, Perry, 1971: Nikitovitch-Winer, 1965: Turkington, Underwood, Van Wyck, 1971.)

Prolactin inhibiting factor

PIF has not been isolated in chemically pure form. However extracts of the hypothalamus from rats, sheep, cattle, pigs and humans have been shown to inhibit prolactin release from pituitaries maintained in vitro. A semi-quantitative assay technique based on this principle is available. Other assays have been based on the effect of injection of hypothalamic extracts on restoring pituitary prolactin content in animals whose pituitary prolactin has been depleted by drugs, or in preventing a stress or suckling-induced fall in pituitary prolactin. It is known that PIF is not identical with LH-RF (Arimura, Saito, Muller, Bowers, Sawano, Schally, 1967: Danon, Dikstein, Sulman, 1970: Debeljuk, Arimura, Schally, 1972: Grosvenor, McCann, Nallar, 1965: Grosvenor, Mena, Maiweg, Dhariwal, McCann, 1970: Kragt, Meites, 1967: Meites, Clemens, 1972: Pasteels, 1961: Schally, Kuroshima, Ishida, 1965.)

In very elegant experiments Kamberi, Mical and Porter have succeeded in cannulating the pituitary stalk vessels in rats. They have been able to demonstrate (PIF activity) in stalk plasma and have also shown that prolactin release may be depressed by infusion of hypothalamic extracts into the stalk vessels. (Kamberi, Mical, Porter, 1970, 1971a, 1971b, 1971c, 1971d.)

Stimuli which can alter hypothalamic PIF content have been extensively studied, notably by Meites and co-workers. Hypothalamic levels of PIF seem to be depleted by three main groups of factors:

1. Environmental stimuli such as suckling, surgery and other forms of stress.

2. Naturally occurring hormones including estrogens, testosterone, progesterone and cortisol.

3. Synthetic hormones and drugs including norethynodrel-mestranol combinations, reserpine, phenothiazines, haloperidol and sodium pentobarbital. (Ajika, Krulich, Fawcett, McCann, 1972: Clemens, Meites, 1972: Danon, Sulman, 1970: Dickerman, Clark, Dickerman, Meites, 1972: Meites, 1972a: Minaguchi, Meites, 1967a, 1967b: Ratner, Meites, 1964: Ratner, Talwalker, Meites, 1965: Sar, Meites, 1968: Wuttke, Gelato, Meites, 1971.)

A more limited group of agents can elevate hypothalamic PIF content. The most notable naturally occurring one is perhaps prolactin itself. The ergot group of drugs, L-dopa and the monoamine oxidase inhibitors iproniazid and pargyline also elevate PIF. Systemic injection of dopamine into rats causes appearance of PIF in the systemic circulation while injection of dopamine into the third ventricle has been shown to increase the amount of PIF released into the pituitary portal vessels. (Chen, Minaguchi, Meites, 1967: Kamberi, Mical, Porter, 1970: Lu, Meites, 1971, 1972: Meites, Clemens, 1972: Voogt, Meites, 1971: Wuttke, Cassell, Meites, 1971.)

Prolactin releasing factor (PRF)

There have been persistent reports that some hypothalamic extracts contain a PRF. One of the first hypothalamic extracts tested initiated lactation in rats although this could have been a non-specific effect. However a mammotropic action of hypothalamic extract was again reported in 1968. When anterior pituitaries from male animals were incubated with median eminence extracts made from normal female rats, prolactin secretion was inhibited during the first four hours of incubation and stimulated during the next eight. If the female rats had been pretreated with either reserpine or estrogen which might be expected to deplete hypothalamic PIF, the inhibitory phase was absent and the median eminence extracts caused only stimulation of the prolactin secretion. In female rats primed with estradiol and progesterone a porcine hypothalamic extract has been reported to elevate plasma prolactin levels within ten minutes of injection. The hypothalamic releasing factor seemed distinct from vasopressin, TRH or LH-RF. In lactating rats hypothalamic extracts containing PIF failed to prevent prolactin secretion in response to suckling. (Amenomori, Meites, 1970: Fiorindo, Nicoll, 1969: Meites, Talwalker, Nicoll, 1960: Mishkinsky, Kazhen, Sulman, 1068: Valverde, Chieffo, Reichlin, 1972.)

Prolactin and TSH-releasing factor (TRF or TRH)

In 1971, Tashjian et al reported that TRH could stimulate prolactin secretion from rat pituitary cells in culture. Gourdji et al observed ultrastructural changes in such cells compatible with secretory activity. No effect of TRH on prolactin release from rat and bovine pituitary tissue (as distinct from cells) could be observed by Convey or by Lu et al although La Bella and Vivian reported a weak effect of TRH on prolactin release by bovine pituitary tissue. (Convey, 1972: Gourdji, Kerdelhue, Tixier-Vidal, 1972: La Bella, Vivian, 1971: Lu, Shaar, Kartright, Meites, 1972: Meites, Clemens, 1972.)

In rats thyroxine treatment elevated pituitary prolactin content without affecting hypothalamic PIF. TRH injections in rats had no immediate effect on pituitary or serum prolactin but when they were continued for six days there were small rises both in pituitary and serum prolactin levels. These rises did not occur in thyroidectomized-parathyroidectomized rats suggesting that they may have been mediated via TSH and thyroid hormones. (Chen, Meites, 1969: Lu, Shaar, Kartright, Meites, 1972: Meites, Clemens, 1972.)

The situation in humans is quite different. Several groups have shown that intravenous doses of as little as 10 μg of synthetic TRH cause elevation of both TSH and prolactin plasma levels within a matter of minutes. Both responses are more pronounced in normal women than in normal men, both are enhanced in hypothyroid patients and both are reduced in hyperthyroid patients. Small amounts of triiodothyronine given to normal individuals suppressed the TSH but not the prolactin response to TRH. Repetition of TRH treatment at 3-hourly intervals in normal individuals tended to lead to a dimimution in the size of the response. Most normal individuals given an adequate dose of TRH elevated prolactin levels 5-12 times within 15-30 minutes. Plasma levels returned to baseline after about three hours. As calculated from plasma levels, the amount of prolactin secreted during the response could probably not have been present in a preformed state within the pituitary suggesting that synthesis as well as release of prolactin was stimulated. (Bowers, Friesen, Folkers, 1972: Bowers, Friesen, Hwang, Guyda, Folkers, 1971: Foley, Jacobs, Hoffman, Daughaday, Blizzard, 1972: Friesen, Guyda, Hwang, Tyson, Barbeaù, 1972: Jacobs, Snyder, Wilber, Utiger, Daughaday, 1971: Kaplan, Grumbach, Friesen, 1972: L'Hermite, Copinschi, Golstein, Vanhaelst, Leclercq, Bruno, 1972: Sachson, Rosen, Cuatrecasas, 1972.)

The mechanism of the response in man is uncertain but its rapidity suggests that the TRH may be directly acting on prolactin-secreting cells. This is supported by the finding that the diurnal rhythm of TSH secretion is very similar to that of prolactin secretion. Chlorpromazine and probably many of the other drugs which release prolactin do not appear to act via TRH since they do not elevate TSH levels. In chlorpromazine treated individuals with elevated plasma prolactin concentrations TRH produced an even further elevation of prolactin. L-dopa produced subnormal responses of both TSH and prolactin to TRH while estrogen treatment penetrated both responses. (Bowers, Friesen, Folkers, 1972: Patel, Baker, Alford, Johns, Burger, 1972: Vanhaelst, Van Cauter, De Gaute, Golstein, 1972.)

Brain amines and prolactin

In rats systemic injection of a wide variety of amines and other substances thought to be involved in neural transmission including adrenaline, noradrenaline, acetyl choline and serotonin can elevate prolactin secretion but since most of these drugs penetrate the blood brain barrier only with difficulty it is now thought that the release of prolactin is merely a stress effect. (Clemens, Meites, 1972: Mittler, Meites, 1967.)

In vitro experiments with anterior pituitaries have shown that moderate concentrations of catecholamines in the medium stimulate prolactin release while higher concentrations inhibit it. The physiological significance of these findings is uncertain since it is unlikely that the catecholamines enter the pituitary portal vessels in any significant quantities. (Birge, Jacobs, Hammer, Daughaday, 1970: Clemens, Meites, 1972: Gala, Reece, 1965: Koch, Lu, Meites, 1970: MacLeod, 1969: MacLeod, Fontham, Lehmeyer, 1970: MacLeod, Lehmeyer, 1972.)

Possibly more significant results have emerged from experiments using drugs which are known to interfere with cerebral amine inactivation or to interfere in one way or another with amine synthesis or amine action at receptor sites. The results will be described species by species, starting with the rat. In this animal monoamine oxidase and catechol-O-methyl transferase inhibitors which interfere with normal amine inactivation both depress serum prolactin levels while at the same time elevate hypothalamic PIF content. In contrast, all the drugs which in some way interfere with amine function including reserpine, chlorpromazine, fluphenazine, perphenazine, amphetamine, guanethidine, α-methyldopa, α-methyl-p-tyrosine and α-methyl-m-tyrosine all increase plasma prolactin levels and reduce hypothalamic PIF content. (Arai, Suzuki, 1971: Arimura, Dunn, Schally, 1972: Ben-David, Danon, Benveniste, Weller, Sulman, 1971: Ben-David, Danon, Sulman, 1970: Fiorindo, Nicoll, 1969: Lu, Amenomori, Chen, Meites, 1970: Lu, Meites, 1971: Meites, 1972a: Meites, Clemens, 1972: Meites, Lu, Wuttke, Welsch, Nagasawa, Quadri, 1972: Ratner, Talwalker, Meites, 1965: Sulman, Winnik, 1956: Superstine, Sulman, 1966: Van der Gugten, Boot, Kwa, 1970: Van Maanen, Smelik, 1968: Yoshida, 1964.)

Injections of L-dopa, the dopamine precursor, in rats inhibited prolactin secretion and elevated hypothalamic PIF content. Dopamine injected into the third ventricle reduced prolactin and elevated LH and FSH secretion while physiological doses of noradrenaline and adrenaline administered by the same route had no effect. Neither dopamine nor noradrenaline nor adrenaline had any effect when infused directly into the anterior pituitary suggesting that the effect of dopamine is mediated by PIF. (Kamberi, Mical, Porter, 1970, 1971a, 1971b, 1971c, 1971d: Lu, Meites, 1971: Meites, 1972.)

The evidence in the preceding paragraph suggests that dopamine rather than adrenaline or noradrenaline may be the amine which regulates hypothalamic PIF secretion. There are two other pieces of evidence pointing to the same conclusion. Pimozide appears able to block dopamine receptors without interfering with noradrenaline receptors significantly. Injection of pimozide into rats produced a marked elevation of prolactin secretion. In contrast disulfiram, which has a preferential action in interfering with noradrenaline action, caused a fall in prolactin levels as compared with controls, raising the possibility that noradrenaline may normally stimulate prolactin release. Selective blockade of noradrenaline biosynthesis with diethyldithiocaramate (DDC) did not alter prolactin levels and did not prevent the fall in prolactin secretion seen with L-dopa, suggesting that the L-dopa effect is not mediated by noradrenaline but by dopamine. However in animals given α-methyl-tyrosine to block catecholamine biosynthesis prolactin levels are high: a further elevation can be brought about by treatment with dihydroxyphenyl serine which normalises noradrenaline synthesis only. The tentative conclusion is therefore that dopamine is the regulator of hypothalamic PIF secretion but that noradrenaline may stimulate prolactin secretion via another pathway, possibly PRF/TRH. (Donoso, Bishop, Fawcett, Krulich, McCann, 1971: Meites, Clemens, 1972.)

Serotonin and melatonin injected into the third ventricle in rats stimulate prolactin and inhibit FSH secretion. Direct infusion into the pituitary has no effect suggesting that the action is mediated by releasing factors. Hypothalamic serotonin levels in rats show a diurnal rhythm with higher levels in the evening than the morning: serum prolactin levels are also higher in the evening than in the morning. Systemic injections of the serotonin precursors tryptophan and 5-hydroxytryptophan both elevate serum prolactin levels significantly. (Kamberi, Mical, Porter, 1971: Lu, Meites, 1971: Meites, Clemens, 1972.)

Other experimental animals have been investigated much less extensively than the rat. Phenothiazines in sheep and reserpine in rabbits have both been shown to elevate prolactin secretion. (Bryant, Connan, Greenwood, 1968: Kanematsu, Hilliard, Sawyer, 1963: McNeilly, Lamming, 1971.)

In humans results have broadly paralleled findings in the rat. Reserpine, methyldopa, amphetamine and the phenothiazines all elevate prolactin secretion while L-dopa and monoamine oxidase inhibitors suppress prolactin secretion. The tricyclic antidepressants which have been reported to facilitate the actions of noradrenaline and adrenaline stimulate prolactin secretion. All the drugs seemed to change prolactin levels within an hour or less of taking an oral dose. On stopping phenothiazine treatment plasma levels may not return to normal for two to three weeks. (Apostolakis, 1968: Apostolakis, Kapetanakis, Lazos, Madena-Pyrgaki, 1972: Fluckiger, 1972: Frantz, Kleinberg, Noel, 1972b: Friesen, Guyda, Hwang, Tyson, Barbeau, 1972: Friesen, Hwang, Guyda, Tolis, Tyson, Myers, 1972: Jacobs, Bauman, Daughaday, 1971: Kleinberg, Noel, Frantz, 1971: Malarkey, Jacobs, Daughaday, 1971: Turkington, 1971c: Turkington, 1972e: Turkington, Ray, Costin, 1972.)

Other drugs and prolactin

Of all the other drugs which may alter prolactin secretion the most potent seem to be the ergot derivatives and in particular 2-bromo-α-ergokryptine (CB 154). Again most studies have been on rats. The main action of the ergot derivatives seems to be a blocking of release of the hormone. The effect seems to be a direct one on the pituitary cells since it occurs irrespective of whether the gland under study is in its normal position, is transplanted to another site such as beneath the renal capsule or is maintained in tissue culture. After brief periods of treatment the secreting cells become loaded with secretory granules and the prolactin content of the gland rises, suggesting an initial effect on release rather than synthesis. Later however, the secretory granules are destroyed by lysosomal activity and synthesis as well seems to be reduced. The effect on prolactin is probably not exclusively due to a direct action on the cells since hypothalamic PIF content may also be elevated by the drugs: it is conceivable, however, that this could be some form of short feedback response to accumulation of prolactin in the gland. Growth hormone secretion does not appear to be altered. (Arai, Suzuki, Masuda, 1972: Arimura, Dunn, Schally, 1972: Ectors, Danguy, Pasteels, 1972: Fluckiger, 1972: Fluckiger, Lutterbeck, Wagner, Billeter, 1972: Fluckiger, Wagner, 1968: Kraicer, Strauss, 1970: Lu, Koch, Meites, 1971: Malven, Hoge, 1971: Nicoll, Yaron, Nutt, Daniels, 1971: Pasteels, 1972: Pasteels, Danguy, Frerotte, Ectors, 1971: Pasteels, Ectors, 1970: Richardson, 1973: Shaar, Clemens, 1972: Shelesnyak, 1954, 1958: Welsch, Squires, Cassell, Chen, Meites, 1971: Wuttke, Cassell, Meites, 1971: Yokoyama, Tomogane, Ota, 1972.)

CB 154 also seems to be effective in suppressing prolactin secretion in sheep, cattle and humans. In humans it has been used clinically for the suppression of both puerperal and non-puerperal lactation. (Besser, Parke, Edwards, Forsyth, McNeilly, 1972: Del Pozo, Brun Del Re, Varga, Friesen, 1972: Niswender, 1972: Schams, Reinhardt, Karg, 1972: Varga, Lutterbeck, Pryor, Wenner, Erb, 1972.)

A wide variety of other drugs has been shown to alter prolactin secretion. Drugs which stimulate secretion include antihistamines, thalidomide, haloperidol, sulpiride, chlordiazepoxide and diazepam. Paraoxon, the organophosphorus choline-sterase inhibitor, gold thioglucose and bipiperydyl mustard elevated pituitary prolactin content but plasma levels were not measured. An ergot derivative, 1-methyl-9,10-dihydro-ergonorcorine appears to be a powerful stimulator of secretion. Drugs which seem to inhibit prolactin secretion include clonidine, frusemide, LSD and piperidendione derivatives. (Cehovic, Dettbarn, Welsch, 1972: Dickerman, Clark, Dickerman, Meites, 1972: Fluckiger, 1972: Gachev, 1968: L'Hermite, Delvoye, Nokin, Vekemans, Robyn, 1972: Locker, Superstine, Sulman, 1971: Quadri, Meites, 1971: Sinha, Van der Laan, 1971: Sulman, 1970: Superstine, Sulman, 1966: Van der Gugten, 1971.)

Hormones and prolactin secretion

In ovariectomised rats prolactin secretion falls to very low levels. In both intact and ovariectomised rats estrogen injections stimulate the secretion of prolactin. The surge of prolactin secretion at proestrus in rats seems to be dependent on estrogens since it can be prevented by the administration of estradiol antiserum on the day before proestrus. (Ajika, Krulich, Fawcett, McCann, 1972: Bishop, Kalra, Fawcett, Krulich, McCann, 1972: Chen, Meites, 1970: Freeman, Reichert, Neill, 1972: MacLeod, Abad, Edison, 1969: MacLeod, Lehmeyer, 1972: Meites, 1972a: Meites, Clemens, 1972: Meites, Lu, Wuttke, Welsch, Nagasawa, Quadri, 1972: Neill, Freeman, Tillson, 1971: Ratner, Talwalker, Meites, 1963: Shani, Givant, Sulman, Eylath, Eckstein, 1971: Swearingen, Nicoll, 1972.)

Estrogens seem to have a dual action in stimulating prolactin secretion. They have been reported to deplete hypothalamic PIF content and median eminence lesions have been reported to prevent prolactin secretion in response to systemic-ally injected estrogen. However estrogen-stimulated prolactin secretion by pituitaries transplanted to the renal capsule and minute implants of estradiol in either the hypothalamus or the anterior pituitary stimulate prolactin secretion.

Hypothalamic extracts from estrogen-treated animals do not inhibit prolactin secretion from pituitary glands in culture suggesting that their PIF has been depleted. Interestingly estradiol and phenothiazines seem to compete for the same hypothalamic receptor sites. Kanematsu and Sawyer on the basis of the differential effects of hypothalamic and pituitary estrogen implants have suggested that the indirect action operating via the hypothalamus is to stimulate synthesis and storage of prolactin while the direct action is to stimulate release. Estrogens added to cultured or incubated pituitary glands in vitro consistently caused prolactin release into the medium. A sex difference has been reported in the response to systemic estrogen treatment. Females ovariectomised when adult and neonatally castrated males respond to estrogen injections by a surge of prolactin secretion. Females treated neonatally with androgen or males castrated when adult have higher baseline levels of prolactin, but do not respond to estrogen injections with a surge of prolactin release. (Ajika, Krulich, Fawcett, McCann, 1972: Ben-David, Dikstein, Sulman, 1964: 1965: Bishop, Kalra, Fawcett, Krulich, McCann, 1972: Chen, Amenomori, Lu, Voogt, Meites, 1970: Chen, Meites, 1970: Fiorindo, Nicoll, 1969: Kanematsu, Sawyer, 1963: Meites, 1972a: Meites, Clemens, 1972: Neill, 1972: Nicoll, Meites, 1962, 1964: Ramirez, McCann, 1964: Ratner, Meites, 1964: Shani, Givant, Sulman, Eylath, Eckstein, 1971.)

In sheep estradiol injections elevated both LH and prolactin release. However, estradiol infusions appeared to depress the release of prolactin while the infusion was continuing: on stopping the infusion there was a surge of prolactin secretion. (Fell, Beck, Brown, Catt, Cumming, Goding, 1972: Fell, Beck, Brown, Cumming, Goding, 1972: Schams, Karg, 1972.)

In humans, estrogen given to males for prostatic cancer caused elevations of prolactin levels in some but not all patients. Estrogens given to females 12 hours post partum had no effect on prolactin secretion. In volunteer normal males, diethylstilbestrol produced a small elevation in plasma prolactin in three and a large one in two. In normal pre-menopausal women estrone elevated prolactin levels for 48-72 hours after a single injection but in post-menopausal women estrone and estradiol depressed prolactin levels: ethinyl estradiol in post-menopausal women with breast cancer elevated prolactin suggesting a possible difference between natural and synthetic estrogens. (Frantz, Kleinberg, Noel, 1972b: Friesen, 1972b: L'Hermite, Delvoye, Nokin, Vekemans, Robyn, 1972, L'Hermite, Stauric, Robyn, 1972.)

There is much less information about the action of progesterone on prolactin secretion. In vitro high doses of progesterone may suppress it but moderate doses have no effect. When injected into rats low to moderate doses of progesterone have been reported to have little effect or to cause some lowering of plasma prolactin levels: they do reduce the prolactin response to estrogen injections. Progesterone implants in the hypothalamus may cause pseudopregnancy which could be due to prolactin secretion and high doses of systemically injected progesterone elevate prolactin secretion. High doses of progesterone (10 mg/day/rat) also deplete hypothalamic PIF. (Ben-David, Dikstein, Sulman, 1964: Chen. Meites, 1970: Khazan, Danon, 1962: Nicoll, Meites, 1964: Pasteels, Ectors, 1968: Pasteels, Gausset, Danguy, Ectors, 1972: Sar, Meites, 1968: Valverde, Chieffo, Reichlin, 1972.)

Testosterone had no effect on prolactin secretion from pituitaries maintained in vitro. When injected into rats it reduced hypothalamic PIF and elevated pituitary prolactin content. Testosterone treatment also appeared to make the pituitary more active in incorporating ^{3}H-leucine in vitro. In human females testosterone treatment produced hypertrophy of prolactin secreting cells. (Ben-David, Dikstein, Sulman, 1964: MacLeod, Abad, Eidson, 1969: Nicoll, Meites, 1964: Pasteels, Gausset, Danguy, Ectors, 1972: Roger, 1970: Sar, Meites, 1968.)

Of synthetic hormones, medroxyprogesterone has been reported to suppress prolactin secretion when injected systemically into rats and to stimulate it when implanted in the hypothalamus. In humans it had little or no effect in ten women but caused a clear elevation in two. Clomiphene had no effect on prolactin levels in sheep. A chlormadinone-ethinylestradiol combination in humans kept prolactin at follicular phase levels without any clear suppression or stimulation. In rats the norethynodrel-mestranol (Enovid) combination depleted hypothalamic PIF content and stimulated prolactin secretion. (Khazan, Danon, 1962: L'Hermite, Delvoye, Nokin, Vekemans, Robyn, 1972: Minaguchi, Meites, 1967: Pasteels, Ectors, 1968: Welsch, Meites, 1969.)

Among the other hormones, thyroxine and triiodothyronine and very high concentrations of cortisol have been reported to stimulate prolactin secretion in vitro. In rats cortisone acetate inhibited the effect of estrogens in stimulating the corpus luteum and it was thought that it might have inhibited prolactin secretion. In rats adrenalectomy caused elevation of basal prolactin levels and greatly potentiated the response of prolactin to perphenazine stimulation. One case has been reported of a woman with primary adrenal insufficiency who presented with amenorrhea and galactorrhea and whose prolactin levels were moderately but consistently elevated. Cortisone acetate therapy restored prolactin levels to normal and led to cessation of galactorrhea and resumption of normal menstruation. (Ben-David, Danon, Benveniste, Weller, Sulman, 1971: Ben-David, Dikstein, Sulman, 1964: Boyns, Cole, Golder, Danutra, Harper, Brownsey, Cowley, Jones, Griffiths, 1972: Johnson, Meites, 1955: Nicoll, Meites, 1964: Refetoff, Block, Ehrlich, Friesen, 1972: Verheyden, 1964.)

Hypothalamus and prolactin secretion

Most of the work in this area has been done on the rat with a much smaller amount in the rabbit. In rats lesions in the medial hypothalamus and median eminence produced a surge of prolactin release and chronically elevated plasma prolactin levels. Lesions in the posterior hypothalamus produced only a small elevation in plasma prolactin and amygdaloid lesions had no effect at all. Complete deafferentation of the hypothalamus produced constant diestrus, with serum prolactin levels typical of normal diestrus and pituitary prolactin content very low. Anterior deafferentation only produced constant estrus with very high serum and pituitary prolactin levels. Estrogen implants in the median eminence increased prolactin secretion but implants in the pre-optic region or globus pallidus had no effect. (Arimura, Dunn, Schally, 1972: Bishop, Fawcett, Krulich, McCann, 1972: Blake, Weiner, Sawyer, 1972: Chen, Amenomori, Lu, Voogt, Meites, 1970: De Voe, Ramirez, McCann, 1966: Meites, Clemens, 1972: Ramirez, McCann, 1964.)

Insertion of electrodes into the ventro-medial hypothalamus with either sham or true stimulation reduced serum prolactin levels. Propranolol doubled serum prolactin concentration and stimulation could not prevent this: phenoxybenzamine also elevated prolactin secretion but this rise could be prevented by stimulation. In contrast other workers reported that both median eminence and basal medial hypothalamic stimulation caused prolactin release. Stimulation of the basal medial hypothalamus caused secretion of both prolactin and LH while pre-optic stimulation elevated LH secretion but depressed prolactin stimulation. (Clemens, Shaar, Kleber, Tandy, 1971: Clemens, Shaar, Tandy, Roush, 1971: Gala, Janson, Kuo, 1972: Kalra, Ajika, Krulich, Fawcett, Quijada, McCann, 1971.)

The endocrine environment seems to have both short term and long term effects on the way in which the hypothalamus regulates prolactin secretion in rats. While in normal rats or in ovariectomised rats treated with estradiol, median eminence stimulation could cause prolactin secretion, it failed to do so in untreated ovariectomised rats. Furthermore male rats castrated at birth and female rats ovariectomised as adults both responded to estrogen treatment with a very striking surge of prolactin release on the third day. Males castrated when adult or females treated with androgens at birth and ovariectomised as adults both failed to respond in this way: these "male type" animals however had higher baseline prolactin levels. In the "female-type" animals the surge could be prevented by a cut separating the anterior from the medial part of the hypothalamus suggesting that it depended on some mechanism in the anterior area. (Clemens, Shaar, Tandy, Roush, 1971: Neill, 1972.)

In the rabbit lesions in the posterior tuberal area initiated lactation but lesions elsewhere did not. In pseudopregnant rabbits the pathway involved in the stimulation of prolactin secretion in response to suckling has been traced by stimulating various parts of the brain and looking for a lactogenic response. The route seemed to go from the mid-brain to the posterior hypothalamus but a number of other areas including parts of the frontal cortex, the lateral hypothalamus and lateral pre-optic area also had lactogenic effects. Estrogen implants in the stria terminalis and amygdala also promoted lactation in pseudopregnant animals. (Cowie, Tindal, 1971: Kanematsu, Hilliard, Sawyer, 1963a, 1963b: Tindal, Knaggs, 1970: Tindal, Knaggs, 1972: Tindal, Knaggs, Turvey, 1967.)

Prolactin, FSH and LH

In humans, galactorrhea is frequently associated with amenorrhea suggesting the possibility that when prolactin secretion is elevated, secretion of FSH and LH may be suppressed. It has been shown in women that spontaneous or drug-induced elevation of prolactin levels was associated with suppression of FSH and LH and that suppression of the prolactin secretion with L-dopa led to an elevation of urinary gonadotrophin excretion and menstruation. In rats, intravenous injection of crude hypothalamic extracts stimulated secretion of LH and simultaneously suppressed prolactin secretion in intact male rats. On castration, plasma prolactin levels initially fell but then later rose to normal: the hypothalamic extracts had no effect in castrated animals with lowered prolactin levels but suppressed prolactin in castrated animals with normal prolactin levels. In this study the FSH levels were not altered. However in another study infusion of hypothalamic extracts into pituitary portal vessels of anesthetised rats reduced secretion of prolactin and elevated secretion of both LH and FSH. In both studies extracts of the cerebral cortex had no effect on any of the three hormones. (Kamberi, Mical, Porter, 1971: Sulman, 1970: Sulman, Winnik, 1956: Turkington, 1971c, 1972c: Watson, Krulich, McCann, 1971c.)

The effects of treatment with drugs and hormones point in the same direction. Melatonin and serotonin injected into the third ventricle in rats suppressed FSH and stimulated prolactin secretion. Methallibure which tends to suppress FSH and LH secretion elevated prolactin secretion. Ovariectomy caused elevation of FSH and LH secretion and suppression of prolactin secretion whereas in spayed animals estrogen treatment lowered plasma FSH and LH and elevated plasma prolactin levels: pituitary levels of all three hormones were elevated indicating the danger of arguing about plasma levels of a hormone on the basis of gland content. The norethynodrel-mestranol combination decreased hypothalamic FSH-RF, LH-RF and PIF content, decreased pituitary FSH and LH content and elevated pituitary prolactin content. Ovarian histology suggested suppression of FSH and LH secretion while mammary histology suggested stimulation of prolactin secretion. Finally, stimulation of the pre-optic area elevated LH and suppressed prolactin secretion. But in contrast, stimulation of the basal medial hypothalamus elevated both LH and prolactin secretion suggesting the possibility that in some natural situations (possibly around the time of ovulation) both LH and prolactin may be secreted together. (Ajika, Krulich, Fawcett, McCann, 1972: Ben-David, Danon, Sulman, 1971: Bishop, Kalra, Fawcett, Krulich, McCann, 1972: Clemens, Shaar, Kleber, Tandy, 1971: Kamberi, Mical, Porter, 1971b: Minaguchi, Meites, 1967.)

Short feedback control of prolactin

Most and probably all the anterior pituitary hormones have a tendency to stabilise their own secretion rates by short feedback loops whereby increases in secretion rate act on the hypothalamus to inhibit secretion of releasing factors. Decreases in secretion rates of the pituitary hormones produce the reverse effect. There is now good evidence to indicate that prolactin is governed by a similar mechanism although whether it operates via PIF alone or PIF plus PRF or TRH is not known.

Minute implants of prolactin in the hypothalamus increased hypothalamic PIF content, reduced pituitary prolactin content and reduced plasma prolactin levels. Such implants caused mammary gland regression, interrupted pregnancy and pseudopregnancy (but only during the first few days) and inhibited lactation. Similar implants in pre-pubertal rats advanced puberty by about six days, presumably due to stimulation of LH and FSH secretion: elevation of FSH release was clearly demonstrated. In rats bearing transplanted pituitaries or prolactin-secreting pituitary tumors, the prolactin content of the in situ pituitary was reduced. If such pituitaries were removed and incubated in vitro, they released much less prolactin than pituitaries removed from normal animals. One report suggested that early pregnancy could be terminated in rats by implantation of minute amounts of prolactin into the pituitary itself: the termination could be prevented by exogenous prolactin injections implying the possibility that prolactin might have a direct effect on the pituitary to inhibit its own secretion. Prolactin implants next to renal pituitary grafts also appeared to reduce prolactin secretion. Effects of prolactin on prolactin secretion in vitro were equivocal. (Averill, 1969: Chen, Minaguchi, Meites, 1967: Chen, Voogt, Meites, 1968: Clemens, Meites, 1968: Clemens, Minaguchi, Storey, Voogt, Meites, 1969: Clemens, Sar, Meites, 1969a, 1969b: MacLeod, Abad, 1968: Mena, Maiweg, Grosvenor, 1968: Spies, Clegg, 1971: Sud, Clemens, Meites, 1971: Voogt, Clemens, Meites, 1969: Voogt, Meites, 1971: Welsch, Negro-Vilar, Meites, 1968.)

The precise mechanism of the feedback remains to be elucidated and it is possible that part of it is due to a direct action on the pituitary cells. However, there do appear to be prolactin receptors in the hypothalamus because in the rabbit it has been shown that intravenous injections of prolactin may increase the firing rate of some hypothalamic neurons, decrease the firing rate of others and leave yet others unaffected. Mass recordings of hypothalamic activity point in the same direction. In normal rats and rats with pituitary tumors which receive hypothalamic prolactin implants, hypothalamic PIF content may be elevated. The possibility that dopamine may stimulate PIF secretion in these animals was raised by the fact that in both normal and castrated male and female rats treatment with prolactin but not with LH, FSH, ACTH or vasopressin produced a dose dependent increase in dopamine turnover in nerve terminals in the median eminence. In female cycling animals dopamine turnover was highest during diestrus when prolactin levels are low and lowest at proestrus when prolactin levels are high. However during lactation when prolactin secretion is high, dopamine turnover was also high, raising the possibility that at this time PRF is important in stimulating prolactin secretion and that this can occur in spite of high dopamine and PIF activity. Prolactin implantation in the hypothalamus in pseudopregnant rats appeared to suppress prolactin secretion yet had no effect on hypothalamic PIF content again indicating the possibility of an effect via PRF. (Chen, Minaguchi, Meites, 1967: Clemens, Meites, 1968: Clemens, Gallo, Whitmoyer, Sawyer, 1971: Faure, Friconneau, 1959: Hillarp, Fuxe, Dahlstrom, 1966: Hokfelt, Fuxe, 1972: Voogt, Meites, 1971.)

Chapter 7

PROLACTIN IN MALE AND
FEMALE REPRODUCTION

In female rats prolactin levels in plasma remained very low until puberty at which time a sharp rise may occur beginning the day before vaginal opening. It is possible that this may be induced by estrogen secretion resulting from the action of FSH and LH on the ovary since estrogen injections can produce a similar rise in prepubertal rats. Similar changes were found in male rats with prolactin secretion paralleling plasma testosterone levels and a sharp elevation just preceding the rapid growth of seminal vesicles at puberty. In young heifers pituitary prolactin content paralleled mammary development, rising rapidly in the first three months and then more slowly until nine months. In humans in contrast, prolactin levels are higher in children than in adults. Levels are very high in cord blood and in infant blood in the first day of life, but then rapidly decline. Prolactin can be detected in the infant's urine in the first few days of life and it has been suggested that this prolactin may be the cause of the "witch's milk" phenomenon when infants lactate in the first few days of life. (Clemens, Minaguchi, Storey, Voogt, Meites, 1969: Dowd, Bartke, 1972: Frantz, Kleinberg, Noel, 1972b: Friesen, Belanger, Guyda, Hwang, 1972: Friesen, Hwang, Guyda, Tolis, Tyson, Myers, 1972: Lyons, 1937: Minaguchi, Clemens, Meites, 1968: Sinha, Tucker, 1969: Voogt, Chen, Meites, 1970: Yamamoto, Taylor, Cole, 1970.)

Old female rats often show constant vaginal estrus and prolactin measurements reveal pituitary levels twice as high as those in young estrous rats. Pituitary LH levels are low but FSH levels are high. Plasma levels of prolactin are at or a little above plasma levels at estrus in normal young rats. It appears that in old animals there may be some change in prolactin regulation. No reports have been made of elevated levels of prolactin in old members of other species. (Clemens, Meites, 1971: Meites, Clemens, 1972.)

Prolactin during the estrous and menstrual cycles

In rats plasma prolactin levels are lowest at diestrus, begin to rise slowly on the morning of proestrus, show a dramatic rise on the afternoon of proestrus and then fall again on the day of estrus. They are still slightly elevated at metestrus.

Pituitary prolactin content is highest on the morning of proestrus and shows a sharp fall in the afternoon. However at estrus it is still higher than at diestrus. Hypothalamic PIF content is lowest on the days of proestrus and estrus. Both synthesis and release of prolactin seem to be elevated at proestrus and estrus. Hypothalamic extract injection can prevent the proestrus surge as can nembutal given at 13.30 hours on the day of proestrus. Ovariectomy and antiestradiol serum given before proestrus both prevent the preoestrus surge. In both cases the surge occurs if the animals are treated with stilbestrol suggesting that the surge depends on ovarian estrogen secretion. (Amenomori, Meites, 1970: Bast, Melampy, 1972: Freeman, Reichert, Neill, 1972: Gay, Midgley, Niswender, 1970: Ieiri, Akikusa, Yamamoto, 1971: Ieiri, Nobunaga, Yamamoto, 1972: Kalra, Ajika, Krulich, Fawcett, Quijada, McCann, 1971: Meites, Lu, Wuttke, Welsch, Nagasawa, Quadri, 1972: Neill, 1972a, 1972b: Neill, Freeman, Tillson, 1971: Sar, Meites, 1967: Spies, Niswender, 1971: Yokoyama, 1971: Yokoyama, Tomogane, Ota, 1971.)

In sheep, cattle and goats findings have been similar to those in the rat with relatively low levels during diestrus and a sharp elevation at the time of proestrus and estrus with the surge slightly preceding the surge of LH release. (Anderson, Peters, Melampy, Cox, 1972: Bryant, Greenwood, 1968: Bryant, Linzell, Greenwood, 1970: Cumming, Brown, Goding, Bryant, Greenwood, 1972: Davis, Reichart, Niswender, 1971: Kann, 1971: Raud, Kiddy, Odell, 1971: Reeves, Arimura, 1970: Reeves, Arimura, Schally, 1970: Threlfall, Martin, Dale, Anderson, Krause, 1972.)

During the human menstrual cycle, older bioassay methods suggested that urinary and plasma levels of prolactin were substantially higher during the luteal phase than during the follicular phase with possible elevated levels at the time of ovulation. The newer radioimmunoassay techniques have as yet failed to show any prolactin peak at the time of ovulation, but this may possibly be because the published reports refer only to single blood samples and if a prolactin surge is very brief it might be necessary to sample very frequently during a day in order to observe it. RI assay has also shown that there is a considerable variation in response between individual women. Many seem to have levels in the luteal phase which are similar to or only slightly higher than those in the follicular phase. Some, however, have a quite different pattern during the luteal phase with highly erratic fluctuations: plasma level may be very high one day and low the next. In view of the probable prolonged tissue half life of prolactin, it seems possible that tissue levels of prolactin in these women may be relatively consistently high during the luteal phase. Using bioassay methods it has been reported that women with menstrual irregularities and abnormalities and the Stein-Leventhal syndrome may have elevated prolactin levels. (Berle, Apostolakis, Link, 1971: Birkinshaw, Falconer, 1972: Friesen, 1971: Friesen, Belanger, Guyda, Hwang, 1972: Friesen, Hwang, Guyda, Tolis, Tyson, Myers, 1972: Gati, Doszpod, Preisz, 1967: Hwang, Guyda, Friesen, 1971: Kowalski, Dabrowski, Stepniewski, 1969: L'Hermite, Delvoye, Nokin, Vekemans, Robyn, 1972: Simkin, Arce, 1963: Simkin, Goodhart, 1960: Talas, 1967: Talas, Stehlikova, Jezdinsky, 1968.)

Effects of coitus on prolactin secretion

In rats, females but not males show dramatic elevations of prolactin, LH and FSH 20 minutes after mating. Ewes and female goats also show prolactin secretion in response to mating. Ejaculation by bulls into an artificial vagina produced a surge of prolactin release, with a smaller effect on growth hormone. In humans sexual intercourse produced an elevation of plasma prolactin levels in some but not all women: there was some indication that orgasm may have been associated with elevated prolactin levels: prolactin levels did not rise significantly in men. The degree of mammary stimulation should be taken into account since in women self-stimulation and stimulation of the nipples by a male partner both produced elevation of prolactin secretion. In men self stimulation of the nipple had no effect but stimulation by a female partner elevated prolactin levels by 2-4 times. (Bryant, Linzell, Greenwood, 1970: Convey, Bretschneider, Hafs, Oxender, 1971: Cumming, Brown, Goding, Bryant, Greenwood, 1972: Kolodny, Jacobs, Daughaday, 1972: Noel, Suh, Stone, Frantz, 1972: Spies, Niswender, 1971.)

Effects of prolactin on the ovary and corpus luteum

This topic has already been partly discussed in the biochemistry chapter where it was shown that in many species prolactin appears capable of facilitating progestin secretion, probably primarily by providing a pool of precursors on which LH can act. This section is mainly concerned with the luteotrophic and luteolytic mechanisms which occur during the estrous cycle and pseudopregnancy. Ergot alkaloids which presumably operate by suppressing prolactin secretion have been reported to have no very obvious effect on the estrous cycle in rats, apart from slight shortening. The ovaries contained large numbers of corpora lutea but vaginal smears suggested that these were not secreting progesterone. One report claimed that ergocornine could prevent ovulation but this was not supported by others. The experiments suggest that in the absence of prolactin corpora lutea fail to produce progesterone but also are not physically destroyed in the usual way. Prolactin injections in CB 154 treated rats caused luteolysis with a restoration of normal ovarian appearance. Prolactin treatment could prevent ovulation in response to LH but apparently only in animals with active corpora lutea. It was thought that the ovulation block was secondary to stimulation of progesterone secretion from the corpora lutea. (Billeter, Fluckiger, 1971: Heuson, Waelbroeck-van Gaver, Legros, 1970: Hixon, Armstrong, 1971: Kraicer, Strauss, 1970: Meites, Lu, Wuttke, Welsch, Nagasawa, Quadri, 1972: Spies, Niswender, 1971: Yokoyama, Tomogane, Ota, 1972.)

In rats sterile coitus or various forms of cervical stimulation at the time of estrus can induce pseudopregnancy which normally lasts for about 14 days. Coitus and cervical stimulation produced a surge of prolactin secretion even in pelvic-neurectomised rats: ergot alkaloid treatment could prevent this surge. However this surge cannot be important in the initiation of pseudopregnancy since the latter did not occur in pelvic-neurectomised rats when the surge was present, yet did occur in ergot-treated rats in which the surge was absent. During the pseudo-pregnancy plasma prolactin levels were elevated for the first 3-4 days, then declined to below diestrus levels and then were elevated again on day 13. Ergot alkaloid treatment or suppression of prolactin secretion by hypothalamic prolactin implants throughout the pseudopregnancy shortened it by only 2-3 days. This suggested that except perhaps at the end of the pseudopregnancy prolactin was not important in maintaining luteal function. In contrast there have been a number of reports, the most convincing involving direct observation of anterior eye chamber ovarian transplants, that prolactin injections or reserpine-stimulated prolactin secretion can maintain active luteal function for up to three weeks. Such prolonged periods of maintenance by exogenous prolactin injections were achieved more easily in hypophysectomised animals. It seems possible therefore that prolactin may have two quite distinct effects on luteal function. When corpora lutea which are in an active state are exposed to prolactin that active state is maintained and the termination of secretion which is associated with a rise in 20α-hydroxysteroid dehydrogenase activity is delayed. On the other hand, once luteal secretion has stopped, prolactin appears to be necessary for the physical dissolution of the old corpora lutea. (Ahmad, Lyons, Ellis, 1969: Averill, 1969: Bast, Melampy, 1972: Billeter, Fluckiger, 1971: Bishop, Orias,

Fawcett, Krulich, McCann, 1971: Browning, Guzman, 1967: Chen, Voogt, Meites, 1968: Clark, 1972: Clemens, Meites, 1968: Choudary, Greenwald, 1967: Everett, 1954: Fluckiger, Lutterbeck, Wagner, Billeter, 1972: Freeman, Neill, 1972: Hashimoto, Wiest, 1969: Heuson, Waelbroeck-van Gaver, Legros, 1970: Hixon, Armstrong, 1971: Kraicer, Strauss, 1970: Macdonald, 1969: Macdonald, Yoshinaga, Greep, 1971: Malven, 1969: Malven, Hansel, Sawyer, 1967: Meites, Lu, Wuttke, Welsch, Nagasawa, Quadri, 1972: Miyakawa, 1972: Rabii, Kragt, 1972: Rothchild, 1960: Saito, Arimura, Sawaro, 1970: Shelesnyak, 1954: Spies, Niswender, 1971: Van Maanen, Smelik, 1968: Wuttke, Meites, 1971: Wuttke, Meites, 1972: Voogt, Meites, 1971: Yokoyama, Tomogane, Ota, 1972: Yoshida, 1964: Zarrow, Brown-Grant, 1964.)

There seem to be considerable species differences in the control of luteal function. In mice, observation of eye grafts indicated that for functional hyperemia to develop in FSH primed follicles, both LH and prolactin were required. After hypophysectomy mouse corpora lutea degenerate and this cannot be prevented by prolactin injections or prolactin-secreting transplants. In intact animals however, prolactin injections prolonged the functional life of the corpora lutea. Much less information is available on the hamster but it suggests that prolactin and FSH are both required for luteal maintenance. Evidence for a luteolytic effect of prolactin has also been obtained in this species. Treatment of cycling animals with ergocornine led to a significant rise in the numbers of corpora lutea found in the ovaries: prolactin treatment restored these numbers to normal. In guinea pigs it has been reported that prolactin alone may prevent the luteal degeneration which normally occurs after hypophysectomy. (Browning, Brown, Crisp, Gibbs, 1965: Grady, Greenwald, 1968: Grandison, 1972: Greenwald, 1967: Illingworth, Perry, 1971: Rowlands, 1962: Turnbull, Kent, 1966.)

In the rabbit hypophysectomy causes luteal regression. A combination of FSH and prolactin seems most important in preventing this although LH has also been reported to have an anti-atrophic action. In sheep, exogenous prolactin injections failed to prolong the life of the corpus luteum during the estrous cycle. After hypophysectomy LH alone had a weak effect in delaying luteal atrophy, but prolactin or FSH alone had no action. (Kaltenbach, Graber, Niswender, Nalbandov, 1968: Karsch, Cook, Ellicott, Foster, Jackson, Nalbandov, 1971: Kilpatrick, Armstrong, Greep, 1964: Rennie, Davies, Friedrich, 1964: Spies, Hilliard, Sawyer, 1968.)

Prolactin and uterine fluid and vaginal mucus

In rats and mice prolactin seems to be the major hormone involved in the stimulation of mucus secretion by the vagina. This may be quantified by studying sialic acid production. In hypophysectomised and ovariectomised rats estradiol alone and progesterone alone failed to increase sialic acid production: together they increased it by 40% but the addition of prolactin increased it by 290%. This suggests that prolactin has an extra-ovarian effect on the vagina not mediated by changes in steroid secretion. Prolactin also had an action on the accumulation of fluid in the uterus, probably by modifying cervical contraction. Estradiol treated ovariectomised rats accumulated uterine fluid for five days after which the cervix relaxed and the fluid escaped. In hypophysectomised, ovariectomised rats, the uterus accumulated fluid continuously and the cervix remained constricted: prolactin treatment then allowed the cervix to relax and the fluid escaped. (Josimovich, Wilson, Leff, 1970: Kennedy, Armstrong, 1972a, 1972b.)

Effects of prolactin on the male reproductive system

Actions of prolactin on the testis have already been discussed in the biochemistry section. It seems to be involved in the provision of a testosterone precursor pool and in the induction of some of the enzymes required for testosterone metabolism. Most other work has concentrated on its effects on the prostate and seminal vesicles, especially in the rat.

Prolactin appeared to be specifically bound to receptors on seminal vesicle tissue but not on prostatic tissue in the rat. However, prolactin stimulated both adenylate cyclase activity and the binding of testosterone in prostatic tissue maintained in culture but reduced the formation of 5-α-dihydroxytestosterone. When prostatic epithelium was maintained for several days in culture, in controls the cells tended to degenerate and become flattened. Prolactin alone had a very slight effect in reducing the degree of atrophy when added in moderate concentrations while testosterone alone had a rather greater effect. The two hormones together completely prevented degeneration and maintained an apparently active epithelium. High doses of prolactin had a reversed action and promoted degeneration. In general, although there have been some negative results, most in vivo experiments have supported the concept that prostate growth and secretion depend on the combined synergistic actions of prolactin and androgens. The diminished response to testosterone seen in hypophysectomised animals may be restored by prolactin treatment. (Boyns, Cole, Golder, Danutra, Harper, Brownsey, Cowley, Jones, Griffiths, 1972: Farnsworth, 1972: Grayhack, Bunce, Kearns, Scott, 1955: Grayhack, Lebowitz, 1972: Lawrence, Landau, 1965: Lostroh, Li, 1957: Ravault, Peyre, 1969: Reddi, 1969: Rosoff, Martin, 1968: Segaloff, Steelman, Flores, 1956: Turkington, Frantz, 1972: Van der Laan, 1953: Walsh, Gittes, 1969.)

The actions of prolactin on rat seminal vesicles may be even more pronounced as might be expected on the basis of receptor binding. Prolactin synergised with testosterone in stimulating seminal vesicle activity and growth both in vivo and in vitro. In castrated, hypophysectomised rats it increased seminal vesicle weights even in the absence of testosterone. (Bengmark, Hesseljo, 1963: 1964: Chase, Geschwind, Bern, 1957: Peyre, Ravault, Laporte, 1968: Turkington, Frantz, 1972.)

Asano has raised the possibility that in rats there may be a prostatic factor modifying prolactin release. After prostatectomy prolactin secretion from and pituitaries incubated in vitro was elevated.   A crude prostatic extract suppressed prolactin release. There have been two other reports of the possibility of some target organ negative feedback mechanism. In a male with galactorrhea mastectomy apparently was associated with elevated prolactin secretion while in pigs this also happened after hysterectomy. Clearly there may be scope for much more work in this area. (Anderson, Peters, Melampy, Cox, 1972: Asano, 1965: Volpe, Killinger, Bird, Clark, Friesen, 1972.)

Dwarf mice seem to have a specific prolactin deficiency: females are sterile and males are sub-fertile. Prolactin treatment by pituitary grafts or injections restored fertility in both sexes, apparently in the case of males by promoting spermatogenesis. In hypophysectomised ordinary mice, prolactin, LH and testosterone all had a small effect in restoring spermatogenesis when given alone. Prolactin augmented the effect of LH but not that of testosterone suggesting that the action of prolactin may have been to provide a precursor pool on which LH could act to stimulate testosterone secretion. (Bartke, 1966, 1967, 1971: Bartke, Lloyd, 1970.)

In castrated guinea pigs prolactin alone had no effect on weight or histology of either prostate or seminal vesicles. It did, however, synergise with testosterone in raising seminal vesicle weight and promoting secretion. Even in combination with testosterone it did not appear to have any prostatic effects. In rabbits, in contrast, injection of prolactin antiserum into adult male animals caused weight decrease and degeneration of both prostate and seminal vesicles. (Antliff, Prasad, Meyer, 1960a, 1960b: Asano, Kanzaki, Sekiguchi, Tasaka, 1971.)

In dogs prostatic atrophy was greater after hypophysectomy than after castration but the pituitary factor responsible was not identified. (Huggins, Russell, 1946.)

In baboons prolactin has been reported to reduce [65]Zn uptake in many tissues but it had no effect on uptake by prostate or seminal vesicles. (Schoonees, De Klerk, Murphy, 1970.)

In humans it has been reported that those with prostatic cancer have higher prolactin levels than those with benign prostatic hypertrophy and that prolactin levels rise as the disease progresses. This will be discussed further in the chapter on cancer. (Asano, 1962. 1965: Farnsworth, 1972.)

Prolactin and reproductive behavior

The role of prolactin in reproductive behavior in non-mammalian vertebrates has been extensively documented but studies in mammals are few. The idea that it might be involved in behaviour is not implausible since it seems to be specifically bound by the cerebral cortex and it is known to alter the behaviour of hypothalamic neurons. (Clemens, Gallo, Whitmoyer, Sawyer, 1971: Faure, Friconneau, 1959: Hokfelt, Fuxe, 1972: Nicoll, Bern, 1972: Riddle, 1963a, 1963b: Turkington, Frantz, 1972.)

In the rabbit prolactin seems to be one of the hormones involved in hair loosening and nest building and it also seems to be required for maternal behaviour in the rat. In both species a combination of prolactin with progesterone and estrogen seems to be required. In male rabbits exogenously administered prolactin has been reported to have a marked inhibitory effect on male copulatory activity: the effect could not be counteracted by simultaneous treatment with testosterone. In male homosexuals, plasma prolactin levels may be slightly elevated. (Farooq, Denenberg, Ross, Sawin, Zarrow, 1963: Hartmann, Endroczi, 1966: Kolodny, Jacobs, Masters, Toro, Daughaday, 1972: Moltz, Lubin, Leon, Numan, 1970: Zarrow, Farooq, Denenberg, Sawin, Ross, 1963: Zarrow, Grota, Denenberg, 1967: Zarrow, Sawin, Ross, Denenberg, Crary, Wilson, Farooq, 1961.)

Chapter 8

PREGNANCY

There appear to be marked differences in prolactin physiology in pregnancy between rodents, ruminants and humans. It is more important than in most areas of physiology to avoid generalising from one species to another without specific evidence.

Rodents

In rats prolactin levels in pregnancy are similar to those in **pseudopregnancy** being elevated for the first 4-6 days, then very low until the last day of pregnancy when a relatively rapid rise takes place on days 20-21. Hypophysectomy, treatment with ergot alkaloids and hypothalamic implantation of prolactin all terminated pregnancy with certainty if carried out during the first week or so. Prolactin injections alone could maintain pregnancy with the last two procedures but in hypophysectomised animals FSH was required as well. Progesterone could maintain pregnancy in the absence of the pituitary hormones, suggesting that the prolactin may have been acting by stimulating the corpus luteum to secrete progesterone. In rats delayed implantation could be achieved by hypophysectomy and pituitary autotransplantation the day after mating. Nidation could then be triggered by estrogen: ergocornine prevented the nidation but the inhibitory effect could be overcome by progesterone. Pelvic neurectomised rats failed to become pregnant unless they received pituitary homografts beneath the renal capsule. Placement of 300 μg exogenous prolactin near the grafts four days after mating terminated pregnancy. All the experiments point to the idea that prolactin is important in the maintenance of pregnancy during the first few days primarily because of its actions on the corpus luteum. (Amenomori, Chen, Meites, 1970: Armstrong, King, 1971: Bast, Melampy, Choudary, Greenwald, 1967: Clemens, Sar, Meites, 1969: Greenwald, Johnson, 1968: Linkie, Niswender, 1972: Meites, Clemens, 1972: Meites, Lu, Wuttke, Welsch, Nagasawa, Quadri, 1972: Schlough, Schuetz, Meyer, 1965: Spies, Clegg, 1971: Spies, Forbes, Clegg, 1971: Varavudhi, Lobel, Shelesnyak, 1966.)

Dwarf female mice with hereditary prolactin deficiency are infertile. They could be made fertile by implanting normal mouse pituitary glands under the renal capsule. Removal of the graft in the first week or so of pregnancy terminated it, but removal later on had no effect. This behaviour which is similar to that of rats suggests that in these species as in humans, there may be a placental lactogen. Rat placental extracts have been reported to have crop sac stimulating activity. Mono-amine oxidase inhibitors which reduce prolactin secretion could also terminate pregnancy much more easily in the first half than the second half: the effect could be overcome by treatment with either progesterone or prolactin. Pregnancy block in mice which may occur on exposure to alien males could be overcome by proges-terone or prolactin. No changes in pituitary prolactin could be detected until the females had been caged with the alien males for 48 hours. (Bartke, 1971: Chapman, Desjardins, Whitten, 1970: Dominic, 1966, 1967: Finn, Martin, 1971: Lindsay, Poulson, Robson, 1963: Nicholson, 1970: Poulson, Robson, 1963: 1964a, 1964b: Shani, Zanbelman, Khazen, Sulman, 1970.)

In rats, estrone increased the deciduoma response of the uterus and stimulated ring A reduction of progesterone by uterine tissue. Prolactin partially inhibited the deci-duoma response in estrone-treated animals and inhibited the ring A reduction of progesterone in progesterone treated rats. (Armstrong, King, 1971.)

In rabbits hypophysectomy in the 2nd week of pregnancy caused degeneration of the corpus luteum. Prolactin and FSH slowed down this process but LH had no additional effect. Treatment with estradiol plus prolactin maintained both corpus luteum and ovarian interstitial tissue in a healthy state and prevented termination. (Spies, Hilliard, Sawyer, 1968.)

Ruminants

After the elevations of prolactin plasma level at the time of mating, prolactin con-centrations in sheep and goats as measured by radioimmunoassay fell progressively until in mid-pregnancy they were below levels seen at diestrus. At this time prolactin levels measured by bioassay were much higher suggesting the possibility of the pre-sence of placental lactogen. About 4-5 weeks before the expected date of parturition levels began to rise slowly and then 30-50 hours before parturition there began a dramatic surge of prolactin secretion which elevated plasma levels 5-10 fold. Levels at parturition were higher than during lactation. There was also a rise of estrogen levels in plasma 1-2 days before parturition: this appeared to start later than the prolactin surge but this might have been accounted for by differences in the sensi-tivities of the two assays. Prolactin could be found in fetal blood only after the 110-135th day of gestation in sheep: levels were always below those in maternal plasma. Prolactin appeared to be absent from the amniotic and allantoic fluid except when the fetal plasma concentration was exceptionally high. Findings in cattle were substantially in agreement with those in sheep and goats. (Alexander, Britton, Buttle, Nixon, 1972: Brumby, Forsyth, 1969: Buttle, Forsyth, 1971: Buttle, Forsyth, Knaggs, 1972: Challis, 1971: Davis, Reichart, Niswender, 1971: Fell, Beck, Brown, Catt, Cumming, Goding,1972: Hart, 1972: Lamming, Moseley, McNeilly, 1972: McNeilly, 1971: Moger, Geschwind, 1971: Ingalls, Hafs, Oxender, 1971: Obst, Seamark, 1972: Oxender, 1972a, 1972b: Oxender, Convey, Hafs, 1972: Schams, Karg, 1970: Schams, Bohms, Karg, 1971.)

Primates

Prolactin physiology in primate pregnancy seems to be quite different from that in other animals. In humans there is a steady but slow rise in plasma prolactin levels reaching a mean of 50 ng/ml in the second trimester. In the third trimester levels rise much more rapidly to a mean of about 200 ng/ml at term (range 35-600). Little change was observed in the last two weeks. Levels in fetal and neonatal blood at term were similar to those in the mother and prolactin appeared in neonatal urine. In one woman with an isolated growth hormone deficiency who was being specially investigated, levels in the umbilical vein were higher than those in the umbilical artery which in turn were higher than those in the uterine vein. In monkeys in complete contrast, plasma prolactin levels remained relatively low throughout pregnancy. It was suggested that this might be related to the low estrogen production during pregnancy in rhesus monkeys: at term a normal human excretes about 25-35 mg estrogens/day while in the same period a monkey excretes about 35 μg. (Berle, Apostolakis, 1971: Friesen, Belanger, Guyda, Hwang, 1972: Friesen, Hwang, Guyda, Tolis, Tyson, Myers, 1972: Hwang, Guyda, Friesen, 1971: L'Hermite, Delvoye, Nokin, Vekemans, Robyn, 1972: L'Hermite, Stauric, Robyn, 1972: Lyons, 1937: Tyson, Hwang, Guyda, Friesen, 1972

Histological studies of the pituitaries taken from women who died during pregnanc confirm the idea that prolactin secretion is much more active at this time. Many more prolactin-secreting cells are found than in the non-pregnant state. (Goluboff, Ezran, 1969: Pasteels, Gausset, Danguy, Ectors, 1972: Pasteels, Gausset, Danguy, Ectors, Nicoll, Varavudhi, 1972.)

The truly remarkable thing about primate pregnancy is, however, the quantity of prolactin to be found in the amniotic fluid. In the first trimester the prolactin concentration in human amniotic fluid is around 2500 ng/ml with a range of from about 1000 to 10000 ng/ml. There is a slow decline until the end of pregnancy when the mean is about 1200 ng/ml, with a range of from about 900 to 2000 ng/ml. These concentrations are of course very much higher than the concentrations of prolactin in plasma. In early pregnancy amniotic fluid prolactin concentration is roughly 80-90 times greater than plasma concentrations and at the end of pregnancy amniotic fluid concentration is about 10 times plasma concentration. Strikingly, although rhesus monkey plasma prolactin levels are so low, amniotic fluid concentrations are even higher than those seen in humans, although for obvious reasons the number of observations so far made is much smaller. Levels after about three months of pregnancy were about 1700 ng/ml but by five months these had doubled or tripled. (Hwang, Guyda, Tolis, Tyson, Myers, 1972: Tyson, Hwang, Guyda, Friesen, 1972.)

The obvious problems raised by these findings are first the source and then the function of this prolactin. It appeared on the basis of a number of physico-chemical and immunological comparisons to be identical with pituitary prolactin and one possibility is that it is pituitary prolactin which is in some way concentrated by the amniotic fluid. However, when ^{125}I labelled prolactin was injected into maternal monkey plasma, it had an initial half life of about 10-15 minutes and virtually none appeared in either fetus or amniotic fluid. [125]I prolactin injected into the amniotic fluid directly appeared to have a half life of several hours indicating that the amniotic prolactin pool was relatively stable. These findings suggest, but do not prove that prolactin in both amniotic fluid and fetal blood could come from somewhere in the feto-placental unit. Since in one human observation umbilical vein prolactin was higher than that in the umbilical artery, a source in the placenta or membranes seems most likely at the moment Incubation of small pieces of amnion, chorion and placenta in Krebs,-Ringer bicarbonate buffer showed that the amnion and chorion but not the placenta released small amounts of prolactin into the medium. On the face of it it seems more likely that this prolactin was bound to the tissues rather than synthesised by them but a definite conclusion awaits further work. (Hwang, Guyda, Tolis, Tyson, Myers, 1972: Tyson, Hwang, Guyda, Friesen, 1972.)

Two hypotheses have been proposed for the role of amniotic fluid prolactin. The first is that prolactin may be playing its ancient role of regulating fluid and electrolyte metabolism and may be important in the control of the amniotic fluid. If this is so then situations in which amniotic fluid regulation is disturbed might be expected to reveal abnormal amniotic fluid prolactin levels. In four human patients with hydramnios prolactin levels were below 200 ng/ml, well below the normal range: in three others prolactin concentrations were normal. This strongly suggests that in some patients there may be a negative correlation between amniotic fluid volume and prolactin concentration. (Friesen, Hwang, Guyda, Tolis, Tyson, Myers, 1972: Tyson, Hwang, Guyda, Friesen, 1972.)

The other hypothesis suggests that the prolactin is in some way delivered to the myometrium and is concerned with the regulation of myometrial activity. It is, of course, not incompatible with the first hypothesis. In rats prolactin has been reported to promote cervical relaxation. In strips of uterine muscle taken from estrogen or estrogen plus progesterone treated rats, oxytocin treatment caused over a period of twelve hours, a steadily increasing pattern of contractile activity. Prolactin added to the bath did not inhibit the basal contractile activity significantly, but it did promote lengthening of the muscle strip and it completely blocked the normal increase in activity. In similar experiments with late pregnant guinea pigs it was shown that prolactin within an hour reduced contractile activity to much less than one half that seen in control strips. An increasing feature of the effect was that after about 25-30 minutes there was a consistent and very abrupt reduction in the amplitude of

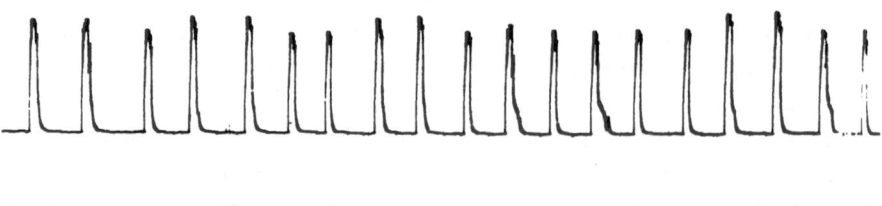

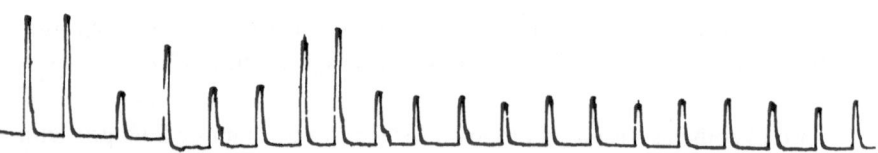

FIG. 1.   A record of oxytocin-stimulated contractions of smooth muscle taken from a guinea pig in late pregnancy. Prolactin in a concentration of 10 microg/ml was added at the arrow. The time marks represent minutes and the lower record follows continuously after the upper one. The characteristic feature is the abrupt change in contraction amplitude. Parallel control strips taken from the same uterus contracted for several hours without significant change in amplitude of contraction.

the contractions (Figure 1). Strips taken from mid-pregnant guinea pigs were less sensitive to this effect while those from early pregnant guinea pigs were inhibited only slightly by prolactin. In recent preliminary experiments using strips of myometrium removed from the edge of the uterine incision during human caesarian section we have shown that in concentrations of 5 μg and 10 μg/ml ovine prolactin could stop oxytocin-stimulated contractions within 30 minutes: control strips without added prolactin went on contracting for hours. Lower prolactin concentrations have not yet been tested. Clearly these observations are only very preliminary but they do indicate that prolactin concentrations within the range found in human amniotic fluid can inhibit myometrial activity in three different species. If amniotic fluid prolactin is important in controlling myometrial activity, this could explain why premature labour is so common with hydramnios (although uterine stretch is clearly a factor here) and why labour is so successfully initiated in most women by rupturing the membranes and allowing the amniotic fluid to drain away. Glucocorticoids appear able to suppress pituitary prolactin secretion: if they suppress prolactin manufacture or concentration by the membranes-amniotic fluid unit, this could account for the initiation of labour in humans by the injection of betamethasone into the amniotic fluid. Clearly much more work must be done in this area. (Horrobin, Lipton, Muiruri, Manku, Bramley, Burstyn, 1973: Mati, Horrobin, Bramley, 1973.)

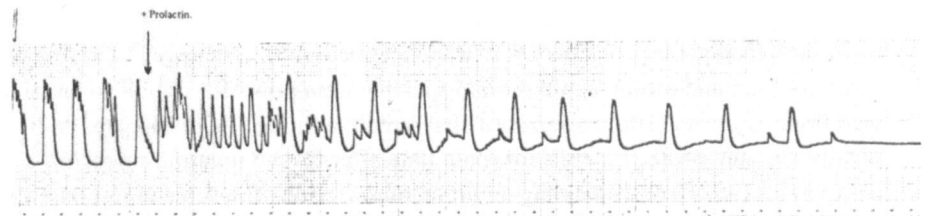

FIG. 2. A record of oxytocin-stimulated contractions in a strip of human smooth muscle taken from the edge of the uterine wound during Caesarian section. Prolactin in a concentration of 10 microg/ml was added to the bath at the arrow. The time marks represent minutes. Prolactin first altered the contraction pattern, then slowed the contractions and reduced their amplitude and finally abolished them altogether.

Chapter 9

LACTATION

The role of prolactin in lactation is the best known of all its actions and has been extensively reviewed many times, notably in the recent book "The Physiology of Lactation" by Cowie and Tindal. For this reason it will be dealt with relatively briefly here and emphasis will be placed on work published in the last two years.

Levels during lactation and suckling

In the rat both pituitary content and plasma levels have been measured during lactation and suckling. Serum prolactin levels were low during pregnancy but rose the day before parturition. During lactation basal plasma levels were elevated so long as the litters were left with the mother but on removal of the litter levels fell to non-pregnant values within a few hours. Suckling consistently caused depletion of pituitary prolactin content and elevation of plasma levels. (Amenomori, Chen, Meites, 1970: Convey, Reece, 1969: Grosvenor, Mena, 1971: Grosvenor, Mena, Schaefgen, 1967: Meites, 1966: Meites, Clemens, 1972: Sar, Meites, 1969: Terkel, Blake, Sawyer, 1972.)

In sheep and goats prolactin levels in the plasma also rose sharply just before parturition. Hand and machine milking and suckling were powerful stimuli to prolactin secretion. After such stimulation levels fell rapidly although there appeared to be slightly elevated prolactin levels for some time after teat stimulation suggesting a more prolonged effect of suckling on prolactin secretion. The surge in response to suckling appeared to be greatest just after parturition and as lactation proceeded the magnitude of the suckling surge declined. (Buttle, Forsyth, 1971: Buttle, Forsyth, Knaggs, 1972: Bryant, Greenwood, 1968: Bryant, Greenwood, Linzell, 1968: Bryant, Linzell, Greenwood, 1970: Fell, Beck, Brown, Catt, Cumming, Goding, 1972: Fell, Beck, Brown, Cumming, Goding, 1972: Lamming, Moseley, McNeilly, 1972.)

Similar results have been obtained in cattle. Again plasma levels rise just before parturition and just afterwards both basal levels and the responses to milking and suckling are at their peak. With prolonged lactation basal levels between milking reach values seen in non-lactating animals and the surges in response to milking and suckling become much smaller. (Joke, 1970: Koprowski, Tucker, 1971: Schams, 1972: Schams, Bohms, Karg, 1971: Schams, Karg, 1970.)

In humans levels of prolactin were high at the end of pregnancy and basal levels during the first few days post partum were of the same order of magnitude, sometimes a little higher than in pregnancy, sometimes a little lower. Basal levels during the post partum two weeks steadily fell but no differences were observed between nursing mothers and those whose lactation had been suppressed by estrogen treatment. After the first two weeks in both groups of women levels were only a little above those seen during normal menstrual cycles and in some lactating women fell to menstrual cycle levels. Suckling produced a sharp rise in plasma prolactin levels: the range of elevation reported by different workers has been from 2-100 fold. Some of the differences in results are undoubtedly due to individual differences between women but some may be due to differences in assay performance with possible non-linearity over part of the range of prolactin concentrations. Tyson et al made a detailed study of the responses to suckling during prolonged periods of lactation. In the first week post partum mean basal levels were about 140 ng/ml rising to about 200 mg/ml after suckling. Up to two months post partum the corresponding figures were 30 and 160 ng/ml and after two months 25 and 60 ng/ml. There were large individual variations and after two months some women showed typical menstrual cycle basal levels with very little response to suckling in spite of the fact that milk production was obviously continuing. The prolactin response to TRH tended to be larger than normal during the post partum weeks although the TSH response to TRH was normal. During late lactation, even in those women who showed little or no response to suckling a normal TRH response was observed. A very interesting observation was that prolactin concentrations in human milk were higher than those in plasma sampled at the same moment suggesting that the breast may be capable of concentrating prolactin. (Bryant, Greenwood, 1972: Frantz, Kleinberg, Noel, 1972: Friesen, 1972c: Friesen, Hwang, Guyda, Tolis, Tyson, Myers, 1972: L'Hermite, Delvoye, Nokin, Vekemans, Robyn, 1972: Tyson, Friesen, Anderson, 1972: Tyson, Hwang, Guyda, Friesen, 1972.)

Mechanism of the response to suckling

The secretion of prolactin in response to suckling seems to depend on stimulation of nipple sensory nerves. Impulses are then carried up to the hypothalamus where prolactin release is stimulated. At least part of the stimulation has been shown in rats to be due to depletion of hypothalamic PIF but doubts have been raised as to whether the dramatic rise in prolactin secretion which occurs could be accounted for solely in terms of removal of inhibition: several workers have felt that such a striking response could be accounted for only by a combination of a rise of releasing factor activity and a fall in inhibiting factor activity. In rats the rise in prolactin secretion in response to ether anesthesia could be blocked by prior injection of rat hypothalamic extracts, presumably containing PIF: the much larger rise in response to suckling could not be so blocked. Bovine and ovine hypothalamic extracts did prevent any fall in rat pituitary prolactin content in response to suckling. Unfortunately there appear to be no studies which have looked at both gland content and blood levels after hypothalamic extract treatment but one possible explanation of the observations is that pr lactin secretion still occurred in response to suckling but in the presence of PIF was insufficient to deplete the gland. (Amenomori, Meites, 1970: Cowie, Tindal, 1971: Grosvenor, 1965: Grosvenor, McCann, Nallar, 1965: Meites, Lu, Wuttke, Welsch, Nagasawa, Quadri, 1972: Mena, Beyer, 1963: Mena, Grosvenor, 1968: Ratner, Meites, 1964: Sar, Meites, 1969: Tindal, Knaggs, 1970, 1972: Tindal, Knaggs, Turvey 1967.)

The fall in pituitary gland prolactin content which occured in response to suckling did not occur in response to a second period of suckling in the rat if the time interval between the first and second suckling was less than two hours. This was true even if prolactin depletion in response to the first suckling period was prevented by a hypo thalamic extract containing PIF. On the other hand, depletion of prolactin content of the pituitary did not occur if the interval between two suckling periods was prolonged to 16 hours. This suggests that there is a refractory period in the mechanism which causes the depletion response to suckling to fail if two suckling periods follow one another too rapidly, but on the other hand that an active response requires regular suckling for its maintenance. Two hours of suckling in rats depleted pituitary prolactin content almost to 10% of the starting level. Normal levels were restored agai after eight hours without suckling. In order to test whether absence of PIF was the only condition required for refilling of the gland, pituitaries were removed immediately after suckling and incubated in vitro. No repletion occurred. This suggests that the main action of PIF is on prolactin release and that some other factor is required to stimulate prolactin synthesis. Rat hypothalamic extracts given to lactating rats after suckling accelerated the rate of reaccumulation of prolactin in the gland. Ovine hypothalamic extracts, rich in PIF, did not alter the rate of reaccumulation. (Convey, Reece, 1969: Grosvenor, Maiweg, Mena, 1970: Grosvenor, Mena, 1971: Grosvenor, Mena, Maiweg, Dhariwal, McCann, 1970: Grosvenor, Mena, Schaefgen, 1967.)

In rats a number of other stimuli apart from suckling appear able to stimulate prolactin secretion. Even if suckling was prevented, the presence of pups or of other lactating rats, but not of male rats, seemed able to stimulate prolactin release. In humans, however, giving her baby to a mother did not appear to stimulate prolactin secretion in the absence of actual suckling. (Frantz, Kleinberg, Noel, 1972b: Grosvenor, 1965: Grosvenor, Mena, 1967: Mena, Grosvenor, 1972: Moltz, Levin, Leon, 1969.)

Benson and Folley in 1956 demonstrated that oxytoxin injections could prevent involution of mammary glands after litter removal and suggested that this indicated that oxytocin could stimulate prolactin secretion. However it is now known that oxytocin may have a direct action on the alveoler cells to retard their rate of involution. Attempts to stimulate prolactin secretion by oxytocin injections in sheep and cattle failed to produce consistent elevations in prolactin secretion except when very large doses which might have been stressful to the animal were used. It therefore seems unlikely that oxytocin is a natural stimulator of prolactin release although it remains conceivable that very high doses of oxytocin given into the blood may be required to simulate the concentrations of oxytocin delivered precisely by nerve cells to a particular hpothalamic site. (Benson, Folley, 1956: Bryant, Greenwood, 1972: Huntingford, 1963: Joke, 1970: Koprowski, Tucker, 1971: Ota, Shinde, Yokoyama, 1965: Schams, 1972: Schams, Bohm, Karg, 1971: Schams, Karg, 1970: Sinha, Tucker, 1969: Thatcher, Tucker, 1970.)

Hormone requirements for mammary function

There is an extensive literature, admirably reviewed by Cowie and Tindal (1971) on the hormonal requirements for mammary development and milk secretion in vivo. While there are considerable species differences, it seems that estrogen, progesterone, glucocorticoids, thyroid hormone, insulin, prolactin and growth hormone are all required for normal lobulo-alveolar growth during pregnancy. The glucocorticoids, thyroid hormone and insulin, probably act mainly as permissive factors. As might be expected with such a complex system there seem to be substantial species differences, not to speak of differences between experimenters working on the same species! It would seem pointless in this book to review again work which has been described so well elsewhere. (Cole, Hopkins, 1962: Cowie, 1964: Cowie, Daniel, Knaggs, 1964: Cowie, Hartmann, Turvey, 1969: Cowie, Tindal, 1971: Cowie, Tindal, Yokoyama, 1966: Djojosoebagio, Turner, 1964: Hartmann, Cowie, 1970: Hartmann, Cowie, Hosking, 1970: Ichinose, Nandi, 1964: Jean, 1971: Meites, 1965: Meites, Hopkins, Talwalker, 1963: Sud, Meites, 1971.)

The main aim of this section is to describe the effects of prolactin on mammary tissue which has been primed by exposure to the other necessary hormones. The first problem to be solved is the precise locus of prolactin action. The biochemical actions of prolactin on mammary tissue were apparently unaltered by binding the prolactin to Sepharose particles larger that the mammary epithelial cells. Provided that the bound prolactin remained attached, this indicates that entry to the cell is not necessary. These observations were supported by the results of autoradiography of rabbit mammary tissue after either intraductal or intravenous administration of prolactin labelled with radioactive iodine. Virtually none of the radioactivity appeared to be within the cells and even after intraductal administration most was found on the boundaries of the alveolar cells adjacent to the vascular supply suggesting the presence of specific prolactin receptors at that site. (Birkinshaw, Falconer, 1972: Falconer, 1972: Turkington, 1970a: Turkington, Frantz, 1972.)

The basic biochemical actions of prolactin, and in particular the interesting way in which prolactin-induced protein kinases may interact with the cyclic AMP system, were described in the biochemistry chapter. These biochemical effects have been studied most precisely in vitro in mammary tissue taken from pregnant mice, rats or rabbits. Cortisol and insulin seem necessary for prolactin to express itself fully in vitro and it also seems that the cells being cultured must undergo one cell division under the influence of the two permissive hormones before prolactin can act on them: the reason for this is unknown. Changes in histone and RNA synthesis and the manufacture of new ribosomes seem to precede the formation of casein, lactose and lipids. The synthesis of all the major componen of milk seems to be stimulated by prolactin, and it seems probable that each mammary cell can make all these components. (Baldwin, Martin, 1968: Barnawell, 1967: Bolton, 1971: Cowie, 1969: Delouis, Denamur, 1972: Denamur, Delouis, 1972: Dilley, Nandi, 1968: Falconer, Fiddler, 1970: Gachev, 1963, 1969: Green, Topper, 1970: Hohmann, Cole, 1971: Kumaresan, Anderson, Turner, 1966: Lockwood, Turkington, Topper, 1966: Marzluff, McCarty, Turkington, 1969: Oka, Topper, 1971, 1972: Simpson, Schmidt, 1971: Sinha, Lewis, Vanderlaan, 1972: Strong, Dils, Forsyth, 1971: Tobon, Josimovich, Salazar, 1972: Topper, 1970: Turkington, 1968a, 1968b, 1968c, 1969a, 1969b, 1970c, 1972a: Turkington, Frantz, 1972: Turkington, Juergens, Topper, 1965: Turkington, Riddle, 1969, 1970: Turkington, Spielvogel, 1971: Turkington, Ward, 1969: Wang, Hallowes, Bealing, Strong, Dils, 1971, 1972: Wang, Hallowes, Smith, Amor, Lewis, 1972.)

The interaction between progesterone and prolactin in the regulation of lactose synthetase synthesis is particularly interesting. Lactose synthetase consists of two components, α-lactalbumin and galactosyl transferase. In late pregnancy there is active synthesis of galactosyl transferase but little manufacture of α-lactalbumin. After parturition there is a dramatic rise of α-lactalbumin activity. Galactosyl transferase alone catalyses the reaction

$$\text{UPD-galactose} + \text{N-acetylglucosamine} \rightarrow \text{N-acetyllactosamine} + \text{UDP}$$

α-Lactalbumin changes the specifity of the enzyme so that it can catalyse the synthesis of lactose

$$\text{UDP-galactose} + \text{glucose} \rightarrow \text{Lactose} + \text{UDP}$$

It seems that progesterone is the hormone which is responsible for the suppression of α-lactalbumin synthesis and that after parturition when progesterone levels fall, the stimulating action of prolactin can be expressed. (Kuhn, 1969a, 1969b: Turkington, Brew, Vanaman, Hill, 1968: Turkington, Hill, 1969.)

Drug suppression of puerperal lactation in humans

Stilbestrol and other synthetic estrogens have been widely used to suppress lactation in humans in the puerperium. Their effect does not appear to depend on inhibition of prolactin secretion since in the first two weeks post partum basal prolactin levels were found to be comparable in both nursing and estrogen suppressed mothers. The inhibiting action is almost certainly directly on the mammary tissue and in animals it has been shown that it can be overcome by large doses of exogenous prolactin. (L'Hermite, Delvoye, Nokin, Vekemans, Robyn, 1972: Meites, 1972: Meites, Sgouris, 1964.)

In pilot studies 2-bromo-α-ergokryptine (CB 154) has been shown to be effective in stopping puerperal lactation in humans by stopping prolactin secretion. Ergot alkaloids are also effective in inhibiting lactation in rats. In cattle although CB 154 suppressed prolactin levels and reduced milk yield it did not suppress lactation completely. (Del Pozo, Brun Del Re, Varga, Friesen, 1972: Fluckiger, Wagner, 1968: Karg, Schams, Reinhardt, 1972: Shaar, Clemens, 1972: Varga, Lutterbeck, Pryor, Wenner, Erb, 1972.)

Chapter 10

PROLACTIN AND THYROID FUNCTION

The subject of the interactions between prolactin and its regulating mechanisms and thyroid hormones and their regulating mechanisms is one which is expanding very rapidly indeed. As yet most of the research has dealt with interactions at the hypothalamus-pituitary level rather than at the thyroid gland-peripheral target organ level.

In amphibians prolactin seems able to stimulate the growth of larval structures by interfering with the thyroid hormones. It does this partly by blocking the effect of TSH on the thyroid gland and partly by blocking the effect of thyroid hormone on the tissues. In mammals thyroid hormones seem to be required as permissive factors in mammary development. In immature rodent mammary glands maintained in culture, low levels of thyroxine synergise with prolactin in stimulating lobulo-alveolar growth while higher levels have an inhibitory effect. (Cowie, Tindal, 1971: Nicoll, Bryant, 1972: Singh, Bern, 1969: Sinha, 1970.)

There have been no direct studies of the effects of prolactin on thyroid function. In lactating rats serum thyroxine levels were inversely related to the intensity of lactation. The reduced serum thyroxine level could not be restored to normal by ten times the normal dietary intake of iodine. In non-lactating rats serum thyroxine levels could not be reduced by treatment with 2 mg prolactin/day for 15 days. In rats bearing prolactin secreting tumours, pituitary content of TSH and thyroid uptake of ^{131}I were reduced suggesting the possibility of a direct suppression of pituitary TSH production. (Lorscheider, Reineke, 1971: MacLeod, Abad, 1968.)

Possibly the most important inter-relationship between the thyroid and prolactin systems was indicated by the finding of Tashjian et al that TSH-releasing hormone (TRH or TRF) could stimulate cultured rat pituitary cells to secrete prolactin. The stimulation was clearly apparent after 4 hours, became maximal (2-5 times control) after 24-48 hours and persisted for at least 20 days in the presence of TRH. A TRH concentration of 0.1 ng/ml had some effect and the maximal response was produced by a concentration of 10 ng/ml. Other workers using rat and bovine anterior pituitaries have had some difficulty in reproducing this effect. In general it seems that a clear effect can be obtained when pituitary cells are cultured but not when pituitary tissue is cultured: it is conceivable that the receptors may be so sited that in the latter preparation prolactin added to the medium may not gain access to them. (Gourdji, Kerdelhue, Tixier-Vidal, 1972: Guillemin, 1972: La Bella, Vivian, 1971: Lu, Shaar, Kortright, Meites, 1972: Meites, 1972: Meites, Lu, Wuttke, Welsch, Nagasawa, Quadri, 1972: Tashjian, Barowsky, Jensen, 1971.)

On attempting to test the effect of TRH on prolactin secretion in vivo and here a clear species difference emerged. In rats when TRH was injected over a period of days, there was a rise in pituitary prolactin and a small rise in serum prolactin. The time scale of the response and the fact that it did not occur in thyroidectomised-parathyroidectomised animals suggest that it may be an indirect phenomenon, mediated by an elevation in thyroid hormone secretion: certainly in vitro both thyroxine and triiodothyronine have been observed to increase prolactin secretion. (Lu, Shaar, Kortright, Meites, 1972: Meites, 1972: Meites, Clemens, 1972: Meites, Lu, Wuttke, Welsch, Nagasawa, Quadri, 1972: Nicoll, Meites, 1963.)

The results in man were quite different. It was soon shown by several groups that injection of as little as 10 μg of synthetic TRH intravenously could elevate prolactin plasma levels within minutes: doses up to 800 μg have been tried and found effective. The rises in plasma levels were 2-5 times control with peak values after about 15 minutes and a decline to normal levels after about 180 minutes. The response was greater in females than males. The rapid and dramatic response makes it unlikely that the effect is mediated via TSH and thyroid hormones although it does not, of course, prove that TRH is a physiological prolactin releasing factor. However, the effects of hypo and hyperthyroidism on prolactin secretion discussed briefly in the next paragraph and more fully in section B of the book make a physiological role for TRH in the regulation of prolactin secretion likely. (Bowers, Friesen, Hwang, Guyda, Folkers, 1971: Friesen, Hwang Guyda, Tolis, Tyson, Myers, 1972: Jacobs, Snyder, Wilber, Utiger, Daughaday, 1971: L'Hermite, Copinschi, Golstein, Vanhaelst, Leclercq, Bruno, 1972: Turkington, Ray, Costin, 1972: Bowers, Friesen, Hwang, Guyda, Folkers, 1971.)

If TRH is a physiological PRF then under conditions of primary hypothyroidism when TSH and probably TRH secretion rates are elevated, prolactin levels might also be elevated. This has been frequently but not always found to be true. In rats made hypothyroid by treatment with propylthiouracil, both TSH and prolactin secreting cells hypertrophied, but on the other hand similar treatment has been reported to reduce pituitary prolactin content and concentration. Cultured pituitaries from rats thyroidectomised some time before sacrifice synthesised more prolactin than controls: triiodothyroxine injections suppressed the increased secretion within three hours. Thyroxine treatment in rats elevated pituitary prolactin content and concentration but at the same time seminal vesicle weight was reduced suggesting the possibility of diminished prolactin secretion. (Chen, Meites, 1969: Doerr-Schott, Stoeckel, Porte, Reville, 1972: Ieiri, 1971.)

In humans there is a rare syndrome in which pre-pubertal primary hypothyroidism is associated with galactorrhea and elevated prolactin levels and precocious puberty. Treatment of the hypothyroidism restored prolactin levels to normal in several patients. In adults there are many reports of a similar syndrome which responded to thyroid treatment. Measurements of prolactin levels in hypothyroid patients without galactorrhea have indicated that they are frequently elevated and the prolactin-secreting cells in the pituitary may be hypertrophied in myxedema. (Arroyo, Aubert, 1971: Clemens, Minaguchi, Storey, Voogt, Meites, 1969: Edwards, Forsyth, Besser, 1971: Forsyth, Besser, Edwards, Francis, Myres, 1971: L'Hermite, Delvoye, Nokin Vekemans, Robyn, 1972: Jackson, 1956: Kinch, Plunkett, Devlin, 1969: Pasteels, Gausset, Danguy, Ectors, 1972: Robyn, 1972: Savely, Modlinger-Odorfer, Szecsenyi-Nagy, 1965: Turkington, Ray, Costin, 1972: Van Wyck, Grumbach, 1960.)

Finally, while the 24 hour secretion patterns of TSH and prolactin are very similar, TSH plasma levels do not rise when prolactin levels rise during suckling. (Friesen, Hwang, Guyda, Tolis, Tyson, Myers, 1972: Nokin, Vekemans, L'Hermite, Robyn, 1972: Patel, Baker, Alford, Johns, Burger, 1972: Sassin, Frantz, Weitzman, Kapen, 1972: Vanhaelst, Van Cauter, De Gaute, Golstein, 1972.)

Chapter 11

PROLACTIN AND CANCER

The demonstration by Huggins that some types of cancer remain dependent on the hormones required for growth and maintenance of the normal tissue of the same organ has stimulated an enormous amount of research. In the case of prolactin the obvious target organ which might generate hormone-dependent tumours is the mammary gland, although increasingly attention is being paid to the prostate as well. Because of the possibility of considerable species differences it seems particularly important in this field to specify the species involved.

Mammary tumors in mice

Many strains of mice develop spontaneous mammary tumors but there are large strain differences in tumor susceptibility. The differences seem to be due to differences at the mammary gland level: certainly it has been shown that similar prolactin levels may be associated with a high tumor incidence in one strain and a low incidence in another strain. The most sensitive strains are those in which both growth hormone and prolactin are equally effective in stimulating the mammary gland. The incidence of the tumors in any strain may be increased by estrogen treatment or by transplantation of extra pituitary glands into an animal, or by prolactin-secreting pituitary tumors. The incidence of development of new tumors may be reduced by treatment with ergocornine or 2-bromo-α-ergokryptine and existing tumors may be reduced in size, strongly suggesting that some at least of these tumors are hormone dependent. Prolactin may potentiate the development of virus-induced tumors. (Boot, 1970: Bruni, Montemurro, 1971: Furth, 1969, 1972: Muhlbock, Boot, 1967: Nagasawa, Yanai, Iwahashi, Fujimoto, Kuretani, 1967: Nandi, Bern, 1960: Yanai, Nagasawa, 1970a, 1970b, 1971, 1972.)

Mammary tumors in rats

There is more information about this species than about any other, partly because several methods are available for reliably obtaining animals with mammary tumors. The most used are the transplantation of tumors from one animal to another, the feeding of 3-methylcholanthrene (3MC) and 7, 12-dimethylbenz(a)anthracene (DMBA) and the induction of prolactin, ACTH and growth hormone secreting (mammotropic) tumors by estrogen treatment or ionizing radiation. Mammotropic tumors may also be transplanted and they produce a high incidence of mammary tumors in the hosts. All the experimental tumors are adenocarcinomas. The DMBA ones tend to be secretory and the 3MC ones to be non-secretory. (Dao, 1968: Furth, 1963: 1969: Furth, Clifton, Gadsden, Buffet, 1956: Hilf, Goldenberg, Michel, Carrington, Bell, Gruenstein, Meranze, Shimkin, 1969: Hilf, Michel, Bell, 1967: Huggins, 1965: Huggins, Briziarelli, Sutton, 1959: Huggins, Grand, Brillantes, 1961.)

The mechanism of cancer induction by the hydrocarbons is unknown. DMBA does not stimulate prolactin secretion. 3MC does stimulate prolactin secretion but whether this is an important part of its action is unknown. Old rats of many strains may develop spontaneous mammary tumors which are usually single and benign. The incidence of these tumours may be increased by median eminence lesions which promote prolactin secretion. Old rats tend to have much higher serum prolactin levels than young ones. (Meites, 1972b: Moon, Young, 1972: Nagasawa, Yanai, Kuretani, 1968.)

It should be stressed that even in rats by no means all of the tumors which occur are hormone-dependent. Some are autonomous and continue to grow irrespective of hormonal manipulations. The discussion which follows refers only to those tumors which show features of hormone dependency.

Stimulation and inhibition of the pre-existing mammary tumors

The hydrocarbon-induced mammary tumors in rats consistently regress after hypophysectomy, ovariectomy and adrenalectomy and can be reactivated by treatment with prolactin or by implantation of a mammotropic tumor. Estrogen administration may reactivate tumor growth after ovariectomy and adrenalectomy but not after hypophysectomy, even if thyroid and adrenal steroid replacement therapy is given. This suggests either that the effect of estrogen depends on stimulation of secretion of a pituitary hormone, possibly prolactin or growth hormone, or that the synergistic effect of a pituitary hormone is required at target organ level. The fact that in intact rats an elevation of prolactin levels can enhance tumor growth is shown by the fact that median eminence lesions which probably reduce secretion of other pituitary hormones apart from prolactin may enhance growth and increase the incidence of both spontaneous and hydocarboninduced tumors. Transplanted pituitaries have a similar effect. Phenothiazines, reserpine and norethynodrel-mestranol also can promote mammary tumor growth. The effects of mammotropic tumors which secrete growth hormone and ACTH as well as prolactin cannot be so specifically related to the concept that prolactin is the key hormone but at least their promotion of tumor growth is not inconsistent with the idea. It is clearly difficult to design experiments which will with certainty distinguish between the possibilities that estrogen promotes tumor growth by stimulating prolactin release, that it does so by synergising with prolactin at target organ level or that it does both of these. In culture DNA synthesis in DMBA induced tumors was not enhanced by estrogen but was enhanced by prolactin. In vivo, in rats with DMBA tumors, ovariectomy produced tumor regression: median eminence lesions which elevated prolactin secretion prevented further regression but did not cause resumption of growth: transplantation of ovaries caused growth to restart. In intact rats median eminence lesions promoted tumor growth: the tumors regressed after ovariectomy even though prolactin levels remained high: ovarian implants caused regrowth. Hypophysectomy of rats with DMBA tumors, however, caused tumor regression which could not be reversed by estrogens. It seems possible therefore that prolactin alone may have some effect in maintaining a tumor while estrogen alone does not: the maximum effect may occur only with estrogen plus prolactin. The evidence is therefore in favour of the concept that estrogen promotes tumor growth partly by synergising with prolactin at the mammary level. (Bates, Milkovic, Garrison, 1962: Clemens, Welsch, Meites, 1968: Dao, Sinha, 1972: Hilf, Bell, Goldenberg, Michel, 1971: Hilf, Bell, Michel, 1967: Huggins, Briziarelli, Sutton, 1959: Ito, Martin, Grindeland, Takizawa, Furth, 1971: Kim, Furth, 1960a, 1960b, 1960c: Kim, Furth, Clifton, 1960: Kim, Furth, Yannopoulos, 1963: Kwa, Van der Gugten, Sala, Verhofstad, 1972: Kwa, Van der Gugten, Verhofstad, 1969: McCormick, Moon, 1967: Meites, 1972: Mizuno, Talwalker, Meites, 1964: Nagasawa, 1971a, 1971b: Pearson, Llerena, Llerena, Molina, Butler, 1969: Pearson, Murray, Mozaffarian, Pensky, 1972: Sterental, Dominquez, Weisman, Pearson, 1963: Takizawa, Furth, Furth, 1970: Talwalker, Meites, Mizuno, 1964: Welsch, Clemens, Meites, 1968, 1969: Welsch, Jenkins, Meites, 1970: Welsch, Meites, 1969, 1970: Welsch, Rivera, 1972: Yokoro, Furth, Haran-Ghera, 1961.)

Other steroids have been studied much less intensively than the estrogens. This is disappointing especially in view of the stimulation of progesterone and adrenal androgen secretion which may be brought about by prolactin. Androgens have been reported to inhibit rat mammary tumor growth possibly by a direct action on the mammary gland. The few reports on progesterone both in vitro and in vivo suggest that it has quite a strong synergistic action with prolactin in stimulating growth of tumor tissue. (Dao, Sinha, 1972: Hilf, Michel, Bell, Freeman, Borman, 1965: Huggins, Briziarelli, Sutton, 1959: Kim, 1965: Koyama, Sinha, Dao, 1972: McCormick, Moon, 1967: Meites, 1972b.)

In contrast to all the reports describing estrogen stimulation of mammary tumor growth, there is an almost equal number describing estrogen inhibition of mammary tumor growth. A relatively consistent pattern has emerged with low to moderate estrogen doses stimulating growth and high estrogen doses inhibiting it even in the presence of high prolactin levels. High doses of progesterone may synergise with estrogen in slowing growth. In most cases, the estrogen inhibition could be overcome with exogenous prolactin injections or with treatments which pushed prolactin levels still higher suggesting the possibility that estrogen was inhibiting competitively a prolactin effect on the target organ. Pregnancy has also been reported to inhibit growth of and even to destroy completely DMBA-induced tumors but may enhance development of 3MC induced tumors. With some transplantable tumor lines, even prolactin itself has been reported to inhibit growth of the tumor: the inhibition occurred at the same time as the stimulation of normal mammary tissue. (Dao, 1971: Hilf, 1972: Hilf, Bell, Michel, 1967: Hilf, Michel, Bell, Freeman, Borman, 1965: Huggins, 1965: Huggins, Grand, Brillantes, 1961: Kim, 1965: Kim, Furth, Yannopoulos, 1963: Meites, 1972a, 1972b: Meites, Cassell, Clark, 1971: Nagasawa, Yanai, 1971, 1972: Pearson, Murray, Mozaffarian, Pensky, 1972.)

Drugs which suppress prolactin secretion, notably the ergot alkaloids, ergocornine and CB 154 have been reported to bring about regression of spontaneous and DMBA-induced tumors and to stop the growth without producing regression of transplanted tumors. Prolactin antiserum also inhibited DMBA tumor growth. (Cassell, Meites, Welsch, 1971: Clemens, Shaar, 1972: Heuson, Waelbroeck-van Gaver, Legros, 1970: Nagasawa, Meites, 1970: Pearson, Murray, Mozaffarian, Pensky, 1972: Quadri, Meites, 1971: Singh, Meites, Halmi, Kortright, Brennan, 1972: Stahelin, Burckhardt-Vischer, Fluckiger, 1971: Van der Gugten, 1971.)

Induction of mammary tumors in rats

There seem to be considerable differences between the effects of hormonal manipulations on the growth of established tumors just discussed and their effects on the induction of new tumors. As might be expected, median eminence lesions and additional pituitary grafts increase the incidence of spontaneous mammary tumors in old rats. Either ovariectomy or hypophysectomy before tumors develop may greatly reduce the incidence of spontaneous or hydrocarbon-induced tumors. Treatment with ergot alkaloids has a similar but smaller effect. Prolactin alone does not appear able to reverse the inhibitory action of ovariectomy on tumor induction but prolactin and growth hormone given together can partially reverse it. Estrogen alone can also partially reverse the ovariectomy effect. These experiments suggest that prolactin, growth hormone, estrogen, and possibly another ovarian hormone (perhaps progesterone) may be required for the induction of hydrocarbon-induced tumors. (Clemens, Shaar, 1972:Heuson, Waelbroeck-van Gaver, Legros, 1970: Meites, 1972a: Stahelin, Burckhardt-Vischer, Fluckiger, 1971: Talwalker, Meites, Mizuno, 1964: Welsch, Jenkins, Meites, 1970.)

In vivid contrast, there exists an impressive series of observations which suggests that while high levels of prolactin stimulate the growth of existing hydrocarbon-induced tumors, if they are present before or at the time of treatment with the carcinogen, the **induction** of tumors is inhibited. In one experiment 95% of rats treated with DMBA developed mammary tumors: median eminence lesions made well after the DMBA treatment enhanced the growth of the tumors but when median eminence lesions were made before DMBA treatment only 30% of the animals developed tumors. With 3MC-induced tumors, pregnancy occurring after treatment enhanced tumor growth but 3MC treatment during pregnancy produced significantly fewer tumors than in controls. Treatment with reserpine or norethynodrel-mestranol or implantation of multiple pituitary grafts had similar effects on DMBA tumors: when given before the DMBA, tumor induction was inhibited but when given after tumor induction growth was stimulated. None of these experiments is completely "clean" in the sense that prolactin can be specifically identified in any one case as the factor responsible for inhibiting tumor induction. However the only thing the various procedures have in common is stimulation of prolactin secretion and this field would seem to deserve more study than has been devoted to it. (Clemens, Welsch, Meites, 1968: Dao, 1971: Huggins, 1965: Welsch, Clemens, Meites, 1968: Welsch, Meites, 1969: Welsch, Meites, 1970.)

Other animal tumors and prolactin

The only other tumors on which the effect of prolactin itself has been studied appear to be liver tumors induced by aniline dye feeding or by tumor cell injections. Prolactin had no effect on the dye induced tumors or on the injected tumors in males. In intact females prolactin increased the size but not the incidence of hepatic tumors following cell injection and in hypophysectomised females it increased both the size and the incidence. (De Prospo, 1967: Fisher, 1963, 1966.)

There are a number of reports of inhibition of tumor growth by chlorpromazine and reserpine but whether this has anything to do with prolactin is a matter for conjecture. In mice reserpine caused regression and even disappearance of leukemic cell tumours: it also caused severe "depression" and loss of appetite. Relief of the "depression" with amphetamine did not affect the anti-tumor action. Starvation of animals not treated with reserpine did not prevent tumor growth. Again in mice, the size and number of mastocytomas developing after malignant mast cell injection were reduced by chlorpromazine. Chlorpromazine inhibited mouse melanoma growth and locally applied chlorpromazine inhibited DMBA-induced cheek pouch tumors in hamsters. Both reserpine and chlorpromazine inhibited growth of implanted mouse sarcomas. (Belkin, Hardy, 1957: Csatary, 1972: Goldin, Burton, Humphreys, Venditti, 1957: Gottlieb, Hazel, Broitman, Zamchek, 1960: Levij, Polliack, 1970: Van Woert, Palmer, 1969.)

Breast cancer in humans

There must obviously be uncertainty as to how far findings on experimental tumors in rats and mice can be applied to man. Unfortunately the majority of rodent tumors are alveolar and may frequently be secretory while most human tumors are ductal and virtually never secretory. However, provided that due caution is applied it would seem appropriate to test in man some of the ideas derived from animal experiments. (Furth, 1972: Llerena, Llerena, Molina, Butler, Pearson, 1969.)

The findings in human breast cancer are highly complex and in the absence of studies using radioimmunoassays and effective doses of prolactin-inhibiting drugs it is difficult to draw any firm conclusions. The main findings seem to be as follows:-

1. There appear to be two main groups of patients who are susceptible to breast cancer. Women with low androsterone and aetiocholanolone excretion, who tend to be infertile, to have anovulatory cycles and low estrogen levels tend to develop tumors which are hormone independent. Women with elevated aetiocholanolone excretion tend to be obese and "feminine" to have high estrogen levels and to

respond to ovariectomy or hypophysectomy. (Bulbrook, Haywood, Spicer, 1971: Bulbrook, Wang, Swain, 1972.)

2. Hypophysectomy appears to give superior results to ovariectomy with or without adrenalectomy. (Atkins, Bulbrook, Falconer, Haywood, Maclean, Schurr, 1968: Murray, Mozaffarian, Pearson, 1972: Pearson, Ray, 1969.)

3. Women with breast cancer tend to have increased sebaceous gland activity. Increased activity may perhaps be produced by prolactin but is more likely to be caused by MSH. However MSH levels and prolactin levels seem to be usually elevated together. (Bulbrook, Wang, Swain, 1972: Friesen, 1972b: Krant, Brandrup, Greene, Pochi, Strauss, 1968: Shuster, Thody, Goolamali, Burton, Plummer, Bates, 1973.)

4. Bioassay using the pigeon crop method has suggested that prolactin levels may be elevated in breast cancer patients but Turkington et al using a different bioassay failed to confirm this. (Berle, Voigt, 1972: Turkington, Underwood, Van Wyck, 1971.)

5. Treatment with L-dopa tends to reduce prolactin levels without suppressing prolactin secretion completely. Several preliminary reports have hinted that L-dopa treatment may produce objective remission in some patients with breast cancer. L-dopa has been reported to be particularly effective in relieving bone pain. (Friesen, Hwang, Guyda, Tolis, Tyson, Myers, 1972: Minton, Dickey, 1972: Murray, Mozaffarian, Pearson, 1972: Papaioannou, 1972: Stoll, 1972.)

6. Normal individuals may respond to prolactin injections by increased urinary excretion of calcium. It has been reported that prolactin injected into women with breast cancer and metastases in bone makes them excrete more calcium than normal if the tumor is hormone-dependent but not if it is hormone-independent. Estrogen has also been reported to increase calcium excretion in women with hormone-dependent tumors. A possible interpretation is that injected prolactin or estrogen-stimulated prolactin increase osteolysis. In contrast another report could find no effect on calcium excretion or on tumor growth following ovine prolactin injections. (Lipsett, Bergenstal, 1960: McCalister, Welbourn, 1962: Pearson, West, Hollander, Treves, 1954.)

7. There is a possibility that long continued estrogen therapy in males may lead to mammary cancer. Some but not all males so treated have elevated prolactin levels. (Friesen, 1972b: Furth, 1972.)

8. Until recently attempts to demonstrate prolactin dependence of human breast cancer tissue cultured in vitro were unsuccessful. However success has been claimed for a new method which uses the activity of the pentose shunt pathway as its end point. Sixteen out of 50 human breast cancers appeared to be prolactin-dependent. If this method can accurately predict the response to hypophysectomy or to prolactin-suppressing drugs it should be a considerable advance. (Barker, Richmond, 1971a, 1971b: Furth, 1972: Salih, Flax, Brander, Hobbs, 1972.)

All that can therefore be said at this stage is that some human breast cancers may be prolactin dependent. But as with hydrocarbon-induced tumors in rats there is some evidence that prolactin may actually have a protective effect against breast cancer. The difference between breast cancer incidence in nulliparous and other women is well-known. When pregnancy occurs subsequent to treatment of human breast cancer, the 5-year survival rate is significantly improved. Pituitary stalk section in mammary cancer frequently leads to objective remission, particularly when the stalk section is followed by galactorrhea. Estrogen treatment may exert part of its effect through stimulation of prolactin secretion. As early as 1954 it was noted that stimulation of normal breast tissue by estrogen might be associated with cancer remission. Lemon has advocated the view that estriol deficiency may be associated with breast cancer: 21% of controls but 62% of untreated breast cancer patients had subnormal estriol excretion. Estriol treatment may produce remission: the effect may be direct but the possibility of an indirect action via prolactin should not be ignored. (Ehni, Eckles, 1959: Huseby, Thomas, 1954: Lemon, 1973: Peters, 1968.)

Prolactin and prostatic cancer

The possibility that the prostate may be one of prolactin's target organs has stimulated thought about the possibility of a role for prolactin in the initiation and growth of prostatic cancer. Bioassay studies of urinary prolactin have been reported as showing elevated levels of excretion in patients with malignant prostatic disease, with more prolactin being excreted the more advanced the disease. Using plasma radioimmunoassay two patients with benign prostatic hypertrophy were found to have normal levels of plasma prolactin pre-operatively while two with prostatic carcinoma had slightly elevated levels: post-operatively levels fell in three of the four patients suggesting the possibility of a stress-induced pre-operative rise. The relative success of estrogen therapy in reducing the death rate from prostatic cancer and improving patient well-being indicates that the rise in prolactin levels does not overwhelm the (presumed) local action of estrogen on the prostate. Again the possibility that prolactin may have an anti-cancer action cannot be excluded: in a group of 47 patients treated with both reserpine and estrogen who might have been expected to have very substantially elevated prolactin levels, the death rate from prostatic cancer was markedly less than in those treated with estrogen alone. (Asano, 1962, 1965: Farnsworth, 1972: Friesen, 1972b: Newball, Byar, 1972: Veterans Administration, 1967.)

Chapter 12

PROLACTIN AND FLUID AND ELECTROLYTE BALANCE AND THE CARDIOVASCULAR SYSTEM

In sub-mammalian vertebrates prolactin seems to be a key hormone in the regulation of fluid and electrolyte balance and there is now substantial evidence that it plays a similar role in mammals as well. (Nicoll, Bern, 1972: Nicoll, Bryant, 1972.)

Lockett and co-workers were the first to draw attention to the renal effect of prolactin in mammals. They used a perfused cat kidney preparation so arranged that the blood could either be excluded from the head of the cat or be allowed to flow through the head. When the blood was allowed to flow through the head aldosterone had its usual action in the kidney of reducing sodium and water excretion. In contrast when the head was excluded from the circuit aldosterone actually increased renal sodium and potassium excretion. In hypophysectomised rats aldosterone also increased sodium and water excretion. The more usual sodium and water retaining action of aldosterone could be restored in both the perfused kidneys and the rats by treatment with prolactin or growth hormone or oxytocin. In the perfused cat kidneys bovine prolactin caused a very transient increase in sodium and water excretion followed by a prolonged period of reduction of sodium, potassium and water excretion. The reduced fluid and electrolyte excretion could not be accounted for by reduction in renal blood flow or glomerular filtration rate since both were increased by the prolactin. (Davey, Lockett, 1960: Lockett, 1965: Lockett, Nail, 1965: Lockett, Roberts, 1963.)

Burstyn et al attempted to reproduce Lockett's findings in intact sheep. They reasoned that if the sodium-losing action of aldosterone were to have any physiological role it should become apparent in animals on a very high salt intake. A basically simple experimental design was used in which urine was collected from the animals from 12.00 to 14.00 and from 14.00 to 16.00 hours each day. On alternate days injections of aldosterone were given by an indwelling jugular venous cannula at 13.30: it was reasoned that since aldosterone takes about 30 minutes to begin its renal effects they would start at about 14.00 hours and the second collection period would be under the influence of aldosterone. Control

saline injections were given on the other days at 13.30: on control days renal
excretion of water, sodium and potassium was very similar during the two
collection periods. During an initial period when the animals were maintained on
a sodium intake of approximately 100 mEq/day aldosterone had its usual sodium
and water retaining effect. On increasing the sodium intake to 400 mEq/day the
sodium retaining action was abolished and in all but one animal aldosterone
actually increased sodium excretion. When the animals were treated with 5 mg
prolactin given as a single intramuscular injection at 08.00 hours, four hours
before the beginning of the first collection period, or with oxytocin given hourly
during the collection period, the sodium retaining effect of aldosterone was restored.
The one animal which failed to respond to the high sodium intake by completely
reversing its response to aldosterone curiously enough had for an unknown reason,
a strikingly elevated jugular venous pressure. (Burstyn, Horrobin, Manku, 1972.)

The sheep treated for 8 days with the very high sodium intake of 400 mEq/day
appeared to cope very satisfactorily with this situation: their total weight gain during
this period was about 2% and was not significant. In contrast, when the single daily
injection of prolactin was added to the regime they put on weight rapidly and
became clinically edematous within two days: after four days their weight was 10%
above its starting level. On stopping the prolactin the excess weight was lost
rapidly: oxytocin stopped the fall but did not reverse it and on stopping the oxytocin
the animals' original weight was regained within 2-4 days. (Burstyn, Horrobin, Manku,
1972.)

Soffer et al demonstrated in the 1940's that in patients with Cushing's syndrome,
DOCA tended to promote salt excretion rather than salt retention. We wondered
whether treatment with high doses of cortisol might reverse the action of aldosterone in sheep. Using an experiment of similar design to the one described in
the last paragraph we treated the sheep with 150 mg cortisol per day instead of
giving them a 400 mEq/day salt intake. Like the high salt intake, the cortisol
treatment reversed the action of aldosterone: again the usual action of aldosterone
could be restored by prolactin. (Horrobin, Manku, Burstyn, 1973: Soffer, Lesnick,
Sorkin, Sobotka, Jacobs, 1944.)

Since ADH does not always exert its expected water-retaining effect we specula-
ted that there might be similar relationships between ADH, cortisol, oxytocin
and prolactin as exist between aldosterone and the other three hormones. Again
a similar design of experiment was used but this time arginine-vasopressin was

injected at 14.00 hours on separate days. In the control period the vasopressin
(15 mμ) exerted its expected water-retaining action but cortisol treatment first

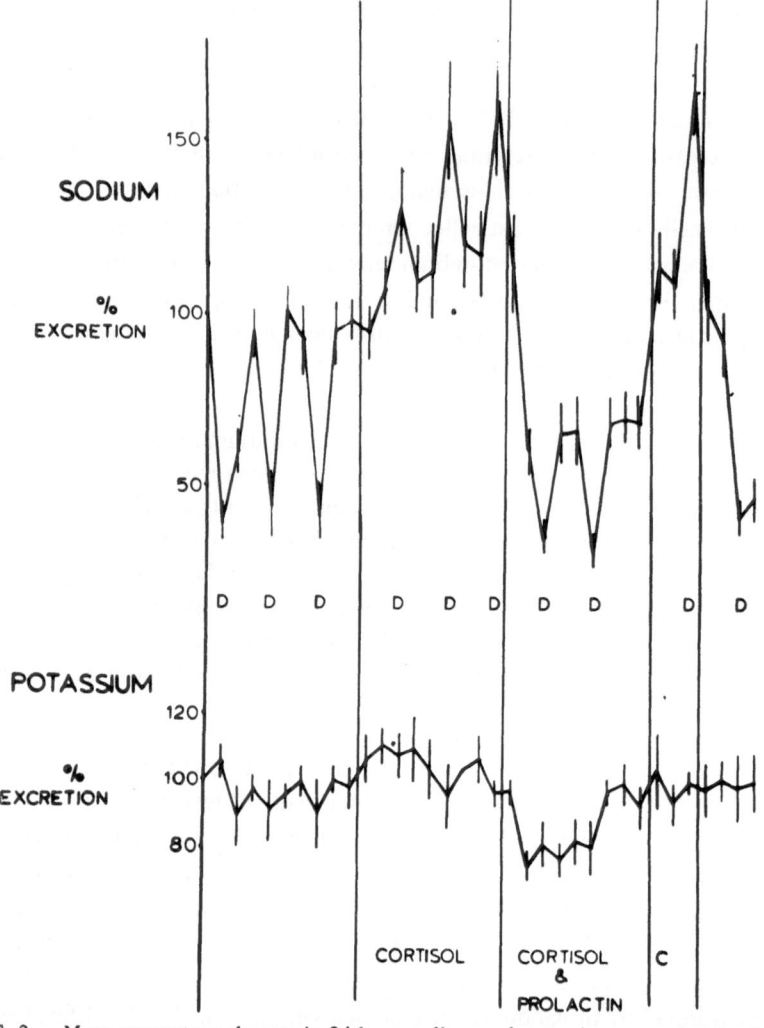

FIG. 3.   Mean percentage changes in 24 hour sodium and potassium excretion in eight rabbits.
For each animal the 100% value was based on mean 24 hour excretion during a two week
preliminary study. Each point represents one day and the bars represent standard errors of
the mean. D indicates a day on which DOCA was injected. C indicates a period when only
cortisol without prolactin was given to the animals. During the first and last periods the
animals received no treatment apart from the test injections of DOCA. Prolactin caused sodium
and potassium retention as well as restoring the "normal" action of DOCA in the cortisol
treated animals.

abolished and then completely reversed this. Both prolactin and oxytocin could restore the water-retaining action of the ADH. (Horrobin, Manku, Robertshaw, 1973.)

The reversal of mineralocorticoid action was also shown in rabbits. This time 24 hour urine collections were made. The experiment started with a 2 week control period and during this time the mean daily water, sodium and potassium excretions were noted for each animal. For each rabbit these mean values were taken as 100% and during the remainder of the experiment daily water, sodium and potassium excretions were expressed as percentages of the control values. Intramuscular injections of 0.5 mg DOCA were given, usually at the beginning of every third collection period. Initially, when the rabbits were not receiving any other treatment, DOCA caused the expected sodium retention. Cortisol treatment (10 mg intramuscularly twice daily) converted DOCA from a sodium-retaining to a saluretic substance. Prolactin restored the sodium-retaining effect and on stopping the prolactin while continuing the cortisol the sodium-losing action again reappeared. On stopping the cortisol the sodium-retaining action of the DOCA was quickly restored. (Horrobin, Manku, Muriuki, Burstyn, 1973.)

In humans the intramuscular injection of prolactin reduced urinary excretion of sodium, potassium and water. Part of the reduction in water excretion appeared to be due to a stimulation of ADH excretion since a substance which was probably ADH appeared in the urine after prolactin injection even in very well hydrated individuals: part of the reduction in water excretion could not be accounted for on this basis. Prolactin produced small but consistent elevations in plasma sodium concentration and plasma osmolality. The first trials of prolactin were carried out on a double blind basis with both experimenter and volunteers unaware as to whether prolactin or saline was being injected. The volunteers were asked to record subjective sensations and four out of five noticed thirst after prolactin but not after control injections: the fifth man experienced a craving for salt. This may have relevance to the increase in water and salt intake which has been recorded in lactating animals and suggests that prolactin could be one of the mediators of the sensations of thirst and appetite. Ovine prolactin has been reported to increase water intake in rats. Four of the five subjects also complained of muscle aches, lethargy and irritability after prolactin injections. (Blair-West, Coghlan, Denton, Funder, Nelson, Scoggins, Wright, 1970: Ensor, Edmondson, Phillips, 1972: Horrobin, Lloyd, Lipton, Burstyn, Durkin, Muiruri, 1971: Manku,

Horrobin, Burstyn, 1972.)

WATER

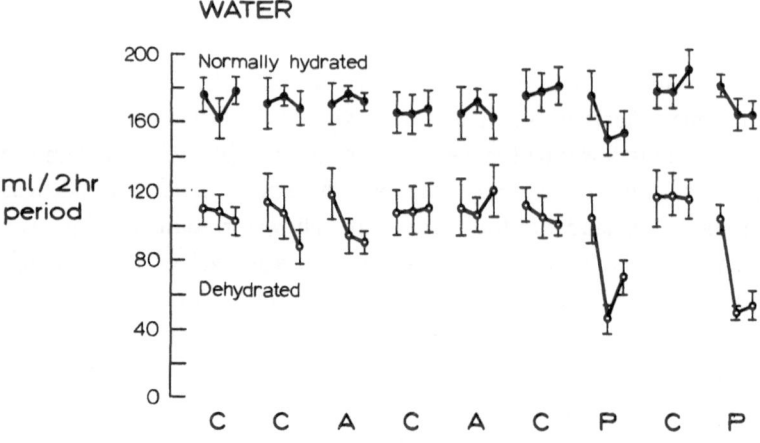

FIG. 4.   Absolute changes in water excretion in six sheep. The "normally hydrated" animals were allowed free access to water while the "dehydrated" ones were maintained in a hot room and allowed only restricted access to water. Each group of three points represents successive two hour collection periods on the same day: in each group of three the first period was without the influence of exogenous hormone, the second two were under the influence of exogenous hormone. Bars represent standard errors of the mean. C indicates a control day when saline was injected, A a day when aldosterone was injected intravenously and P a day when prolactin was injected intramuscularly.

SODIUM

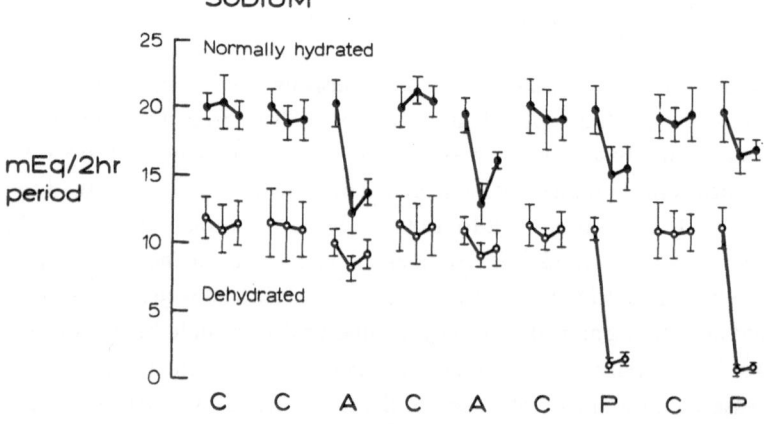

FIG. 5.   Absolute changes in sodium excretion in six sheep. Details as for fig. 4. Note the reduced sodium excretion in the dehydrated animals with the complete absence of overlap in absolute excretion between the two groups.

The relative effects of aldosterone and prolactin on renal excretion have been compared in normally hydrated sheep with free access to water and in sheep maintained in a hot room (30°C dry bulb and 20°C wet bulb temperature) with limited access to water. On each day urine collections were made for three successive 2-hour periods. On successive days injections of either saline (1ml IV intravenously 1.30 hours after the start of the first collection period), aldosterone (500 μg IV 1.30 hours after the start of the first collection period) or prolactin (5 mg IM 1 hour after the start of the first collection period) were given Previous experience with sheep had indicated that intravenous aldosterone has a demonstrable effect on renal function only after about 30 minutes while the effect of intramuscular prolactin takes an hour to develop: the idea was that renal actions of both hormones should begin at the start of the second collection period. The control injections had no effect on sodium, potassium or water excretion in either normally hydrated or dehydrated animals. Aldosterone had no significant effects on water or potassium excretion: in the normally hydrated animals it caused clear cut sodium retention but this action was barely apparent in the dehydrated sheep. Prolactin had no significant effect on potassium excretion although there was a tendency for this to be reduced. It caused a very small reduction

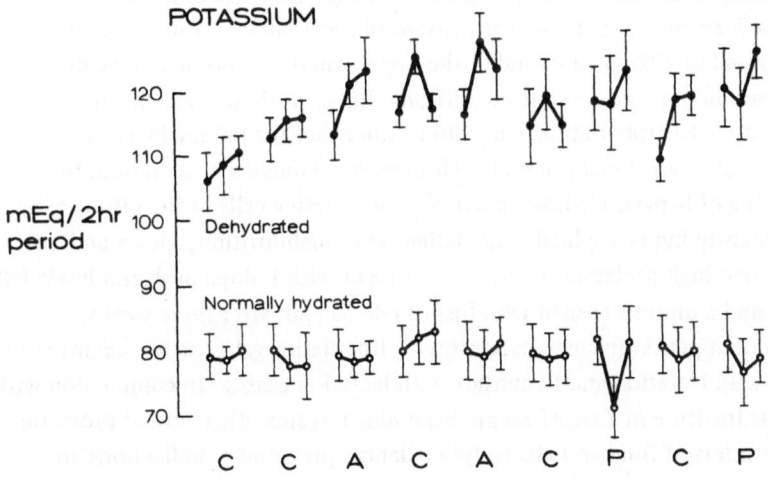

FIG. 6.   Absolute changes in potassium excretion in six sheep. Details as for fig. 4. Note the increased potassium excretion in the dehydrated animals which with their reduced sodium excretion strongly suggests elevated levels of aldosterone secretion.

of water excretion in the normally hydrated animals but had a much greater effect in the dehydrated animals. It reduced sodium excretion by a small amount in the normal animals but virtually stopped sodium excretion in the dehydrated animals. The main observations to be explained are therefore the loss of effect of aldosterone on sodium excretion in the dehydrated animals and the enhancement of the actions of prolactin on both water and sodium excretion. We feel that in the dehydrated animals aldosterone levels may have been so high (unfortunately we were not in a position to measure them) that all renal receptors were saturated and therefore the additional exogenous aldosterone had no effect. We also feel that while prolactin may have some renal actions in its own right, the major part of its effect is due to the modulation of the actions of aldosterone and ADH at renal level. If this is so then the higher the renal concentrations of aldosterone and ADH the greater effect should prolactin have. In rats it has been shown that dehydration causes a reduction in pituitary prolactin content suggesting release of the hormone. Water deprivation in cows has been reported to raise serum prolactin levels. (Ensor, Edmondson, Phillips, 1972: Manku, Horrobin, Robertshaw, 1973: Raud, Kiddy, Odell, 1972.)

Information about the role of prolactin in human disorders of fluid and electrolyte balance is scanty. In patients with advanced renal failure serum prolactin was grossly elevated in 20% of cases and at the upper end of the normal range in .others. Hemodialysis produced no significant change in these levels but they usually fell after transplantation, suggesting either that the kidney inactivates prolactin or that some renal product such as renin stimulates its secretion. In patients dying of hepatic cirrhosis the prolactin-secreting cells of the pituitary were consistently hypertrophied. One patient with malnutrition, edema and loss of appetite had high prolactin levels: on treatment with L-dopa prolactin levels fell to normal, and a diuresis ensued with loss of edema and, after three weeks, restoration of appetite. In some patients with fluctuating galactorrhea edema seems to develop with lactation and to subside with lactation ceases. In conjunction with the Tenovus Institute in Cardiff we are beginning a systematic study of prolactin levels in disorders of fluid and electrolyte balance: preliminary indications are that prolactin plasma levels are elevated in patients with edema due to congestive cardiac failure or liver failure. It is conceivable that the edema which occurs in some patients on reserpine could be related to stimulation of prolactin secretion. (Fries, Hwang, Guyda, Tolis, Tyson, Myers, 1972: Jarvik, 1970: Lunn, Cole, Boyns, Nassar, Horrobin, 1973: Pasteels, Gausset, Danguy, Ectors, 1972: Turkington, 1972c, 1972d.)

As yet there have been few reports on the effects of prolactin-suppressing drugs on fluid and electrolyte balance. L-dopa has been reported to increase fluid and electrolyte excretion in a human. In rats 2-bromo-α-ergokryptine increased urinary excretion of sodium, potassium and water and in preliminary experiments in sheep we have shown that it appears to convert aldosterone from a sodium-retaining to a sodium-losing hormone. (Manku, Horrobin, 1973: Richardson, 1973: Turkington, 1972c.)

Effects of prolactin on cardiac output and blood pressure

Bryant et al reported that in rats 2.5 mg/day of prolactin given for three weeks reduced arterial pressure by about 20% and increased blood volume by about the same amount. Also in rats removal of pups from a lactating mother led to a fall in cardiac output which could be completely prevented by a single injection of 3 mg prolactin given at the time of separation. Prolactin elevated cardiac output in virgin rats. These doses were, of course, enormous since 5 mg prolactin in man or sheep can produce effects on renal functions which last for 12-24 hours. In decerebrate rabbits, very much smaller amounts of prolactin elevated arterial pressure when given by intravenous infusion. 10 μg/kg/hr produced a mean 8% rise after 4 hours, 20 μg/kg/hr produced a mean 19% rise and 50 μg/kg/hr produced a mean 42% rise. Clearly much more work is required in this area. (Bryant, Douglas, Ashburn, 1971: Hanwell, Linzell, 1972: Horrobin, Manku, Burstyn, 1973).

Chapter 13

OTHER EFFECTS OF PROLACTIN

Prolactin has been observed to have effects on a number of other systems but as yet the information in each case is relatively sparse.

Red and white blood cells

In lactating mice red cell volume and erythropoietin activity are elevated. In non-pregnant mice, whether intact or castrated, prolactin stimulated red cell synthesis and the incorporation of radioactive iron into red cells. It appeared to potentiate the effect of erythropoietin. In dwarf mice, which are anemic and prolactin deficient, prolactin also stimulated red cell synthesis. It has been suggested that fetal hemoglobin synthesis may be partially under the control of prolactin. In adult hamsters both prolactin and perphenazine treatment led to the synthesis of small amounts of fetal hemoglobin.: growth hormone had an equivocal effect and human placental lactogen had no effect. In rats prolactin was reported to elevate neutrophil and eosinophil counts and to decrease lymphocyte counts. (Davis, Bull, 1971: Jepson, Lowenstein, 1964, 1965, 1967: Martinazzi, Baroni, 1962: Stupnicki, Stupnicka, Domanski, 1960.)

Gut

I have been able to find only one paper on the effect of ovine prolactin on the mammalian gut although in some fish it seems to be established that prolactin can decrease gut absorption of water and ions. In rats everted sacs were prepared from various levels of the small intestine for incubation in vitro. Prolactin (0.5 mg) was injected into the animals 24 or 48 hours before removal of the intestinal segments: it seemed to potentiate water uptake and the more proximal segments were more sensitive. After bilateral adrenalectomy/nephrectomy the prolactin was effective at all levels of the gut. Prolactin had no effect when added in vitro, suggesting that the action may be long term. (Ramsey, Bern, 1972.)

Arthritis

In hypophysectomised or adrenalectomised rats growth hormone given alone had no effects on joints while prolactin produced a mild arthritis. Prolactin given with growth hormone, however, consistently produced severe arthritis after 10-20 days treatment. The periarticular tissues became edematous and inflamed with infiltration of white cells, mostly mononuclear phagocytes. The synovial membranes sometimes protrude into the joint cavity. Any joint could be affected but the small joints especially those of the paws, were most consistently attacked. (Jasmin, Bois, 1959a, 1959b.)

In contrast, Ingvarsson has reported favorably on the use of prolactin in rheumatoid arthritis. Some patients seemed to respond dramatically to prolactin injections but in some the disease was exacerbated and one patient developed hematuria. The trial design did not exclude a placebo effect. (Ingvarsson, 1969.)

Prolactin and albuminuria

In old rats there is a tendency to develop a form of nephrotic syndrome with severe albuminuria. A similar but much more dramatic condition occurs in younger animals with prolactin-secreting tumors. In old rats there is a tendency for prolactin levels to be high. Prolonged treatment of rats with 2-bromo-α-ergokryptine has been reported to reduce greatly the incidence and severity of the spontaneous kidney lesions and albuminuria. In contrast, prolactin has been reported to exert a protective action on the renal damage in rats which may follow total renal ischaemia for 1 hour. (Clemens, Meites, 1971: Furth, Clifton, Gadsen, Buffet, 1956: Kohnlein, Bianchi, Biermann, 1966: Richardson, 1973.)

Prolactin and calcium metabolism

It has been known for some time that humans given injections of prolactin may respond by increased calcium excretion in the urine. Rats may also respond the same way and chronic treatment with 2-bromo-α-ergokryptine, the prolactin suppressing drug, reduced urinary calcium excretion. Possible other connections with calcium metabolism are found in sarcoid, and in metastatic breast and prostatic cancer: in all these conditions elevations of both plasma calcium and prolactin levels have been reported. In breast cancer it has been suggested that a large hypercalciuric response to injections of ovine prolactin may indicate hormone responsiveness of the tumor. It has been usually assumed that in both prostatic and breast cancer elevated prolactin levels may play a causative role. However if prolactin increases calcium excretion it is conceivable that it could help to prevent excessive rises in plasma calcium in patients with osteolytic lesions. In this case the elevated prolactin levels might be a response to the bony involvement rather than a cause of the disease. (Asano, 1962: Farnsworth, 1972: McCalister, Welbourn, 1962: McGarry, Beck, 1962, 1972: Schussler, Verso, Nemoto, 1972: Richardson, 1973: Turkington, MacIndoe, 1972.)

Prolactin and polyarteritis nodosa

About 10% of old rats develop lesions which are virtually indistinguishable from those of human polyarteritis nodosa. In old rats prolactin levels are elevated. Similar lessions may be provoked in young rats by estrogen treatment which also elevates prolactin secretion. The possibility that prolactin is involved in the formation of these lesions should therefore be considered. (Clemens, Meites, 1971: Cutts, 1966.)

Prolactin and the immune system

There seems to be an almost total absence of any work on prolactin and the immune system. Prolactin, like growth hormone, oxytocin, parathyroid hormone and vasopressin has been reported to stimulate mitotic activity of rat thymocyte populations in vitro. Antiserum to placental lactogen has some anti-lymphocytic action. There is of course a vast literature on the effect of pregnancy and of drugs like the phenothiazines and reserpine on the immune response but so far the possibility that prolactin may be involved does not appear to have been tested. (Whitfield, Perris, Youdale, 1960: Yamini, Chard, Blake, 1972.)

Prolactin and the pineal

The pineal is the major source of melatonin and light has been shown to be one of the factors controlling melatonin manufacture: darkness seems to promote melatonin synthesis and light to inhibit it. Melatonin injected into the 3rd ventricle of rats stimulated prolactin secretion: melatonin had no effect when infused directly into the anterior pituitary suggesting that its effect was mediated by releasing or inhibiting factors. Pinealectomy produced a transient elevation of prolactin levels in the pituitary and a fall in plasma prolactin: the effect lasted less than 4 weeks when 3-week old rats were pinealectomised, and less than 8 weeks when 8-week old rats were pinealectomised. Constant illumination of intact rats produced similar changes to those seen after pinealectomy while constant darkness produced a fall in pituitary prolactin content and a rise in plasma prolactin concentration. Pinealectomy prevented the effect of constant darkness. Blinding of rats also depressed pituitary prolactin levels and the effect was prevented by pinealectomy. Thus it seems that pineal melatonin may stimulate prolactin release.

Since darkness stimulates melatonin synthesis and prolactin release and since high levels of prolactin as a result of primary hypothyroidism may lead to precocious puberty, it is conceivable that this mechanism may be involved in the earlier age of menarche observed in blind girls. (Donofrio, Reiter, 1972: Kamberi, Mical, Porter, 1971: Relkin, 1972a, 1972b: Relkin, Adachi, Kahan, 1972: Wurtman, Axelrod, Chu, 1963.)

Prolactin and sebum

The possibility has been raised that prolactin may be involved in sebum production. However, at least in the intact and hypophysectomised rat no sebotrophic effect of prolactin has been found. (Nikkari, Valavaara, 1970: Shuster, Thody, Goolamali, Burton, Plummer, Bates, 1973.)

Section B: Prolactin and Human Disease

Chapter 14

INTRODUCTION - HORMONES AND DISEASE

The aim of the first section of this book was to present a concise factual review of our current knowledge of the physiology and effects of prolactin in mammals. As far as possible speculation was avoided and little attempt was made to apply to man findings made in animals. This second section is quite different in purpose. Because prolactin secretion fluctuates so dramatically in response to a number of stimuli and because it has such widespread actions on physiological systems it seems possible that it may play a role in a number of diseases which are not yet very well understood. Unfortunately at present knowledge of prolactin is limited to a small group of people many of whom have little interest in clinical applications (except in so far as they may be used to generate financial support for a project!) The aim of this section is therefore to review a number of diseases in which prolactin may perhaps be involved. In a few of these its importance has already been clearly established but in others the evidence is as yet fragmentary. In many, however, consideration of the possible role of prolactin brings a completely new element into research areas where progress may charitably be described as slow. I have not hesitated to be frankly speculative in the hope that medical scientists in a whole range of disciplines in which prolactin is now never considered may be encouraged to investigate its role. In contrast to much speculative effort, almost all the hypotheses suggested are testable by methods currently available. Scientists who do decide to look at prolactin may also be encouraged by the fact that if either high or low levels are found to be important in a particular disease process, then safe, orally effective drugs are already available for stimulating or suppressing prolactin secretion. This fact adds an almost unique aspect to research on prolactin.

In looking for possible clinical roles of prolactin I have considered particularly the following factors:

1. The physiology and effects of prolactin as described in the first section of this book. Knowledge of these immediately suggests some diseases where prolactin may be important.

2. The use of drugs such as phenothiazines and estrogens which are known to stimulate prolactin secretion. Diseases in which these drugs are helpful might be suppressed or prevented by the high prolactin levels. The high prolactin levels might also be involved in syndromes precipitated by use of these drugs.

3. The use of drugs such as L-dopa, glucocorticoids, monoamine oxidase inhibitors and ergot derivatives which are known to suppress prolactin secretion. Prolactin might be involved in the diseases in which these drugs are helpful and absence of prolactin might be a factor in syndromes occurring during treatment with these drugs.

This section of the book is so written that it can be read alone without the first section. However the first section will be referred to repeatedly as a source of information about both the physiology of prolactin and the original papers which deal with each subject. For the most part only references not mentioned in section A of the book will be specifically referred to here.

Hormones and disease

Before considering the various clinical syndromes individually it seems to me to be necessary to consider the roles which hormones may play in disease. In particular I should like to consider the validity of the phrase seen so often in clinical reports "Levels of hormone X were normal", with its implied conclusion" "and therefore we can rule out the possibility that hormone X may be playing a part in this patient's disease".

Crudely speaking there are two extreme types of disease causation. At one end of the spectrum are conditions like sickle cell disease which will occur in all individuals of a particular constitution irrespective of the environment to which they are exposed. At the other end are conditions like plague which for practical purposes can be said to occur in all individuals irrespective of constitution into whose bodies the bacillus gains access: plague will not occur in any individual who does not harbour the organism. But as every medical student knows (or ought to know) the great majority of diseases fall into neither of these two extreme categories. In most there is a dynamic interaction between an environmental factor (such as exposure to an infective or physical or a chemical agent) and an individual constitution on which the environmental factor acts. "Constitution" itself is of course partly determined by genetic and partly by other environmental factors. Well known examples of this are the facts that of the population who at some time act as host to the tubercle bacillus only a proportion develop tuberculosis or that of the population of heavy smokers only a small number will develop lung cancer. There can be little doubt that in practical terms heavy smoking often leads to the development of lung cancer. Yet one could never come to this conclusion by looking only at a heavy smoking population. There would be no obvious differences between the majority of heavy smokers who do not get lung cancer and the minority who do. The relationship between smoking and lung cancer is apparent only when we compare the occurrence of the disease in heavy smokers, moderate smokers, light smokers and non-smokers. **Within** each of these groups the disease free person may have precisely the same smoking habits as the diseased one.

The relationship between smoking and lung cancer was relatively easy to prove because the "abnormal" population of smokers could be readily compared with a "normal" population of non-smokers of the same race living in the same country. But in some respects a doctor working in say North America or Europe may no longer be able to compare "normal" and "abnormal" populations because the "normal" population no longer exists. Changes in lighting, in physical activity and in diet are all known to produce changes in endocrine status. These changes are so universal in, say, the USA or the UK, that the so-called "normal" levels of hormones in the population are almost certainly different from those in populations of similar races who were alive one thousand years ago. Which one calls "normal" is largely a semantic problem but there can be little doubt that the two are different.

This type of approach is undoubtedly more familiar to those doctors who have worked in the developing countries. For example, in the industrialised world a great deal of emphasis is placed on the importance of genetic factors in diabetes mellitus. Yet the doctor in Africa is much more concerned with environmental ones for he is often fortunate enough to be able to observe two populations from the same tribe. One retains the traditional way of life and in this group diabetes is very rare: the other has adopted a "Western" style of living and the incidence of diabetes is rising rapidly. By looking at an industralised society alone, the importance of environmental factors in diabetes is not very easy to prove conclusively. By looking at changing African societies it can be made obvious. In Europe and North America clearly almost everyone is exposed to a "diabetogenic" environment: but only those of a particular constitution will develop diabetes.

In some ways endocrinologists are the most sophisticated of clinical scientists but in others their conceptual framework is primitive. For the most part they are limited by a view of endocrine disease as being something like the plague: a patient who has a particular hormone level must have endocrine disease: another patient with another hormone level cannot have endocrine disease. This may, of course, be true but as yet it must be recognised that it is not the self-evident gospel it so often appears but is a hypothesis which remains to be proven. It is in fact probably true for practical purposes in the diseases which are now conventionally called endocrine. But it may not be true for a host of other diseases where endocrine factors are now not normally considered but which may in the future prove to have a hormonal base. It is therefore perhaps worth spelling out some of the factors which must be considered before endocrine factors can be implicated or eliminated in disease in the same way as smoking is implicated in lung cancer.

1. The fact that levels of hormone X in sufferers from the disease are within the normal range seen in those who are free from the disease does not mean that hormone X is not playing a part in the disease process. If all adults were heavy smokers, most would not get lung cancer and there would be no difference in smoking habits between those seen in lung cancer patients and the "normal" levels seen in disease-free individuals. No one doubts that chloramphenicol can "cause" marrow aplasia even though it does so in only a minute fraction of those exposed to the drug. A disease which occurs in only 0.1% of the population exposed to a particular level of a hormone may still be "caused" by that hormone.

2. If a hormone is playing a part in a disease the disease is likely to become commoner as hormone levels rise: if the hormone is preventing a disease the reverse will be true.

3. If a hormone is playing a part in a disease, the disease should become less

common if the hormone levels are lowered as part of a therapeutic manoeuvre: if the hormone is helping to prevent a disease the disease will become more common in this situation.

If the possible roles of hormones in disease are not to be missed it is vital for endocrinologists to be fully aware of these concepts. They are obviously valid when considering infectious diseases or side effects of drugs yet for reasons which I do not really understand they often appear to be greeted as totally revolutionary in an endocrine context.

"Normal" hormone levels

Hormones come to the attention of clinicians because of their effects on the tissues. It is the tissue effects which are important and it is therefore the level of hormone present in the target tissue which is of most concern. Unfortunately as yet we have no clinically applicable method of measuring the tissue concentration of any hormone in any target organ. It is therefore necessary to resort to less desirable alternatives.

Often when a hormone is first studied the methods available are totally inadequate for the estimation of the small amounts present in plasma. In the urine there are often larger amounts of the free hormone and still greater quantities of its metabolites. It is therefore common to progress from estimations of urinary excretion of metabolites to estimates of urinary excretion of the free hormone. Only after great refinement of methodology does it become possible to reach the Holy Grail which most endocrinologists seek, the ability to measure physiological quantities of the hormone in a few millilitres of blood. Increasingly, however, this consummation is being achieved, usually by means of radioimmunoassay. Unfortunately it is also increasingly apparent that this apparently ultimately desirable end may be less helpful than had been anticipated. With almost all hormones, measurements of plasma levels every ten minutes or so over a 24 hour period have yielded disturbing results: in entirely normal individuals values fluctuate dramatically and the plot of the results looks like a cross-sectional relief map of a continent with dramatic peaks, deep troughs and some plateaus. It is increasingly apparent that while a plasma or serum level which is grossly abnormal is of value, it is impossible to assess the significance of a single reading which appears to be within or only a little outside the "normal" range. Unless one knows whether the sample was taken at a peak or during a trough or during a plateau interpretation is fraught with hazard. The importance of this point can be appreciated only by considering relationships between plasma half life and tissue half life and the ways in which hormone secretion may be controlled.

Half lives

Some hormones, notably the catecholamines, are rapidly destroyed in the tissues. The half life of the hormone in the tissues is little longer than its half life in the plasma: plasma peaks will usually be associated with tissue peaks and plasma levels will usually be an accurate reflection of tissue levels. With other hormones however, there is a marked discrepancy between tissue half life and plasma half life. The hormone is bound by the tissues, there are no specific enzyme systems for its destruction and its action may be very prolonged. The contrast between tissue and plasma half life is very marked in the case of prolactin. Plasma half life ranges from about two to twenty minutes depending on the species and the physiological state of the individual. In contrast the tissue half life in rabbit mammary tissue has been reported as being of the order of 40-50 hours. In humans a single prolactin injection has been shown to have actions on the kidney which are demonstrable for at least 12-18 hours. In consequence, a single plasma prolactin peak which is over within a few minutes may have actions on target organs which may last for hours or even days.

Regulation of hormone secretion

Almost all hormones seem to be regulated by the actions of other hormones or of metabolic factors operating in the context of a negative feedback system. Two extreme models for the operation of such a feedback system may be considered: they provide a surprising amount of insight into clinical and experimental situations. In order to use a non-emotive example I will illustrate these by reference to two types of thermostatically controlled water bath with three basic components, a thermometer for measuring the water temperature, a control system and a heater for heating the water. In this example, heat is equivalent to a hormone level. The heat output of the heating system is equivalent to the plasma level which is the source from which the tissues receive their hormone. The heat content of the water (i.e. its temperature) is equivalent to the tissue level of the hormone. In a good, well-insulated water bath, the heat will be lost only slowly, i.e. the tissue half life will be prolonged.

With simple thermostats, the control switch is on and the heater is on if the temperature of the bath is below the set level and the switch is off when the temperature is above. The operation of the system is all-or-nothing: the heater is off or it is on with no grades in between. Provided that insulation is good, the relationship between the heat output from the heater and the temperature of the bath will be as shown in fig.7 a. When the temperature falls below the set level the heater will turn on and will quickly elevate the bath temperature. The heater will then turn off and the added heat will be very slowly dissipated. The heat content of the bath will thus be kept very nearly constant even though the heater is turned on for only brief periods with long intervals when it is completely off.

If the thermostat is then switched to a higher setting so that a temperature 5°C higher is required, then the sequence of events shown in the figure will occur. While the temperature of the bath is being elevated to the new level there will be a sustained period of heat output. Once the new desired temperature

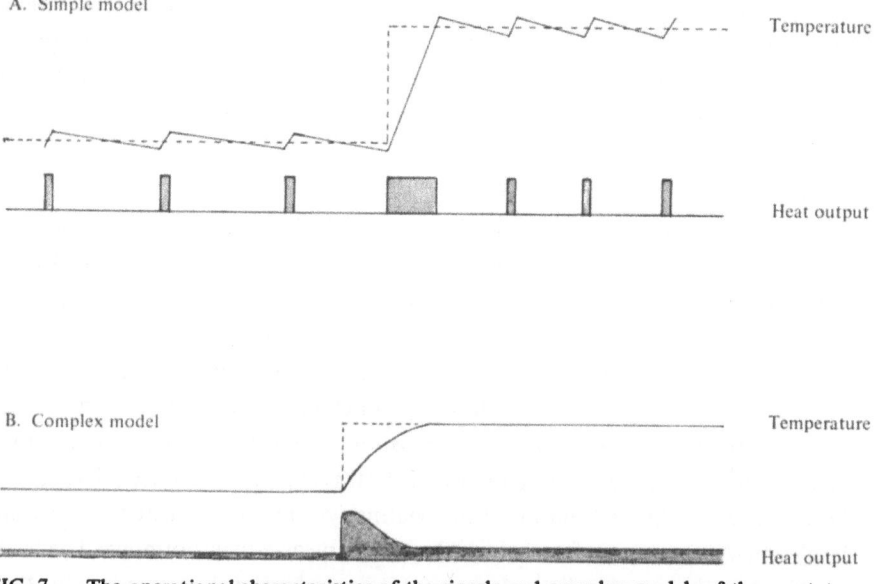

A. Simple model

Temperature

Heat output

B. Complex model

Temperature

Heat output

FIG. 7.   The operational characteristics of the simple and complex models of thermostats discussed in the text. Scales and slopes are entirely arbitrary and have no quantitative significance. The dotted line indicates the desired temperature and the complete line the actual temperature of the water. With the complex model the actual and desired temperatures are the same in the steady state. These models can be used to consider the relationship between the plasma level of a hormone and its tissue level with the heat output being equivalent to the plasma level and the temperature being equivalent to the tissue level.

has been attained, however, the pattern of heater function will return to one very similar to the one before. The only difference will be that the higher bath temperature will result in a slightly greater rate of heat loss. This means that the heater will have to be turned on a little more frequently than before.

The second much more sophisticated thermostat has an infinitely variable control switch with an equally variable heating system. The heater output is proportional partly to the difference between the desired bath temperature and the environmental temperature and partly to the difference between the desired bath temperature and the actual bath temperature. If the unit is very sophisticated then the relationship between bath temperature and heat output will be as in figure 7b. Fluctuations will occur but they will be so small as to be undetectable on the scale shown. The steady heat loss from the bath will be precisely balanced by a low but steady heat production. On switching the thermostat to a higher desired temperature, heat production will initially rise rapidly but will then fall progressively as the bath temperature approaches the desired level. Eventually the new higher bath temperature will be maintained by a new slightly elevated level of heat output. The higher level of heat output will be necessary to compensate for the greater heat loss which will occur as the result of the greater difference between bath and environmental temperatures.

If the regulation of hormone secretion is similar to the first simple model then the following conclusions may be drawn:

1. The tissue level of the hormone will depend only on the **frequency** of pulses of secretion and on the **height** of each pulse.

2. Plasma hormone levels in between pulses will be low and no guide whatsoever to tissue hormone levels.

3. If the setting of the feedback system is changed so that a higher tissue level of the hormone is required there will be a period of sustained hormone secretion with plasma levels continuously in the region of those seen at the peak of the individual pulses.

4. Once the new tissue level has been reached there will be a reversion to transient pulses of secretion. Neither the basal plasma level between pulses nor the

height of each individual pulse will be changed: a single plasma determination will therefore be totally unable to indicate the new higher tissue level of the hormone. The change in tissue level will be indicated **only** by the increase in the **frequency** of pulses of secretion. If a hormone has a tissue half life of many hours apparently small changes in pulse frequency may be able to produce large changes in tissue concentration. The main point to be emphasised is that a high hormone plasma level is needed only during the period when tissue levels are being raised: once the elevation has been achieved it can be maintained by an increase in hormone supply just sufficient to compensate for the increased rate of hormone loss. It is even possible that with a biological system the rate of hormone loss may not be altered when tissue levels are elevated: if this is so then after the transient period of change the new elevated tissue levels will be maintained by the same secretion rate as before.

If the second model is followed, the conclusions will be as follows:

1. In the steady state, the tissue hormone levels will be proportional to plasma hormone levels and the latter will be a good guide to the former.

2. If the setting of the feedback system is changed as before than there will be a period during which the secretion rate is markedly elevated in order to raise the tissue concentration to the new desired level.

3. As the desired tissue concentration is approached plasma levels of the hormone will fall but this fall will **not** indicate a fall in tissue concentration. Once the right concentration has been reached, then plasma levels, although they will be higher than before, will be elevated only sufficiently to compensate for any increased rate of tissue hormone loss occurring as a result of the increased tissue concentration.

There has in the past been a tendency to assume that the second more complex model is a relatively accurate picture of the feedback systems by which most hormones are regulated. But increasingly, determinations of many hormones made several times per hour over a 24 hour period are showing a pattern of spikes and troughs rather than a steady plateau. This picture looks much more like the simple model than the complex one. As almost always truth is likely to lie at neither extreme and regulation of hormone secretion may turn out to have features of both models. However the current evidence clearly points to the idea that the control systems are closer to the simple on/off all-or-nothing model than to the more complex sustained release infinitely variable one. For the sake of simplicity in the discussion I have not discussed the effects of changes in metabolic clearance rate and plasma half life but these do not affect the principles involved and can relatively easily be incorporated in the scheme. Broadly speaking an increase in the metabolic clearance rate and a shortening of the plasma half life will tend to increase the discrepancies between plasma and tissue levels: prolongation of the metabolic clearance rate will have the reverse effects.

The most important conclusions which follow from this discussion are as follows:

1. With either model a sustained elevation of tissue hormone concentration can be achieved by a transient period of obviously elevated plasma levels followed by a period when although hormone secretion rate may be elevated this will not be easily detectable by current techniques. In the steady state a particular tissue concentration can be maintained by a pattern of plasma levels which is sufficient only to replace loss. It seems probable that the higher the tissue concentration the higher will be the rate of loss but the difference between rates of tissue loss is unlikely to be dramatic, especially when the tissue half life is prolonged. If the first model is near-valid then basal plasma levels before and after the tissue level change will be virtually the same and the only change will be an increased frequency of peaks. Even if the second model is correct the plasma levels before and after a change in tissue level are unlikely to be dramatically different except during the period of change itself. In practice the difference between the two steady states is likely to be apparent only if plasma levels are precisely monitored in an individual over a prolonged period before and after the change. Single plasma levels are likely to appear within the normal range since it is now obvious that the normal range for a population is much wider than the normal range for an individual within that population.

2. Single plasma samples are very unlikely to give any real indication of hormone tissue levels unless the values are grossly abnormal. This is especially true if the first model is anything like correct and if the frequency of plasma level peaks rather than absolute plasma values is more important in determining tissue concentrations. It is likely that many individuals whose plasma values seem within the normal range have elevated tissue levels. The value of single plasma

determinations is relatively high when the plasma half life and tissue half life are comparable but decreases sharply if a short plasma half life is associated with a prolonged tissue half life.

3. Ideally when investigating an individual's endocrine status plasma samples should be taken several times an hour over a 24 hour period. This is possible only as a research and not as a routine clinical procedure. A poor man's alternative may be to estimate the 24 hour urinary excretion of the hormone. Provided that renal function is near normal this may well give a better indication of endocrine status than single plasma samples. The value of this approach has already been demonstrated with urinary free cortisol determinations and accurate methods for looking at urinary excretion of other hormones, including prolactin, are urgently required.

4. Even more satisfactory would be a method of measuring target organ tissue concentration suitable for routine clinical use but as yet we seem to be very far from this.

5. The considerations discussed here should be applied to all aspects of endocrine physiology and pathophysiology. One particularly striking example is the hypertension which follows renal artery clamping. There is a brief period when renin-angiotensin-aldosterone levels are obviously elevated but they then return almost back to normal. It is therefore frequently stated that the renin-angiotensin-aldosterone system plays little part in chronic renal hypertension but if the analysis presented here is at all correct this conclusion could be completely false. Tissue hormone levels might well be elevated even during the chronic phase.

Tissue activity of hormones

Unfortunately, even when accurate ways of measuring the tissue concentrations of hormones become available the end of the road will not have been reached. The effect of a particular tissue concentration of the hormone is not constant. It may vary very considerably depending on the constitutional make-up of the individual, on the biochemical and metabolic environment and in particular on the overall pattern of endocrine function. It is increasingly clear that it is almost meaningless to study one hormone in isolation. The endocrine system functions as an integrated whole with each hormone having its own actions but simultaneously modifying the effects of other hormones. Prolactin, for example, is involved in some of the most dramatic effects of this type. Aldosterone "normally" reduces renal sodium excretion. Treatment with a high salt intake, with cortisol or with the suppressor of prolactin secretion, 2-bromo-α-ergokryptine all first of all abolish the action of aldosterone on renal function and then revese it so that aldosterone becomes a hormone which promotes sodium loss. Prolactin will then restore the "normal" salt-retaining effect. Thus depending on the biochemical and endocrine environment the same amount of exogenous aldosterone may cause sodium retention, have no effect on sodium excretion or cause sodium loss. In this sort of situation it is therefore meaninless to say simply the plasma or tissue level of aldosterone was X ng/ml in the belief that this figure will give some indication of what aldosterone is doing to renal function in that individual. X ng/ml may cause sodium loss, have no effect or cause sodium retention. What is therefore required is not only an estimate of tissue concentration but also an estimate of the biological activity of the hormone in the particular system under consideration in the individual from whom the sample was taken. In the case of aldosterone, for example, it might be possible to take a tissue or a blood sample and then to inject a dose of the hormone in order to estimate the biological effect of a standard amount. Ideally also a standard amount of a specific aldosterone inhibitor should also be tested in order to investigate the effects of both lowering and raising the effective concentration of the hormone. Since there are presumably a finite number of hormone receptors on a tissue, one which was saturated with a hormone would fail to respond to an exogenous addition of the same hormone but would show a clear response to an inhibitor.

Thus by measuring tissue level of a hormone, the effect of adding exogenous hormone and the effect of inhibiting endogenous hormone one might be able to derive an expression which indicated the true effective level of hormone activity in that individual. In the meantime all one can say is that if the current tests such as plasma and urine sampling indicate that hormone levels in these fluids are abnormal, then tissue hormone levels will almost certainly also be abnormal. The reverse is not true. A body fluid hormone level within the "normal range" is no guarantee of normal tissue levels or normal tissue activity.

Conclusions

The main conclusions of this chapter may be summarised as follows:

1. It is possible that some forms of endocrine-mediated disease will prove to be

similar to diseases produced by exposure to many infective agents, environmental factors or drugs. If this is so, then even in a group exposed to precisely the same hormone levels (which may be within the so-called normal range) some individuals will develop the disease and others will not. However, as with smoking and lung cancer, groups exposed to different levels of the hormone would be expected to have different incidences of the disease. The relationship between the hormone and the disease may not become readily apparent by looking for differences in hormone levels between those who have the disease and those who do not. An approach more likely to achieve results will be to look for differences in disease incidence between populations with high and low levels of the hormone. Final proof of a relationship will require the demonstration that deliberate therapeutic manipulation of hormone levels in the appropriate direction will lower the incidence of the disease.

2. Because the concept is much simpler it is sensible not to discard the hypothesis that members of the population with a particular disease will, if the disease is endocrine-mediated, have different hormone levels than members of the same population without the disease. In fact, with the diseases which are now classified as "endocrine" this is obviously the case. Patients with Cushing's syndrome have obviously overactive adrenals and patients with myxedema have obviously underactive thyroids. There may however be other diseases whose causes are as yet unknown and which are now not thought of as "endocrine" in which the hormone-disease relationship described in the first paragraph may be valid.

3. All measures of hormone functions are at the moment inadequate and likely to remain so for some time. As an over-simplified generalisation it may be stated that if a hormone function test gives an abnormal result then an abnormality of tissue function is very likely. In contrast a normal test result cannot exclude an abnormality of hormone function at the tissue level.

Chapter 15

TESTS OF THE PROLACTIN
SECRETING SYSTEM

If possible, it is desirable to be able to test the various components of the system which controls the synthesis and secretion of a hormone. A prerequisite for such testing is an understanding of the control mechanisms which regulate secretion of the hormone. In the case of prolactin we already know enough to be able to carry out useful tests but most of these are still in the early stages of development.

The basic mechanisms regulating prolactin secretion in humans have been extensively discussed in chapter 6. The main points to be noted are as follows:

1. Prolactin secretion in humans is under the control of a prolactin-inhibiting factor (PIF). Animal experiments, primarily in the rat have shown that hypothalamic PIF levels are regulated by dopamine with the more dopamine being present the higher being hypothalamic PIF levels. Animal experiments have also shown that there is a short feedback loop whereby high prolactin levels elevate PIF levels.

2. TRH injections in humans stimulate prolactin secretion. The response is so rapid that it is probably a direct action of TRH on pituitary cells. That TRH may naturally stimulate prolactin secretion is suggested by the fact that in primary hypothyroidism when TSH and presumably TRH secretion are high, prolactin plasma levels are also frequently elevated. It is possible that as with other releasing factors high prolactin secretion may inhibit TRH secretion by a short feedback loop.

3. In lactating humans suckling produces a sharp rise in prolactin secretion with no change in TSH secretion. Since the response seems to be too rapid to be accounted for entirely on the basis of hypothalamic PIF depletion with removal of inhibition of prolactin release, it is possibly mediated by a prolactin releasing factor as well. Since TSH levels do not change, this releasing factor is presumably distinct from TRH and here will be termed PRF. Again there may be a mechanism whereby prolactin can inhibit secretion of PRF.

4. Relatively little has been done on control of the synthesis as distinct from the release of prolactin in humans. However, the amount of prolactin secreted during a TRH response appears to be greater than could be accounted for by release of pre-existing hormone, suggesting that it stimulates synthesis. The same is probably true of the response to suckling during lactation and since TRH does not appear to be involved here, PRF can presumably also stimulate synthesis.

5. There is some evidence that in animals serotonin and noradrenaline may stimulate prolactin secretion, possibly through the intermediary of one of the releasing factors.

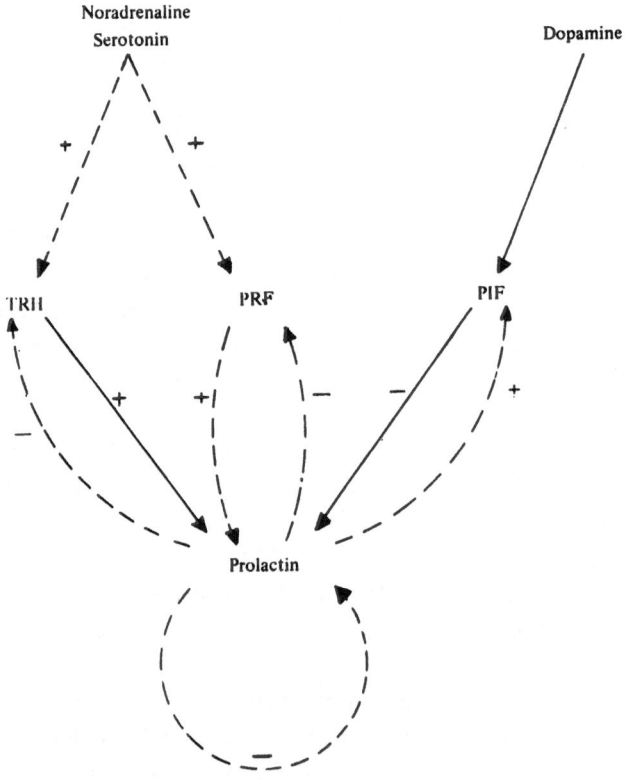

FIG. 8. Mechanisms of control of prolactin secretion. Heavy lines represent relatively well established pathways, dotted lines represent probable but not yet firmly established ones. Plus signs indicate stimulate of secretion, minus ones inhibition of secretion.

6. There is also evidence from animals that prolactin may inhibit its own secretion by acting directly on the prolactin cells.

These observations are summarised in figure 8. The heavy lines represent pathways which have been reasonably well established in humans. The dotted lines represent pathways whose existence in humans has not yet been proved but which seem likely to be present.

TRH, TSH and prolactin

Since the TRH test has been so widely used now in thyroid disease it seems appropriate to begin this section by a brief review of what has been established as far as the TSH response to TRH is concerned. The main points are:

1. Like the prolactin response, the TSH response to intravenous TRH is very rapid with peak levels being reached after 20-30 minutes. Daily testing may blunt the response but testing on alternate days does not seem to do this.

2. The response is greater in females than in males and in both sexes may be exaggerated by estrogen treatment.

3. In patients with primary hypothyroidism and elevated TSH levels before testing, the response to TRH is exaggerated and prolonged.

4. In patients with hyperthyroidism and suppressed TSH levels due either to thyroid disease or treatment with thyroid hormones the response is depressed and may be absent altogether.

5. In patients with hypothyroidism due to failure at pituitary level the response is absent.

6. In patients with hypothyroidism due to hypothalamic failure presumably with absent or reduced TRH secretion, the TSH response may be normal or exaggerated. In some such patients the response may be considerably delayed suggesting the possibility of a time when TRH-mediated TSH synthesis may occur.

7. In a patient with hyperthyroidism which appeared possibly due to excess TRH secretion, TSH did not respond to TRH.

8. L-dopa and glucocorticoids both inhibit the TSH response to TRH. High levels of prolactin due to prolactin-secreting tumors or to chlorpromazine treatment do not appear to alter it.

9. In patients with depression the TSH response to TRH is also depressed even though there is no evidence that depressed individuals may be hyperthyroid.

(Andersson, Bowers, Kastin, Schalch, Schally, Snyder, Utiger, Wilber, Wise, 1971: Emerson, Utiger, 1972: Foley, Jacobs, Hoffman, Daughaday, Blizzard, 1972: Foley, Owings, Hayford, Blizzard, 1972: Friesen, 1972a: Haigler, Pittman, Hershman, Baugh, 1971: Hall, 1973: Hall, Ormston, Besser, Cryer, McKendrick, 1972: Kastin, Ehrensing, Schalch, Anderson, 1972: Ormston, Garry, Cryer, Besser, Hall, 1971: Ormston, Kilborn, Garry, Amos, Hall, 1971: Pittman, Haigler, Hershman, Pittman, 1971: Prange, Wilson, Lara, Alltop, Breese, 1972: Rybakowski, Sowinski, 1973: Sachson, Rosen, Cuatrecasas, 1972: Spaulding, Burrow, Donabedian, Van Woert, 1972.)

The TRH test may therefore be useful in the diagnosis of hypothyroidism and hyperthyroidism although depression may be a complicating feature since depressed hypothyroid patients probably have a diminished TRH response. It may also be used to distinguish between TSH disorders of pituitary and hypothalamic origin. The changes in the response in the various clinical conditions have not been adequately explained. The only exception is primary failure of the TSH secreting cells: if the cells are not there they obviously cannot respond. The failure of response in a patient with high TSH levels, possibly due to excess hypothalamic TRH secretion, might be explained by saturation of the pituitary TSH receptors by TRH: that this explanation may perhaps be valid is supported but not confirmed by the reduction in the TSH response which may occur with frequent testing at short intervals. In primary hyperthyroidism, presumably TRH and TSH levels in the hypothalamus and putuitary are low. However it seems unlikely that the pituitary contains no TSH at all. The alternative possibility that the response may fail in the absence of "tonic" stimulation of the pituitary by TRH is not supported by the exaggerated, though often delayed, response which occurs in patients who appear to have hypothalamic failure. The delay in these patients may possibly be due to the need to stimulate TSH synthesis before it can be secreted. The depressed response in hyperthyroidism also cannot simply be explained by an action of excess circulating thyroid hormones since a diminished response also occurs in depressed patients who are certainly not hyperthyroid and may be hypothyroid. Conversely the exaggerated response in hypothyroidism cannot be accounted for by low levels of thyroid hormones since these are also present in depressed individuals in whom the response is diminished. The reduction in the response with L-dopa therapy has not been explained.

There is therefore no explanation based on TRH, TSH and thyroid hormones alone which can account for all the changes. Another possibility which does not appear to have been so far considered is that as with prolactin, TSH is regulated by both releasing and inhibiting factors. I feel that there is a good case for postulating the existence of a TSH-inhibiting factor (TIF). A factor which tonically exerted an inhibiting effect on TSH release might be able to allow increased release

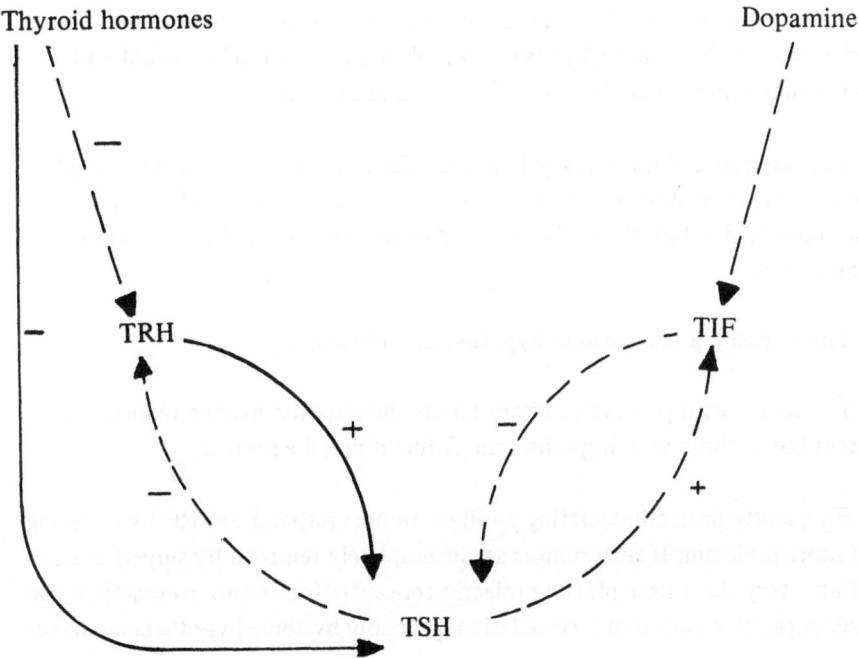

FIG. 9.   Mechanisms of hypothalamic control of TSH secretion. Heavy lines represent well-established pathways, dotted lines indicate ones which are not yet certain. Plus signs indicate stimulation of secretion, minus signs inhibition.

or to block release completely. A tentative scheme for the hypothalamic regulation of TSH secretion is therefore shown in figure 9. Again short feedback loops whereby increased TSH levels would diminish TRH and elevate TIF are shown. The proposal that a TIF exists would make particular sense in the suppression of the TRH response by L-dopa since L-dopa is known to elevate hypothalamic MSH-IF and PIF and might have a general effect on hypothalamic inhibiting factors.

TRH and prolactin secretion

There can now be no doubt that even quite small doses of TRH given orally or intravenously to human beings may produce a dramatic prolactin secretory response which probably involves stimulation of both release and synthesis. As yet the response has been much less extensively tested than the TSH response but all the evidence so far indicates that similar factors affect both.

1. Even though baseline levels are similar the response is greater in females than males. Most males respond by elevating prolactin plasma levels 2-4 fold within 15 minutes while in females 4-10 fold elevations are usual.

2. The response is diminished in hyperthyroid individuals or in normal people taking thyroid hormones. With increasing hyperthyroidism the TSH response is extinguished before the prolactin response but eventually the latter dissappears as well.

3. The response is enhanced in hypothyroid individuals.

4. In patients with primary pituitary failure the response may be reduced or absent but in those with hypothalamic failure it may be normal.

5. Frequently prolactin-secreting pituitary tumors respond to TRH by secreting yet more prolactin. If such tumors are incompletely removed by surgery then within a very short time plasma prolactin concentrations return to pre-operative levels suggesting continuous stimulation, probably by some hypothalamic factor.

Tests which primarily involve PIF

It would be desirable to be able specifically to increase or diminish hypothalamic PIF secretion in order to test the prolactin secretory response in individuals with various disorders. Reserpine and chlorpromazine both seem to increase prolactin secretion primarily by reducing secretion of PIF, although other mechanisms involving releasing factors have not been categorically excluded. In contrast, L-dopa seems to inhibit prolactin secretion by increasing the dopamine effect on PIF. So far chlorpromazine and L-dopa have been tried as possible clinical tests, with the following results:

1. In normal individuals an intramuscular dose of 25 mg chlorpromazine reliably elevated prolactin secretion with a peak after about 60 minutes. The response is therefore considerably slower than the response to intravenous TRH. As with TRH the response seems to be greater in females than in males.

2. Chorpomazine had no effect on TSH. TRH in chlorpromazine treated individuals elevated both TSH and prolactin.

3. L-dopa suppressed prolactin levels with a nadir 2-4 hours after a 500 mg oral dose. Treatment with L-dopa suppressed both the prolactin and TSH responses to TRH. In the case of prolactin there is little doubt that this suppression is due to elevated PIF which therefore strengthens the case for a hypothalamic TIF.

4. Patients without functioning anterior pituitary tissue as expected showed no response either to chlorpromazine or to L-dopa. Patients with primary anterior pituitary hypofunction showed subnormal responses.

5. Many patients with prolactin-secreting anterior pituitary tumors showed reduced prolactin levels after L-dopa but no increase in response to chlorpromazine. If surgical removal of such tumors was not complete plasma prolactin levels rapidly returned to pre-operative values. This suggests that these patients may have tumors secondary to hypothalamic stimulation. It is interesting that in normal individuals a high rate of prolactin secretion should be associated with peak levels of PIF because of the short negative feedback loop. The absence of any response to chlorpromazine suggests that in these individuals PIF may already be very low instead of high and that a low PIF, possibly coupled with a high PRF, may be a primary factor in initiating the syndrome.

6. Many patients with prolactin-secreting pituitary tumours responded to TRH with a further increase in secretion.

7. A patient with elevated prolactin levels because of a craniopharyngioma failed to respond to L-dopa.

(Bowers, Friesen, Folkers, 1972: Bowers, Friesen, Hwang, Guyda, Folkers, 1971: Friesen, 1972b: Friesen, Hwang, Guyda, Tolis, Tyson, Myers, 1972: Friesen, Guyda, Hwang, Tyson, Barbeau, 1972: Jacobs, Bauman, Daughaday, 1971: Friesen, Webster, Hwang, Guyda, Munro, Read, 1972: Turkington, 1971b, 1972c, 1972g, 1972h.)

Direct effects on pituitary prolactin secreting cells

Ergot derivatives inhibit prolactin secretion partly by increasing hypothalamic PIF secretion but more importantly by a direct inhibition of the pituitary prolactin-secreting cells. The most potent one seems to be 2-bromo-α-ergokryptine (CB 154) which is now undergoing clinical trial in humans. Other ergot derivatives may have a direct effect on pituitary cells to stimulate prolactin secretion. (Del Pozo, Brun del Re, Varga, Friesen, 1972: Fluckiger, 1972: Varga, Lutterbeck, Pryor, Wenner, Erb, 1972.)

Chapter 16

DRUGS WHICH ALTER
PROLACTIN SECRETION

The aim of this chapter is to summarise information on the drug effects on prolactin secretion which have been reported in mammals. The data has been extensively discussed in section A of this book, mainly in chapter 6. Only the references to statements which may be controversial are given in this chapter.

Steroid hormones

Estrogens have a dual and possibly triple effect in stimulating prolactin secretion. They deplete hypothalamic PIF and stimulate the prolactin-secreting pituitary cells directly. There is some evidence that they may also act via a releasing or synthesis-stimulating factor as well. Hypothalamic estrogen implants appear to promote pituitary prolactin synthesis. Also estrogens have a greater effect on prolactin secretion from in situ pituitaries in PIF-depleted, chlorpromazine-treated animals than on secretion from pituitaries transplanted into the abdominal cavity. There is also a suggestion that the natural estrogens, estrone and estradiol, may actually inhibit prolactin secretion in post-menopausal women while the synthetic estrogen ethinyl estradiol stimulates it. The response to estrogen is greater in women than in men. (Kanematsu, Sawyer, 1963: Kwa, Van der Gugten, Sala, Verhofstad, 1972: L'Hermite, Delvoye, Nokin, Vekemans, Robyn, 1972.)

Low to moderate doses of progesterone may have no effect on prolactin secretion or may suppress it. Very high doses of progesterone may deplete hypothalamic PIF and stimulate prolactin secretion.

Testosterone may reduce hypothalamic PIF and in humans cause hypertrophy of the prolactin-secreting cells.

Medroxyprogosterone may elevate prolactin secretion in some individuals but have little or no effect in others. A chlormadinone-ethinylestradiol combination left prolactin at follicular phase levels in humans without any clear suppression or stimulation. The norethynodrel-mestranol combination (Enovid) has been reported to elevate plasma prolactin levels.

Glucocorticoids suppress prolactin secretion.

Monoamine oxidase inhibitors

Iproniazid, pargyline and phenelzine appear to suppress prolactin secretion probably by potentiating the effect of dopamine which stimulates PIF secretion.

Tricyclic antidepressants

The tricyclic antidepressants imipramine and amitriptyline both elevate plasma prolactin levels in man. Since they seem to be operative only in the presence of intact catecholamine stores and may potentiate catecholamine effects it is unlikely that they work by reducing PIF levels which would, in fact, be increased if the effect of dopamine were potentiated. A more likely explanation is that they potentiate the effect of noradrenaline which may operate by stimulating PRF or TRH secretion.

Phenothiazines

All the phenothiazines tested including chlorpromazine, promazine, perphenazine, fluphenazine and thioridazine have been reported to stimulate prolactin secretion. They deplete hypothalamic PIF and this is believed to be their main mode of action.

Tranquillizers and anti-histamines

Chlordiazepoxide, diazepam, butyrophenones (the "peridol" group of drugs) thalidomide, sulpiride, some antihistamines and a variety of other experimental tranquillising agents have been reported to elevate prolactin secretion in animals. Haloperidol appears to be the only one of the group where the effect has been documented in man. (Sulman, 1971: Fluckiger, 1972.)

Drugs which act on amine metabolism

Methyltyrosines which block the biosynthesis of dopamine, noradrenaline and adrenaline elevate prolactin secretion: dihydroxyphenyl serine which normalises noradrenaline synthesis only produces a further elevation in prolactin secretion suggesting that noradrenaline stimulates TRH or PRF secretion. L-dopa which is a precursor of both dopamine and noradrenaline elevates PIF secretion and reduces prolactin secretion. Blockade of noradrenaline synthesis with diethyldithiocarbamate, which does not affect dopamine synthesis, leaves unchanged the suppression of prolactin secretion seen with L-dopa. It therefore seems that dopamine is the catecholamine which inhibits prolactin secretion via PIF.

Methyldopa leads to the synthesis of methyldopamine and methyl noradrenaline which are both "false transmitters". The lack of dopamine seems to be more important than the lack of noradrenaline: PIF levels fall and prolactin secretion rises. Reserpine and guanethidine deplete catecholamine stores in different ways and probably also act primarily by preventing the normal effect of dopamine on PIF: reserpine seems to be by far the more potent of the two which is probably because guanethidine does not readily cross the blood-brain barrier.

d-Amphetamine may act partly because of a competitive effect with dopamine or depletion of dopamine resulting in lowered PIF. There is no evidence as yet that it does in fact deplete PIF and my own opinion is that a stimulation of PRF because of the sympathomimetic effects of amphetamine is probably part of the explanation for its action.

Tryptophan, 5-hydroxytryptophan and serotonin have all been reported to elevate prolactin secretion, probably by acting on PRF or TRH.

LSD has been reported to inhibit prolactin secretion.

Ergot derivatives

Almost all the ergot derivatives, including ergotamine, seem able to suppress prolactin secretion primarily by a direct action on the prolactin secreting cells but partly also by increasing hypothalamic PIF secretion. 2-Bromo-α-ergokryptine (CB 154) seems to be the most effective agent, a single oral dose suppressing prolactin secretion for as long as 12 hours. Another ergot derivative, however, 1-methyl-9,10-dihydroergonorcornine appears to be able to stimulate prolactin secretion, (Fluckiger, 1972.)

Other drugs

Clonidine which has been used as a hypotensive and also in migraine suppresses prolactin secretion, (Fluckiger, 1972.)

Frusemide (furosemide) has been reported to block lactation in rabbits, thus raising the possibility that it may either compete peripherally with prolactin or may suppress prolactin secretion. The possibility of peripheral competition is a particularly interesting one at the renal level as many of its actions could be accounted for in terms of a blocking effect on the renal effects of prolactin. If this is so then during frusemide treatment aldosterone should become a salt-losing substance. Strangely enough, long before we became interested in prolactin, Lloyd and I demonstrated in frusemide-treated rabbits that progesterone reduced rather than increased sodium excretion. Since progesterone is believed to increase sodium excretion by acting as a competitive inhibitor of aldosterone, this reversal of progesterone action would be expected if aldosterone had also reversed its action. Ethacrynic acid presumably has a similar action to frusemide. (Gachev, 1968: Horrobin, Lloyd, 1970.)

Lithium

There have been no studies on prolactin secretion during lithium treatment but some at least of the actions of lithium are compatible with the concept that in some way it reduces prolactin secretion. On beginning therapy there is a loss of sodium, potassium and water in the urine and some individuals on lithium treatment became resistant to the renal actions of ADH. The interpretation of the electrolyte changes is however complicated by the fact that after the initial fluid and electrolyte loss, aldosterone secretion may also be markedly stimulated with development of spironolactone-sensitive edema. The antidiabetic actions of lithium are compatible with a suppression of prolactin secretion. This is also true for the good results claimed in the premenstrual syndrome which may perhaps be caused by prolactin. Lithium has also been reported to be effective in migraine, a condition in which all the known effective drugs are suppressors of prolactin secretion. (Angrist, Gershon, Levitan, Blumberg, 1970: Baer, Platman, Fieve, 1970: Demers, Henniger, 1970: Lee, Jampol, Brown, 1971: Maletzky, Blachly, 1971: Mannisto, Koivisto, 1972: Mellerup, Plenge, Vendsborg, Rafaelsen, Kjeldsen, Agerbaek, 1972: Murphy, Goodwin, Bunney, 1969: Ramsay, Mendels, Stokes, Fitzgerald, 1972: Sletton, Gershon, 1966: Tupin, Schlagenhauf, Creson, 1968: Van der Velde, Gordon, 1969.)

Chapter 17

PUERPERAL LACTATION
AND GALACTORRHEA

As might be expected from the history of our knowledge of prolactin, the clinical areas where its role has been shown to be unequivocal are in puerperal lactation and in galactorrhea of many different types. The role of prolactin in puerperal lactation has been discussed in the previous section of the book. At this point it is interesting to note that especially in late lactation, prolactin plasma levels in between periods of suckling may be within the normal range. This is a striking demonstration of the concept that where the tissue half-life of a hormone is prolonged while its plasma half-life is short, plasma levels may need to be elevated only intermittently in order to maintain the activity of the hormone at its target site. The action of estrogens in blocking puerperal lactation is probably a peripheral one, and is not dependent on interference with prolactin secretion. CB 154 in contrast can interfere with puerperal lactation by blocking prolactin secretion. (Besser, Parke, Edwards, Forsyth, McNeilly, 1972: L'Hermite, Stauric, Robyn, 1972: Tyson, Hwang, Guyda and Friesen, 1972.)

Galactorrhea and gynecomastia

Prolactin levels do not appear to be elevated in gynecomastia. In galactorrhea in contrast, prolactin levels are almost always raised: it seems probable that 24 hour sampling would reveal elevated levels even in those whose prolactin appears to be within the normal range when judged on the basis of a single sample. On the other hand, many individuals with elevated prolactin levels do not have galactorrhea, indicating that prolactin is only one of a complex of hormones required to induce milk secretion. Galactorrhea can occur in both non-puerperal females and males, but in the presence of similar hormone levels it seems, not surprisingly, to be more frequent in women of reproductive age. (Besser, Edwards, 1972: Forsyth, Besser, Edwards, Francis, Myres, 1971: Hwang, Guyda, Friesen, 1971: L'Hermite, Delvoye, Nokin, Vekemans, Robyn, 1972: Turkington, 1971c, 1972f: Volpe, Killinger, Bird, Clark, Friesen, 1972.)

Drugs

Galactorrhea may be associated with treatment with any of the drugs which can elevate prolactin levels. The phenothiazines appear to be the commonest offenders but this may merely be because they are more widely used than the others. Cessation of drug therapy usually results in termination of the lactation although this may not happen for two or three weeks (Apostolakis, Kapetanakis, Lazos, Madena-Pyrgaki, 1972: Frantz, Kleinberg, Noel, 1972b: Polishuk, Kulesan, 1956: Turkington, 1972: Winnik, Tennenbaum, 1955.)

Oral contraceptives

A small number of women taking oral contraceptives develop galactorrhea. Some do not appear to be aware of this until manual expression of milk is attempted. Other women may have persistent amenorrhea and galactorrhea after stopping oral contraceptive treatment. There do not appear to be any systematic reports of prolactin levels in women on the pill, but it would not be surprising if many had some elevation of prolactin secretion. There is a possibility that ethinyl estradiol may be a more effective stimulator of prolactin secretion than the natural estrogens. Medroxyprogesterone may also elevate human prolactin levels (Gambrell, Greenblatt, Mahesh, 1971: Halbert, Christian, 1969: L'Hermite, Delvoye, Nokin, Vekemans, Robyn, 1972: Shearman, 1971.)

The effects on prolactin secretion of the steroids contained in oral contraceptives have not been systematically studied in animals. There is evidence in rats that the norethynodrel-mestranol combination elevates pituitary prolactin content and secretion (Kahn, Baker, 1966: Minaguchi, Meites, 1967: Welsch, Meites, 1969.)

Post-partum galactorrhea (Chiari-Frommel syndrome)

Post-partum galactorrhea in women not being suckled is usually known as the Chiari-Frommel syndrome. In some women it is associated with a pituitary tumor. The prolactin levels may be suppressed and galactorrhea terminated by treatment either with L-dopa or CB154. Unfortunately cessation of the drug therapy often allows the return of the galactorrhea. (Besser, Parke, Edwards, Forsyth, McNeilly, 1972: Hwang, Guyda, Friesen, 1971: L'Hermite, Delvoye, Nokin, Vekemans, Robyn, 1972: Lutterbeck, Pryor, Varga, Wenner, Erb, 1971: Malarkey, Jacobs, Daughaday, 1971: Turkington, 1971a.)

Occasionally the Chiari-Frommel syndrome may be an indicator of hypothyroidism or adrenal insufficiency (Kinch, Plunkett, Devlin, 1969: Savely, Modlinger-Odorfer, Szecsenyi-Nagy, 1965: Refetoff, Block, Ehrilich, Friesen, 1972.)

Pituitary tumors

Galactorrhea may occur in association with a number of types of pituitary tumor. This syndrome has been given a number of names but Forbes-Albright is perhaps the most widely used. In some cases the tumor appears to secrete prolactin alone, in some cases prolactin and growth hormone. In others the tumor itself may not secrete prolactin but may disturb hypothalamic-pituitary relationships so that prolactin secreting cells are released from the inhibitory influence of PIF. With some tumors the prolactin secretion seems autonomous but with others it may respond to L-dopa, suggesting persistence of hypothalamic control (ref. as in previous section plus Argonz, Del Castillo, 1953: Forbes, Henneman, Griswold, Albright, 1954: Forsyth, Besser, Edwards, Francis, Myres, 1971: Friesen, Webster, Hwang, Guyda, Munro, Reed, 1972: Nasr, Mozaffarian, Pensky, Pearson, 1972: Peake, McKeel, Jarrett, Daughaday, 1969: Turkington, 1971.c)

Surgery

There are a number of reports of lactation occurring following surgery. Initially this wa thought to be due to stimulation of mammary afferents following thoracic operations, but it is now apparent that other forms of surgery may be associated with galactorrhea. It seems more likely that the most important factor is the sharp rise in prolactin secretion which may be seen in surgical patients. This is apparent pre-operatively, presumably because of psychological stress, and during the operation itself there may be a dramatic rise in prolactin levels. Such prolactin secretion occurring in an individual whose endocrine environment permits mammary development could presumably lead to overt lactation. (Frantz, Kleinberg, Noel, 1972b: Friesen, Belanger, Guyda, Hwang, 1972: Grossman, Buchberg, Brecher, Hallinger, 1950: Lavoie, 1968: Noel, Suh, Stone, Frantz, 1972: Quinlan, 1968: Shield, Charme, 1969.)

Starvation

Galactorrhea does not occur during starvation itself but may occur during refeeding. The best reports of this syndrome relate to American prisoners of war in the Far East in World War II. About 10% of PoWs developed gynecomastia but only a small proportion of these showed galactorrhea as well. One possibility is that refeeding produced elevation of secretion of all the hormones necessary for breast development. Another is that reduction of LH and FSH secretion during starvation led to elevated prolactin secretion and that in some men this persisted for long enough to allow lactation when other hormone levels returned to normal on refeeding. It would seem worthwhile to measure prolactin levels in human starvation as famine edema could conceivably be partly accounted for by elevated prolactin levels. (Hibbs, 1947: Jacobs, 1948.)

Galactorrhea, precocious puberty and hypothyroidism

In this rare syndrome it has recently been demonstrated that prolactin levels are elevated. The primary disturbance seems to be in thyroid regulation because treatment with L-thyroxine corrects the hypothyroidism, lowers plasma prolactin levels, abolishes the galactorrhea and lowers the high gonadotrophin levels. In rats prolactin implants in the median eminence can cause precocious puberty and by a short feedback mechanism can elevate hypothalamic PIF levels. Since high PIF levels are often associated with increased release of LH and FSH and vice versa, resulting normally in a reciprocal relationship between prolactin secretion on the one hand and LH and FSH secretion on the other, it is possible that high prolactin levels act on the hypothalamus to elevate levels of gonadotrophin releasing factors. If this is so then the sequence of events in this unusual syndrome might be as follows:

1. The hypothyroidism is primary.

2. Low thyroid hormone levels lead to elevated TRH secretion and increased responsiveness of prolactin secreting cells to TRH.

3. Elevated prolactin levels act via the hypothalamic releasing factors to increase secretion of FSH and LH and galactorrhea and precocious puberty occurs (Clemens, Minaguchi, Storey, Voogt, Meites, 1969: Turkington, Ray, Costin, 1972.)

Sarcoidosis

It has long been known that the hypothalamus may be involved in sarcoidosis but the extent of the relationship has only recently been revealed. In 11 out of 34 patients with sarcoid, prolactin levels were consistently elevated but no elevation was noted in 18 patients with pulmonary tuberculosis. Some of the patients had galactorrhea. L-dopa consistently lowered prolactin levels.

One of the patients with prolactin elevation died and post mortem examination revealed granulomata in the median eminence. It is possible that all patients with elevated prolactin levels have such granulomata but in view of the very high incidence of elevated prolactin secretion the possibility of some other disturbance of prolactin secretion in sarcoid should be considered.

The effects of prolactin on calcium metabolism and the disturbance of calcium metabolism in sarcoid raise the possibility that the two may be related. However in four patients, lowering of plasma calcium levels by cortisone was not associated with a fall in prolactin secretion. This does not exclude an interaction between steroids and prolactin at target organ level and the subject is worth further exploration. (Turkington, MacIndoe, 1972.)

Male hypogonadism

There is one report in the literature of a young male with reduced testosterone secretion, slight testicular atrophy and elevated prolactin secretion. L-dopa reduced prolactin levels while TRH elevated them. Interestingly, mastectomy seemed to be associated with a further rise in prolactin secretion raising the possibility of a feedback from the breast. (Volpe, Killinger, Bird, Clark, Friesen, 1972.)

Ectopic prolactin production

Prolactin must now be added to the list of hormones which may be produced ectopically by tumor tissues. Apparently normal human prolactin was produced by an undifferentiated bronchial carcinoma and by a hypernephroma. In the case of the lung tumor irradiation lowered plasma prolactin levels. With the hypernephroma, on removal of the tumor plasma prolactin levels fell to normal and prolactin secretion was demonstrated by fragments of the tumor tissue in vitro. (Turkington, 1971b.)

Conclusions

Galactorrhea, but not gynecomastia, is an almost certain indicator of elevated prolactin secretion. Treatment with a drug which elevates prolactin secretion is probably the commonest cause with persistent post partum prolactin secretion and secretion in association with a pituitary tumor next on the list. However, hypothyroidism, adrenal insufficiency, sarcoid and malignant disease are all important in the differential diagnosis because their identification will have an important bearing on treatment.

Chapter 18

PREMENSTRUAL SYNDROME AND PREGNANCY TOXEMIA

Both these relatively common syndromes have eluded satisfactory explanation. They have at least some features in common and it therefore seems appropriate to consider them together in this chapter.

Premenstrual syndrome

The premenstrual syndrome has been frequently described. It is characterised by cyclical changes in mental state and fluid and electrolyte balance. The abnormalities occur during the luteal phase of the menstrual cycle and are most pronounced just before menstruation. Relief normally occurs at the time of or within 24 hours of the onset of menstrual flow. A wide variety of mental changes has been described but the most consistent seem to be lethargy, irritability and the features characteristic of a neurotic personality. No obvious abnormalities in hormone levels have been described and the syndrome is not convincingly explained by the known physiological properties of any of the hormones which are elevated in the luteal phase of the menstrual cycle. Of course, if the analysis presented in chapter 14 is at all correct, then differences in hormone levels between those who suffer from the syndrome and those who do not are not necessarily to be expected. Suppose that hormone X has a moderate tendency to provoke neurotic behaviour: in one woman with a very stable personality an increase in the level of hormone X may be quite unable to provoke overt neuroticism: another woman with neurotic tendencies who is stable in the absence of hormone X may become overtly neurotic in the presence of the hormone. In the second woman, because of her constitution the hormone causes overt neurotic behaviour and if the elevation of hormone levels is prevented, the neurotic behaviour will not occur. Therefore even though hormone levels in the two women may be the same, the hormone will clearly be causing the syndrome in one woman though not in another.

Although the hormone involved has not been identified the regular cyclic nature of the disorder has led most investigators to believe that some hormonal

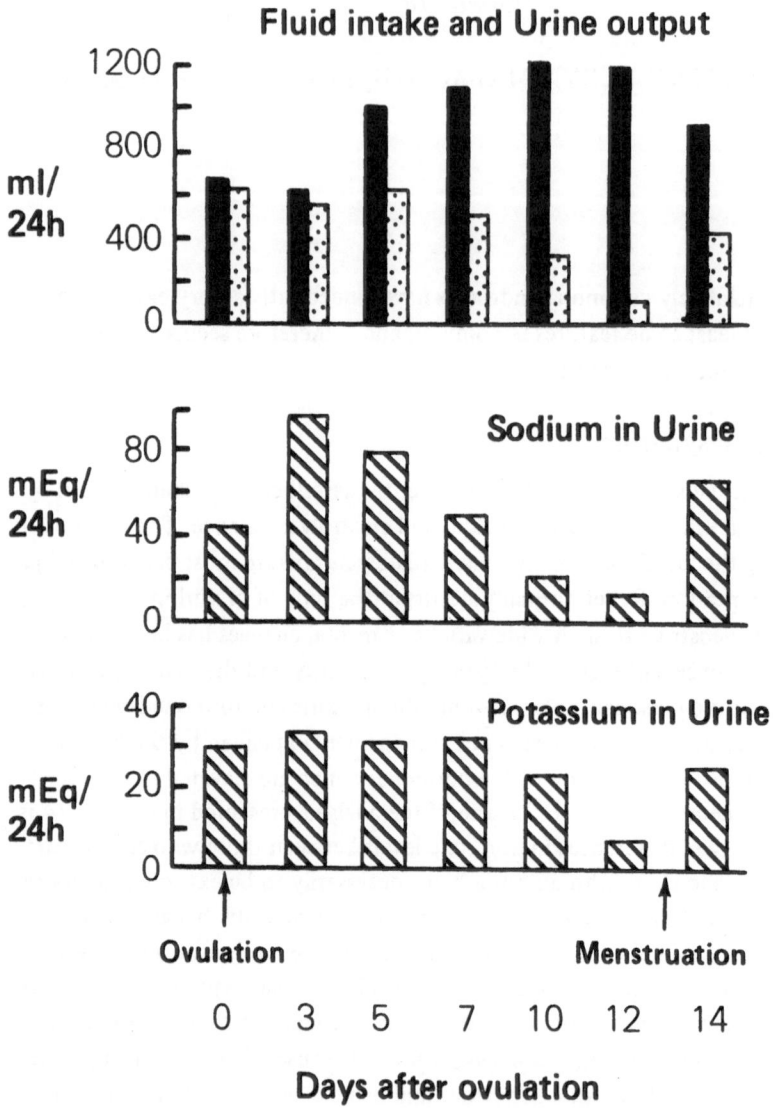

FIG. 10. 24 hour fluid intake and urine output, urinary sodium output and urinary potassium output in a woman with severe premenstrual syndrome (see text). The black bars represent fluid intake and the dotted bars the volume of urine.

basis must be present. There is no consensus of opinion as to whether the electrolyte and the mental changes are both independently caused by a hormone or whether the electrolyte changes cause the mental changes. There is no doubt that the use of diuretics prevents the fluid accumulation in most women but while some may find that this is all they need, many find that their mental symptoms are not helped by diuretic treatment. No controlled trial of any form of therapy has been carried out but two forms of treatment do seem to have been successful. The fact that they are successful in the severest forms of the condition in women who have proved resistant to diuretics, tranquillizers and psychotherapy suggests that they cannot be accounted for on a placebo basis. The two are.treatment with lithium or with high doses of progesterone itself: the synthetic progestins seem to be less successful although good results have been claimed for oral contraceptives which, of course, completely destroy the normal endocrine picture.

Because the premenstrual syndrome is rarely disabling and frequently affects busy women in middle life it is not normally possible to ask patients to come into hospital for prolonged periods in order to study their fluid and electrolyte balances throughout a cycle. Some studies have been carried out in psychotic patients, but in view of the fact that psychoses themselves may alter fluid and electrolyte balance their value is uncertain. We were recently fortunate enough to be able to study a woman whose illness was very nearly disabling. Each month in the ten days or so before menstruation she put on 10-15 pounds in weight, losing it again just after starting menstruation: she also experienced marked lethargy and irritability and a very strong sensation of thirst during the premenstrual week. We were able to ask her to come onto a metabolic ward during the luteal phase of her cycle where she was maintained on an approximately constant electrolyte intake. She was asked to restrict her fluid intake to 800 ml per day. She came in on the day of ovulation (as indicated by the rise in basal temperature) and the changes in 24 hour urinary water, sodium and potassium excretion are shown in fig. 10. The collections were made on alternate days. She found it impossible to keep to an intake of only 800 ml because of intense thirst and her fluid input climbed to about 1200 ml. Simultaneously her urine volume progressively fell as did her sodium excretion. Potassium excretion was markedly reduced in the few days immediately preceding menstruation. Unfortunately she was unable to stay in hospital for more than one post-menstrual day but at that time her sensation of thirst had almost gone and excretion of sodium, water and potassium were all rising again.

It seems to me that there is a strong case for considering the possibility that prolactin may be a key factor in the premenstrual syndrome.

1. There seems to be retention of sodium and potassium and water. Prolactin unlike the mineralocorticoids retains all three.

2. There may be a strong sensation of thirst. Injection of prolactin into humans consistently produced a sensation of thirst.

3. The first time I injected prolactin into myself my wife accused me of being lethargic and irritable, i.e. "premenstrual"! This first aroused my interest in the syndrome. There is a considerable amount of evidence suggesting that prolactin may be capable of altering cerebral function. It is bound to cerebral cortical tissue, it alters neuronal activity and may produce behavioral changes in animals.

4. While some women show relatively little difference between prolactin levels in follicular and luteal phases, others after having normal stable levels in the follicular phase show a highly erratic pattern in the luteal phase with some high and some normal values. Given the fact that prolactin has such a short half life and that all studies so far have utilised once daily sampling it seems probable that in the second group tissue levels may be considerably elevated in the luteal phase. The woman whose electrolyte changes have just been described showed this erratic pattern.

5. Progesterone in moderate doses seems able to suppress prolactin secretion in animals. In humans lithium has some effects which suggest that it may suppress prolactin secretion.

I should like therefore to propose that prolactin causes both the mental and the renal changes which occur in the premenstrual syndrome and that the two are to a large extent, independent of one another, so that a woman may have severe mental changes but only minor renal changes and vice versa. I also suggest that the syndrome occurs in those women who show an erratic pattern of elevated and normal prolactin levels in the luteal phase of the cycle. However, because of wide variations in individual susceptibility not all women who show this erratic pattern will develop the syndrome. Nevertheless I predict that suppression of prolactin secretion in the luteal phase, perhaps using 2-bromo-α-ergokryptine, will produce a striking improvement in women with the syndrome. (Bruce, Russell, 1962: Dalton, 1964: Evered, Horrobin, Nassar, 1973: Greene, Dalton, 1953: Maletzky, Blachly, 1971: Reeves, Garvin, McElin, 1971: Shabanah, 1963: Sletton, Gershon, 1966: Sundsfjord, Aakvaag, 1970: Sutherland, Stewart, 1965: Torghele, 1957).

The premenstrual syndrome is also interesting because of the light it may throw on other conditions not normally thought of in relation to the hormones whose levels vary during the menstrual cycle. The main ones are as follows:

1. Headache. This is one of the most consistent features of the syndrome. In many patients it takes on the form of a typical migraine attack.

2. Asthma. It has been reported that in about one third of female asthma sufferers attacks repeatedly occurred in the premenstrual period.

3. Constipation is frequent but diarrhea is unknown. This suggests that there may be an inhibition of smooth muscle activity. In this connection the inhibitory effect of prolactin on uterine muscle may be relevant. Varicose veins have been reported to be worse premenstrually.

4. There may be spontaneous bruising. Cutaneous capillary resistance is consistently reduced in many women during the premenstrual period.

5. Basal blood glucose levels rise during the luteal phase of the menstrual cycle and glucose tolerance falls in parallel. In some individuals attacks of diabetic coma may consistently occur premenstrually and far more women than expected have been reported to go into diabetic coma premenstrually.

6. A number of conditions though to have some immune response component in their pathology may regularly flare up premenstrually. They include rheumatoid arthritis, ulcerative colitis, rhinitis, various skin lesions and Behcet's syndrome.

7. Some women with peptic ulcer report a regular premenstrual exacerbation.

8. Glaucoma may occur premenstrually.

9. Patients with mitral sterosis have been reported to deteriorate premenstrually with increased incidences of pulmonary edema and features of right ventricular failure. A few women with apparently normal cardiovascular function may show transient premenstrual elevations of blood pressure and albuminuria.

10. Epileptic attacks may occur consistently premenstrually. (Brewer, 1938: British Medical Journal, 1970: Clark, 1953: Cramer, 1942: Dalton, 1964: Philbert, 1962: Rivlin, 1955).

Toxemia of pregnancy

The main features of pre-eclampsia are albuminuria and hypertension. Edema often accompanies these but also occurs in many normal women. Eclamptic fits occur in the severest cases. There seems to be an association between the premenstrual syndrome and pre-eclampsia, women who are susceptible to the one being also susceptible to the other.

The causes of the fluid and electrolyte and blood pressure changes in pre-eclampsi (and indeed of those which occur in normal pregnancy) are quite unknown. This is not the place for an extended discussion of the syndrome and all I would like to do here is to suggest that there are some sound reasons for considering the possibility that prolactin may play a part:

1. Prolactin levels in the plasma rise progressively during pregnancy, reaching their highest levels in the third trimester. There have been no studies as yet comparing prolactin levels in normal and pre-eclamptic pregnancies.

2. In both normal pregnancy and pre-eclampsia there is retention of sodium and water and potassium. The potassium retention cannot be accounted for by the action of mineralocorticoid hormones. It has recently been shown that aldosterone and deoxycorticosterone levels are unequivocally lower in pre-eclamptic than in normal pregnancy and so these mineralocorticoids by themsleves cannot account for the sodium and water retention. The action of aldosterone modulated by prolactin might do so.

3. Prolactin can elevate arterial pressure and increase cardiac output in animals. Renin and angiotensin levels are below normal in patients with pre-eclampsia

and therefore they alone cannot account for the elevated arterial pressure.

4. There is some evidence that prolactin may be able to cause renal damage with proteinuria (chapter 20).

5. There is some evidence that high levels of prolactin may be associated with epileptic attacks (chapter 28).

6. There is indirect evidence that high levels of salt intake may suppress prolactin secretion. One of the few large scale controlled trials ever carried out in pre-eclampsia showed that in about a thousand women advised to take a high salt intake throughout pregnancy the rates of pre-eclampsia and perinatal mortality were considerably less than those seen in a thousand women not so advised. These results seemed so absurd at the time that they have been completely ignored in spite of the significant difference in perinatal mortality between the two groups which could hardly be accounted for on the basis of problems of diagnosis. The effect of the high salt intake might logically have been explained on the basis of suppression of renin-angiotensin-aldosterone secretion but since levels of these are now known to be well below normal in pre-eclampsia an effect due to suppression of prolactin secretion might possibly be worth consideration.
(Burstyn, Horrobin, Manku, 1972: Dalton, 1964: Horrobin, 1971: Robinson, 1958: Tampan, Sundaram, Chanukattam, 1956: Weir, Brown, Fraser, Kraszewski, Lever, McIlwaine, Morton, Robertson, Tree, 1973).

Oral Contraceptives

There are no systematic published reports on the effects of oral contraceptives on human prolactin levels. However, estrogens stimulate prolactin secretion while progestins tend to reduce prolactin secretion in low to moderate doses and so the two might be expected partially to cancel out. One might expect, however, that some women at least would show elevated prolactin levels while on the drugs and this is supported by the occasional occurrence of galactorrhea (chapter 17). Relatively high levels of prolactin may be required to produce galactorrhea and it is therefore possible that a much larger number of women have more moderately elevated prolactin levels. It might be expected that the pills with the higher estrogen contents would be more likely to stimulate prolactin secretion. Certainly in animals there is no doubt that the norethynodrel-mestranol combination can elevate prolactin secretion.

Of the reported side effects of oral contraceptives, migraine (chapter 24), changes in glucose tolerance (chapter 27), depression (chapter 31), fluid retention (chapter 19) and hypertension (chapter 23) might conceivably be considered in the prolactin context. In a double blind cross-over trial in four women who developed a clearly elevated blood pressure while on oral contraceptives, it was shown that the blood pressure could be reduced by increasing salt intake. In rabbits treated with high doses of progesterone an elevated blood pressure developed which was responsive to a rise in salt intake. These effects might possibly be explained by salt suppression of an elevated prolactin secretion. Again the evidence is no more than fragmentary but the possibility that prolactin might be involved in some of the side effects of the pill should at the very least, reach the consciousness of the many people carrying out research in this area. (Adams, Rose, Folkard, Wynn, Seed, Strong, 1973: Bolton, Hampton, Mitchell, 1968: British Medical Journal, 1969: Committee on Safety of Drugs, 1970: Dear, Jones, 1971: Fisch, Freedman, Myatt, 1972: Grant, 1968: Harris, 1969: Heefner, 1973: Horrobin, 1968: Horrobin, Lloyd, 1970: Irey, Manion, Taylor, 1970: Laragh, 1970: Mears, Grant, 1962: Ndeti, Horrobin, Burstyn, Hopcraft, 1972: Oliver, 1970: Phillips, 1968: Vessey, Doll, 1969: Weir, Briggs, Browning, Mack, Naismith, Taylor, Wilson, 1971: Waxler, Kimbiris, Van der Broek, Segal, Likoff, 1971: Weiss, 1972: Winston, 1969: Woods, 1967).

Chapter 19

DISORDERS OF FLUID AND
ELECTROLYTE BALANCE

The effects of prolactin on fluid and electrolyte balance were reviewed in chapter 12. The most important points appear to be:

1. Prolactin can act on the kidney to reduce sodium, potassium and water excretion. It may act on the proximal tubule.

2. The sodium and water retaining effects depend at least in part on interaction with aldosterone and ADH. It seems that in the absence of prolactin, oxytocin and growth hormone, aldosterone and ADH lose their normal sodium and water retaining actions and may even promote renal loss of sodium and water. Prolactin can restore the "normal" actions.

3. Prolactin may stimulate ADH secretion.

4. Prolactin may cause a sensation of thirst.

5. A high salt intake and high levels of glucocorticoids appear to suppress prolactin secretion. Low levels of glucocorticoids and of thyroid hormones may be associated with excess prolactin secretion.

6. Prolactin secretion has a diurnal rhythm being maximal during the night, especially the later part.

So for there is no conclusive evidence that any of these effects plays any part in any clinical fluid and electrolyte disorder. However the suggestive evidence is strong and appears to throw light on a number of areas where current explanations are unconvincing.

24 hour rhythm of urinary excretion

As yet there is no satisfactory explanation for the nocturnal reduction in urine output. It could however be explained by the nocturnal secretion of growth hormone and of prolactin, growth hormone secretion being highest just after sleeping and prolactin being elevated later in the night. It is interesting that the normal urinary 24 hour rhythm is lost in thyrotoxicosis when nocturia is frequently present. In thyrotoxicosis the response of prolactin secretion as well as of TSH secretion to TRH is lost. This raises the possibility that the nocturnal secretion of prolactin depends on TRH. It has already been mentioned in chapter 6 that the 24 hour secretion patterns of TSH and prolactin are similar. (Tucci, Lauler, 1972.)

Disorders of the adrenal gland

Some of the characteristics of fluid and electrolyte disorders in Cushing's syndrome and Addison's disease may in part be explained by changes in prolactin secretion since it is known that in adrenal failure or after adrenalectomy prolactin secretion may increase and it is probable that glucocorticoids suppress prolactin secretion. The main possibilities are as follows:

1. Addison's disease may be associated with hyperkalemia and Cushing's syndrome with hypokalemia. These phenomena are usually attributed to the reduced and increased steroid kaliuresis respectively. However it is possible that an excess of prolactin may play a part in potassium retention and a deficiency in potassium loss. The enhancement of the kaliuretic effect of aldosterone by glucocorticoids could be explained by suppression of prolactin secretion.

2. In patients with Addison's disease and in animals after adrenalectomy there is a great increase in the sensitivity of the kidneys to the sodium-retaining effects of aldosterone: this could be explained by potentiation of the aldosterone by prolactin. The increased excretion of sodium loads in Cushing's syndrome and the failure of patients with Cushing's syndrome to retain sodium in response to DOCA could be accounted for by prolactin lack.

3. The reduced ability to excrete a water load in adrenal insufficiency could be accounted for by prolactin excess as could the tendency of adrenalectomized but not normal animals to become edematous in response to injections of DOCA. The change in the osmotic threshold for ADH release in Addison's disease might also be partially accounted for by excess prolactin secretion as might the increased plasma ADH levels, which can be restored to normal by glucocorticoid therapy. (Ahmad, George, Gonzalez-Auvert, Dingman, 1967: Aubry, Nankin, Moses, Streeten, 1965:

Barger, Berlin, Tulenko, 1958: Black, 1972: Davis, Howell, Hyatt, 1955: Green, Harrington, Valtin, 1967: Kriss, Futcher, 1949: Horrobin, Manku, Burstyn, 1973: Horrobin, Manku, Muriuki, Burstyn, 1973: Horrobin, Manku, Robertshaw, 1973: Mulrow, Boyd, 1972: Ragan, 1940: Soffer, Gabrilove, 1952: Soffer, Gabrilove, Jacobs, 1949: Soffer, Lesnick, Sorkin, Sobotka, Jacobs, 1944: Tucci, Lauler, 1972.)

The escape phenomenon, saluretic hormone and edema

It is clear in various experimental situations which may have in common a very low prolactin secretion rate, that mineralocorticoid hormones can promote renal salt loss. This in no sense denies the existence of other saluretic hormones but it does suggest that at least some of the evidence such as that involving saluretic hormone assay in animals with congenital diabetes insipidus does require re-examination. It may well be that at least some of the experiments could be interpreted on the basis of a reduction of prolactin secretion or a competitive inhibition of prolactin at the renal tubular level. The possibility of such inhibition is discussed in the section on diuretics at the end of this chapter.

The escape phenomenon itself could be accounted for by a reduction in prolactin secretion to levels where mineralocorticoids ceased to have any sodium-retaining action. The association of escape with potassium loss while obviously partly explained by excess mineralocorticoid action might also be partly explained by low levels of prolactin. This suggestion gives a good reason for the lack of escape from the kaliuretic effect. The belief that escape is primarily a proximal tubular phenomenon fits in with Lockett's suggestion that prolactin acts mainly on the proximal tubules.

Most of the situations where escape does not occur may also be accounted for in terms of a failure of reduction in prolactin secretion. The best documented are perhaps congestive cardiac failure, cirrhosis with edema and ascites, pregnancy, the nephrotic syndrome and experimental procedures involving ligatures on the vena cava close to the heart. It is known that in pregnant humans plasma prolactin levels are elevated and there is preliminary evidence that this is also true in humans with renal failure, congestive cardiac failure and hepatic failure. A sheep with high jugular venous pressure of unknown origin failed to reverse the action of aldosterone while on a high salt intake. It may be relevant that in the clinical situations where escape does not occur mineralocorticoid treatment is not associated with excess renal potassium loss and this could of course be explained by high levels of potassium-retaining prolactin.

Escape usually fails to occur in situations when edema develops. In sheep it was shown that they could readily tolerate a 400 mEq/day salt intake without becoming distressed or suffering a rapid rise in body weight. Addition of a single daily injection of 5 mg prolactin to the regime produced a rapid rise in body weight with gross clinical edema within 3-4 days. It is therefore possible that edema may occur in situations when a high salt intake, a reduced cardiac output or excess mineralocorticoid secretion are not accompanied by suppressed secretion of prolactin (and perhaps also of growth hormone and oxytocin). The improvement of hepatic and cardiac edema with glucocorticoid therapy might be due to prolactin suppression. It is interesting to note that mineralocorticoid treatment of intact animals does not readily make them edematous while similar treatment of adrenalectomized animals does. The edema which sometimes occurs in patients on reserpine therapy might be associated with excess prolactin secretion. Edema occurring in the pre-menstrual syndrome and pre-eclampsia was discussed in the last chapter.

(August, Nelson, Thorn, 1958: Biglieri, Schambelan, Slaton, Stockigt, 1970: Black, 1972: Brenner, Berliner, 1969: Burstyn, Horrobin, Manku, 1972: Cirksena, Dirks, Berliner, 1965: Davis, Howell, Hyatt, 1955: Davis, 1964: De Wardener, Mills, Clapham, Hayter, 1961: De Wardener, 1969a, 1969b: Dirks, Cirksena, Berliner, 1965: Earley, 1972: Friesen, Hwang, Guyda, Tolis, Tyson, Myers, 1970: Jarvik, 1970: Levinsky, Lalone, 1963, 1965: Lockett, 1965: Lockett, Noel, 1965: Lockett, Roberts, 1963: Lunn, Cole, Boyns, Nassar, Horrobin, 1973: Mulrow, Boyd, 1972: Nelson, August, 1959: Pasteels, Gausset, Danguy, Ectors, 1972: Perera, 1948: Ragan, 1940: Rovner, Conn, Knopf, Cohen, Hsueh, 1965: Sealey, Laragh, 1971: Strauss, Earley, 1959: Swingle, De Vanzo, Glenister, Osborne, Wagle, 1960: Tompson, Edmonds, 1971: Tucci, Lauler, 1972: Turkington, 1972c, 1972d: Vesin, 1972: Weston, 1972: Williams, Lauler, 1972.)

ADH and diabetes insipidus

It seems probable that the kidney may escape from ADH in the same sort of way that it escapes from mineralocorticoids. Prolactin and oxytocin in animals both restore the water-retaining action of ADH. It is possible that water loading should be added to the list of potential stimuli which may suppress prolactin secretion. An interaction between ADH and prolactin may help to explain some of the water retention which occurs in edema. The precise balance between water and sodium retention would be determined by levels of ADH, aldosterone and prolactin. It is not difficult to conceive of a situation where water retention might relatively exceed sodium retention leading to the hyponatremia which sometimes occurs.

The hyponatremia and hypernatriuria which may follow cerebral injury and which have perhaps wrongly been associated with inappropriate secretion of antidiuretic hormone might be accounted for by lack of prolactin: these patients are often clinically dehydrated. In true inappropriate ADH secretion when over-hydration does occur this could lead to suppression of prolactin secretion with consequent failure of mineralocorticoid acitvity and a renal loss of sodium. The excess renal sodium loss has been one of the most puzzling features of the syndrome.

It is possible that prolactin may be able to throw some light on the mechanism of the improvement in diabetes insipidus which can occur in patients treated with tolbutamide or chlorpropamide. It seems possible since prolactin has some "diabetogenic" effects that treatment with an anti-diabetic drug might by some feedback mechanism promote prolactin secretion. In one patient on tolbutamide we have found moderately elevated prolactin levels but unfortunately we do not know what pre-treatment levels were. If prolactin levels are elevated by these drugs then they should both stimulate ADH release and potentiate the renal actions of ADH: they might be expected to be of little effect in the total absence of ADH. All these findings have of course, been made. Prolactin could therefore perhaps explain what has been a most puzzling phenomenon. It might even play a part in the diuretic-induced improvement of diabetes insipidus if sodium loss elevates prolactin secretion as seems possible.

It is conceivable that the role of prolactin should be investigated in the diabetes insipidus-like syndromes associated with lithium therapy and with divalent cation disturbances.

The improvement in diabetes insipidus which has several times been recorded during pregnancy might be attributed to prolactin secretion occurring at the time.

The fluid and electrolyte retention occurring in response to surgery and trauma may also perhaps be partially explained by the release of prolactin which occurs at this time. (Angrist, Gershon, Levitan, Blumberg, 1970: Gupta, 1971:

Horrobin, Lloyd, Lipton, Burstyn, Durkin, Muiruri, 1971: Horrobin, Manku,, Robertshaw, 1973: Irvin, Modgill, Hayter, McDowall, Goligher, 1972: Kleeman, 1972: Leaf, Bartter, Santos, Wrong, 1953: Lunn, Cole, Boyns, Nassar, Horrobin, 1973: Manku, Horrobin, Burstyn, 1972: Moses, Numann, Miller, 1973: Orloff, Hutchin, 1972: Ramsay, Mendels, Stokes, Fitzgerald, 1972: Schwartz, Bennett, Curelop, Bartter, 1957: Taylor, 1971: Tupin, Schlagenhauf, Creson, 1968: Weissman, Shenkman, Gregerman, 1971.)

Diuretics and prolactin secretion

There do not appear to have been any studies on the effects of diuretics on prolactin secretion. Sodium excretion might be expected to stimulate prolactin secretion and the possible association between prolonged diuretic use and reduced glucose tolerance could perhaps partly be accounted for on this basis. However this association may have been much exaggerated since few of the published studies looked at glucose tolerance before starting diuretic therapy. It is now known that many of the hypertensives to whom diuretics are prescribed have reduced tolerance before treatment.

One interesting possibility is that frusemide (and therefore perhaps also ethacrynic acid) may be a competitive inhibitor of prolactin at the renal level. Gachev reported that frusemide could inhibit lactation in rabbits: this could be explained in a number of ways, one of which is a suppression of prolactin secretion and another an inhibition of prolactin action at mammary tissue level. At the renal level, of course, frusemide acts within minutes and if an interaction with prolactin is involved it could only be at the level of the renal tubules themselves. Certainly the actions of frusemide on the kidneys would not be inconsistent with the idea that they were reversals of prolactin effects. More direct evidence that frusemide may have this type of action is that in rabbits progesterone given in the presence of frusemide seemed to cause sodium retention rather than the expected sodium loss. Progesterone seems to be a competitive inhibitor of aldosterone and so if aldosterone were causing sodium retention, progesterone should cause sodium loss but if aldosterone were causing sodium excretion progesterone should cause sodium retention. The sodium retention observed in rabbits raises the possibility that during frusemide treatment the blocking of prolactin actions on the kidney could lead to mineralocorticoids having a sodium-losing effect. This possible prolactin antagonism could account for the massive diuretic effect and also for the serious potassium loss which can occur. It might also help to explain the phenomenon whereby once equilibrium has been reached and fluid and electrolyte balance achieved at one frusemide dose (possibly by increasing prolactin secretion) a further diuresis and saluresis may be obtained by increasing the dose. The need for and effectiveness of very high doses of frusemide in edema and renal failure when prolactin levels are almost certainly elevated also suggests a competitive effect.

Oxytocin in situations where prolactin secretion has probably been suppressed can act with mineralocorticoids to cause sodium retention. In other more normal circumstances oxytocin may cause sodium excretion. These apparently paradoxical effects could be explained if oxytocin could activate the prolactin receptors on the kidney but was less effective than prolactin itself. In the absence of prolactin oxytocin would then have a prolactin-like effect but in the presence of prolactin it might reduce the effectiveness of prolactin by competing with it for receptors. (Chan, Sawyer, 1961: Dieterle, 1968: Earley, 1972: Gachev, 1968: Graybiel, Sode, 1971: Horrobin, Lloyd, 1970: Kohner, Dollery, Lowy, Schumer, 1971: Weston, 1972.)

Potassium

Of all the actions of prolactin on fluid and electrolyte balance it is possible that the most important one may prove to be the action on potassium metabolism. It is the only one which does not appear to be imitated by any other hormone. At the renal level prolactin seems to be unique in promoting potassium retention which is, of course, the complete opposite of the effect of aldosterone. At the cell membrane, the effect of aldosterone seems to be to stimulate the exchange of sodium outwards for potassium inwards: it thus promotes an increased intracellular potassium concentration. If prolactin opposes the effects of mineralocorticoids at the cell membrane as at the renal level, then its effect will be to promote a movement of potassium out from cells. If this occurs the two effects will combine to produce hyperkalemia. The hyperkalemia will deliver an increased potassium load to the renal tubules and this may partly or even completely overcome the potassium-retaining effect. In the absence of prolactin the reverse changes may occur with a movement of potassium into cells, a loss of potassium in the urine and hypokalemia.

It is possible that the so-called "sick cell syndrome" may be attributable to excess levels of prolactin with or without excess levels of mineralocorticoids. The syndrome tends to occur in situations such as severe hepatic or cardiac failure where both hormones may be elevated together. An abnormally high prolactin level will tend to allow potassium to escape from cells: if enough escapes it will overcome the potassium-retaining effect of prolactin and be lost in the urine. However, if mineralocorticoids are present in adequate amounts they may tend to stimulate and aggravate the renal potassium loss.

The effects of prolactin on potassium movements across the membranes of nerve and muscle fibres may also be important. If the changes are as described, with potassium moving out of the cells, this will tend to produce a depolarisation. Initially this will make muscle fibres and neurons more excitable but if the process continues far enough they will be inactivated. The overall effect on the nervous system will be complicated by the reduced sizes of the action potentials which will tend to release smaller amounts of transmitter and so even in the early stages there may be some depression of activity, coupled with an over-responsiveness to stimuli such as epileptogenic ones. In the later stages there would be unequivocal neural depression.

The actions on muscle would also be interesting with again an initial excitation followed by depression if enough prolactin were present. A pattern like this certainly appears when prolactin in concentrations at the upper end of the physiological range is added to human uterine smooth muscle (fig. 2) with an initial flurry of activity followed by a more prolonged depression. At the heart, these changes might produce various forms of arrhythmia perhaps followed by blocks in the conducting system. In this context it may be relevant to point out that all the reported cases of hypoaldosteronism have been characterised by hyperkalemia and some form of arrhythmia, usually complete heart block. In this syndrome it seems very possible that sodium balance may be maintained by the effect of hypersecretion of prolactin.

Finally it should perhaps be noted that prolactin may be a complicating factor in studies of glucose tolerance simply because of its effect on potassium, quite apart from any other metabolic actions. Reduced intracellular potassium levels seem to be associated with decreased glucose tolerance. Potassium repletion alone may restore glucose tolerance to normal. (Black, 1972: Horrobin, Manku, 1972: Earley, 1972: Graybiel, Sode, 1971: Horrobin, Lloyd, Lipton, Burstyn, Durkin, Muiruri, 1971: Lunn, Cole, Boyns, Nassar, Horrobin, 1973: Pasteels, Gausset, Danguy, Ectors, 1972: Williams, Lauler, 1972.)

Chapter 20

THE NEPHROTIC SYNDROME

There are, of course, many varieties of nephrotic syndrome and many different causes of albuminuria. In some of these it is possible that prolactin may play a role but in others it is very unlikely to be involved.

The best evidence for the role of prolactin in a nephrotic-type syndrome comes from work in the rat. In many strains of rat old animals are liable to develop glomerular lesions and albuminuria: old rats tend to have much higher levels of circulating prolactin than young rats. When prolactin-secreting tumors are transplanted into rats, the renal lesions are more florid and develop in virtually all the animals. Many die of a syndrome characterised by massive albuminuria. Even more strikingly, it has very recently been demonstrated that prolonged treatment of rats with 2-bromo-α-kryptine, the drug which seems to have a highly specific action in blocking prolactin secretion, can virtually completely prevent the development of the nephrotic-type syndrome in old rats. This is therefore very strong evidence that in rats this type of albuminuria cannot develop in the absence of prolactin.

There is of course nothing remotely like this evidence in relation to the human forms of albuminuria. At best there are only a few scattered hints, the main ones being as follows:

1. The failure of many patients with the nephrotic syndrome to "escape" from the sodium-retaining effects of mineralocorticoids is consistent with the possibbility that they have elevated prolactin levels. (chapter 19).

2. The response of some patients with nephrotic syndrome to steroid therapy is also consistent since some forms of elevated prolactin secretion are clearly steroid suppressible.

3. Diabetic nephropathy tends to occur in that group of diabetics who are also

susceptible to retinopathy. These patients have increased cutaneous capillary fragility which may perhaps be due to prolactin. (chapter 27)

4. High cholesterol levels which occur in the nephrotic syndrome also occur in patients on prolonged chlorpromazine therapy and in those with myxedema in whom prolactin levels are elevated. (chapter 21)

5. There is some very indirect evidence (chapter 19) that frusemide may be a competitive inhibitor of prolactin. This might explain its relative success in mobilising edema of renal origin. (Clemens, Meites, 1971: Furth, Clifton, Gadsen, (Clemens, Meites, 1971: Furth, Clifton, Gadsen, Buffet, 1956: Richardson, 1973.)

THYROID DISEASE

The relationship between prolactin and the thyroid is now well established although much remains to be done. TRH can stimulate the release of both TSH and prolactin in man. The 24 hour rhythm of prolactin secretion is similar to that of TSH with elevated levels during the night, particularly the later part. High levels of circulating thyroid hormones and also L-dopa treatment suppress the response of both TSH and prolactin to TRH. Interestingly in thyrotoxicosis the 24 hour rhythm of TSH secretion is lost as is the 24 hour rhythm of fluid and electrolyte secretion: this suggests that the nocturnal secretion of prolactin may also be abolished (chapter 23) and that the nocturnal secretion of both TSH and prolactin may depend on TRH. The surges of prolactin secretion in response to suckling and surgery are not accompanied by surges of TSH secretion suggesting that TRH cannot be involved in these events.

Two clinical syndromes have now been clearly shown to relate primary hypothyroidism (and therefore probable TRH hypersecretion) with excess prolactin secretion. These are the association of galactorrhea, amenorrhea and primary hypothyroidism in post-pubertal individuals and of precocious puberty, galactorrhea and primary hypothyroidism in children. Both syndromes have already been discussed in chapter 10. Both respond to treatment of the hypothyroidism which abolishes the galactorrhea. It has recently been confirmed that in both prolactin plasma levels are elevated and that thyroid treatment lowers these to normal. The presumed mechanism is the release of prolactin brought about by high TRH secretion rates which are in turn a response to primary hypothyroidism. The precocious puberty may possibly be related to that which has been demostrated in rats following hypothalamic prolactin implants. The presumed mechanism is elevation of the secretion of the releasing factors which govern FSH and LH secretion.

The question of whether prolactin levels are elevated in hypothyroidism in the absence of galactorrhea has not yet been settled. Most results have shown only marginally elevated plasma levels although one group claimed that five out of nine hypothyroid patients had clearly elevated plasma prolactin levels and another two had levels at the upper end of the normal range. In severe myxedema there is good evidence that the pituitary prolactin-secreting cells are markedly hypertrophied. It seems to be probable that as yet the definitive experiments have not been performed. If it is the nocturnal prolactin secretion which is primarily TRH-dependent then it will be the nocturnal levels (or at least those in the very early morning) which will be elevated. However, because of the very long tissue activity of a single surge of prolactin elevated nocturnal secretion alone would be sufficient to produce sustained tissue prolactin elevations.

Reports of prolactin levels in hyperthyroidism have suggested nothing unusual. However since daytime levels are normally low, since none of the work has involved nocturnal or early morning sampling, and since patients with hyperthyroidism do not reduce to a normal extent their nocturnal fluid and electrolyte secretion, it seems possible that the nocturnal surge may be absent. If this is so it is possible that tissue prolactin levels may be abnormally reduced even though daytime plasma levels may be near normal.

In amphibians prolactin seems able to inhibit the response of both the thyroid gland to TSH and of the tissues to thyroid hormones, but as yet this possible aspect of the interaction has not been specifically investigated in man. It is conceivable that the reversible hypothyroidism seen in Addison's disease and which responds to adrenal replacement therapy alone could be partly due to excess prolactin secretion. This might suppress TRH secretion by the hypothalamic short feedback loop and also exert an inhibitory effect at both thyroid and thyroid hormone target organ levels.

If prolactin tissue levels are elevated in myxedema this raises the interesting possibility that some of the features of myxedema usually attributed to lack of thyroid hormone may in fact be caused by prolactin excess alone, or by the combination of prolactin excess and thyroid lack. Perhaps the most likely candidates for this type of explanation are the elevated secretion of ADH and increased renal responsiveness to ADH which have been reported in myxedema (chapter 19). The increased capillary permeability of myxedema may also be prolactin dependent (chapter 27). The "edema" itself may be prolactin-associated since a similar type of edema with increased binding of water to conncetive tissue mucopolysaccharides has been reported in response to estrogens which, of course, stimulate prolactin secretion. The possibility that some of the mental sluggishness may be related to prolactin is discussed in chapter 31. One possibly important idea is that the high cholesterol levels seen in myxedema may be in part prolactin-dependent. Similar high levels occur in the nephrotic syndrome in which prolactin levels may be elevated and cholesterol levels are also elevated by phenothiazine therapy which stimulates prolactin secretion.

Similarly it is conceivable that some of the features of hyperthyroidism may be due partly to prolactin lack and partly to thyroid hormone excess although here the possibilities are less obvious. The agitation is perhaps the one that deserves most attention.

In conclusion as with most areas of prolactin physiology and pathophysiology, a great deal remains to be done but the possibilities, to say the least, look interesting.

(Arroyo, Aubert, 1971: Chesley, 1972: Clemens, Minaguchi, Storey, Voogt, Meites, 1969: Edwards, Forsyth, Besser, 1971: Emerson, Utiger, 1972: Foley, Jacobs, Hoffman, Daughaday, Blizzard, 1972: Forsyth, Besser, Edwards, Francis, Myres, 1971: Gharib, Hodgson, Gastineau, Scholz, Smith, 1972: Jackson, 1956: Jacobs, Snyder, Wilber, Utiger, Daughaday, 1971: Kinch, Plunkett, Devlin, 1969: Lange, 1944: L'Hermite, Delvoye, Nokin, Vekemans, Robyn, 1972: Mulrow, Boyd, 1972: Nicoll, Bryant, 1972:. Nokin, Vekemans, L'Hermite, Robyn, 1972: Pasteels, Gausset, Danguy, Ectors, 1972: Patel, Baker, Alford, Johns, Burger, 1972: Pittinger, Talner, Ferris, 1965: Robyn, 1972: Sassin, Frantz, Weitzman, Kapen, 1972: Savely, Modlinger-Odorfer, Szecsenyi-Nagy, 1965: Spaudling, Burrow, Donabedian, Van Woert, 1972: Turkington, Ray, Costin, 1972: Vanhaelst, Van Cauter, De Gaute, Golstein, 1972: Van Wyck, Grumbach, 1960.)

Chapter 22

DISEASES OF THE ADRENAL CORTEX

Much of the material relevant to the theme of this chapter has already been reviewed in chapters, 4, 12 and 19. In summary the main factual points which are known are as follows:

1. Prolactin modifies the effect of aldosterone on the renal tubules. In the absence of prolactin (and of growth hormone and oxytocin) aldosterone promotes sodium loss: prolactin restores the sodium-retaining effect of aldosterone. The effect does not appear to be of the "all-or-nothing" variety and the renal action of aldosterone may be increased or reduced by altering the prolactin concentration. The effects of prolactin on aldosterone secretion or of aldosterone on prolactin secretion have not been explored.

2. In the absence of adrenal steroids prolactin secretion rises: it is possible that lack of either mineralocorticoids or glucocorticoids may have this result but there is no clear evidence on this point. Elevated levels of glucocorticoids can suppres prolactin secretion. It is probable that elevated mineralocorticoid levels can do so also although whether directly or via the intermediary of sodium metabolism is unknown.

3. Prolactin may act on the adrenals to provide a precursor pool on which other agents such as ACTH and angiotensin may act. It may also have a particular effect in stimulating adrenal androgen secretion. The nocturnal prolactin secretion could help to provide precursors for the morning cortisol surge.

The known renal actions of prolactin may partially explain the increased excretion of salt, the failure to respond normally to DOCA and the potassium loss which can occur in Cushing's syndrome. They may help to account for the failure to excrete a water load and the hyperkalemia of adrenal failure (chapter 19).

An isolated deficiency of aldosterone is a rare but interesting disease often characterised by marked hyperkalemia. This could perhaps partly be explained by high levels of prolactin attempting to compensate as a sodium-retaining hormone for the aldosterone lack and in the process causing severe potassium retention.

Of the non-electrolyte disturbances in adrenal diseases a possible role of prolactin in eosinophilia and eosinopenia might be worth exploring. Prolactin has been reported to cause an eosinophilia on injection into animals but it is possible that this could have occurred as part of a reaction to foreign protein and the lack of correlation of the eosinophil count in humans with elevated prolactin levels in many situations makes a key role in the regulation of eosinophils unlikely.

Prolactin is certainly involved in the galactorrhea which has been reported in adrenal failure. In one case this was shown to be associated with elevated prolactin levels. The galactorrhea disappeared and the elevated prolactin levels returned to normal on treatment of the primary hypoadrenalism. An interesting possibility is that prolactin could be involved in the hypothyroidism which sometimes occurs in adrenal failure and which responds to treatment of the adrenal disease without any thyroid treatment. The hypothyroidism may be a failure of the gland to respond to TSH since thyroid hormone levels are low, the gland is enlarged and in the one patient in whom it was measured the plasma TSH level was high. This may simply be due to a requirement of thyroid cells for adrenal steroids but since blocking of the effect of TSH on the thyroid is one of the established effects of prolactin in lower vertebrates, this should be considered.

(Gharib, Hodgson, Gastineau, Scholz, Smith, 1972: Retetoff, Block, Ehrlich, Friesen, 1972: Stupnicki, Stupnicka, Donanski, 1960.)

Chapter 23

HYPERTENSION

As mentioned in chapter 12, the evidence relating prolactin to the regulation of blood pressure is conflicting. In decerebrate unanesthetised rabbits prolactin intravenous infusions at rates as low as 10 μg/kg/hr produced a clear cut elevation of arterial pressure within 4 hours: 50 μg/kg/hr infused for four hours produced a mean elevation of about 40%. In contrast, 2.5 mg/day (i.e. about 12,500 μg/kg) given to rats for about three weeks led to a fall in arterial pressure of about 20%. Similar doses given to rats rapidly elevated cardiac output. At present no sense can be made of these observations apart from saying that the rabbit doses were in the physiological range while the rat doses were grossly abnormal. In preliminary experiments using a mesenteric artery preparation Manku (1973) has recently shown that the high rat doses abolished the response of the pre-paration to noradrenaline.

However it is possible to make some speculations on the assumption that the physiological doses are more likely to be relevant. If prolactin is involved in the elevation of arterial pressure, the most likely circumstances for this to happen would be in pre-eclampsia, in women on oral contraceptives and in those women who experience a clear elevation of prolactin levels during the luteal phase of the menstrul cycle. There is of course no direct evidence relating prolactin and elevated blood pressure in any of these situations, but the concept is not implausible. One interesting finding which might be explained by this is Miall's demonstration that in women of reproductive age those with higher salt intakes had slightly but definitely lower blood pressures. Since there is good evidence that a high salt intake may be able to lower prolactin secretion then if prolactin were involved in the maintenance of arterial pressure in women of this age group, those with higher salt intakes should have lower pressures. A similar explanation might account for the observations that increasing salt intake could lower arterial pressure in women with elevated pressures as a result of taking oral contraceptives and that it could partly prevent the development of preeclampsia. This last

piece of work by Robinson has been ignored and derided largely because it is so
out of sympathy with the work of the last three decades on salt intake and hypertension. She studied approximately 2000 consecutive antenatal patients and
instructed one group of 1000 to take a high salt diet with salt supplements and
the other group to keep salt intake down. The high salt group had something
like half the pre-eclampsia and half the perinatal deaths (when gross congenital
malformations were excluded) of the low salt group. If results of that sort had
been obtained using an expensive drug, that drug would now be universally
used and her trial would be quoted as a model of a large controlled trial. But
because the drug was salt and because (to quote several obstetricians) her
results simply cannot be true (!) no attempt has been made to repeat her trial
and test her results, let alone put them into practice, However, if prolactin is
involved in pre-eclampsia, her findings may be satisfactorily explained and she
may yet be vindicated.

Other evidence for a possible role of prolactin in blood pressure regulation
comes from the use of L-dopa in Parkinsonism. One of the more common side
effects is hypotension, although hypertension is occasionally reported. Experiments
using monamine oxidase inhibitors to facilitate the conversion of L-dopa to
catecholamines and extracerebral or intracerebal decarboxylase inhibitors to
block selectively conversion to catecholamines at either intracerebral or extracerebral sites, have shown that L-dopa may indeed be either hypotensive or
hypertensive. Its hypertensive action depends on extracerebral stimulation of
catecholamine synthesis presumably mainly at sympathetic nerve endings. Its
hypotensive action depends on a CNS effect but the precise mechanism remains
unknown.

One possible candidate for a hypotensive effect brought about by increased
CNS catecholamine activity is the suppression of prolactin secretion which has
been clearly shown with L-dopa. Since prolactin does seem able to alter neuronal
excitability in the hypothalamus and other places, it is not inconceivable that
prolactin could in some way be involved in the hypothalamic regulation of
arterial pressure.

If prolactin were a part, albeit a minor one, of the pressure regulating mechanism
and if the effect of prolactin were to elevate pressure, then it would not be surprising if there were a mechanism whereby elevated pressures suppressed prolactin

secretion. As far as prolactin was concerned there would then be two types of hypertension, those in which prolactin was a primary agent and in which prolactin levels might be elevated and those in which prolactin was not a primary agent and in which prolactin secretion might be suppressed. The main types of hypertension which seem likely to be related to elevated prolactin secretion have already been discussed. A possible additional one is the so-called labile or borderline hypertension in which cardiac output is elevated, which in some individuals seems to be related to a stressful life situation and in which the circulatory pattern suggests a "hypothalamic" origin.

The electrolyte disturbances in hypertension are interesting to interpret in the light of the possibility that in many forms of hypertension prolactin secretion may be suppressed. It seems not improbable that the normal nocturnal reduction of fluid and electrolyte excretion while in part due to hemodynamic changes may in part be due to the nocturnal secretion of prolactin. If this is so then disappearance of this normal cycle with the appearance of nocturia might, among other things, be attributed to suppression of prolactin secretion. More convincingly, many hypertensive patients show a response to a salt load which is similar to that shown by patients with Cushing's syndrome: they excrete it considerably more rapidly than normal individuals. Again hemodynamic factors may be part of the explanation for this but they are unlikely to be the full one. In sheep a Cushingoid renal function may be produced by cortisol treatment but may be substantially restored by prolactin even though the cortisol is continued, strongly suggesting that part of the renal effect is due to suppression of prolactin secretion. If the rapid Cushingoid excretion of a salt load can be accounted for by prolactin lack then it is at least worth considering that the similar phenomenon in hypertensives may also be due to reduced levels of prolactin. The possibility of a prolactin deficiency should also be considered in that large group of hypertensives who show some degree of potassium loss without any very obvious mineralocorticoid hypersecretion.

Further evidence of possible low prolactin levels in some types of hypertension comes from studies on the effect of DOCA administration to patients with hypertension. When given to normotensives, DOCA produced sodium retention and weight gain before escape occured after 5-9 days. When given to 36 hypertensives of various types (essential, renovascular, primary aldosteronism, pheochromocytoma) 16 showed no change or a rise of less than 0.5 kg in weight and 20 actually lost weight. These results are consistent with the concept that many hypertensives may have subnormal prolactin levels. Also consistent is the finding that frusemide has a greater effect in normal individuals than in hypertensives. If frusemide is a competitive inhibitor of prolactin (chapter 19) then it would be expected to have a smaller effect if the renal tissue concentration of prolactin were already low.

One very interesting phenomenon is the high rate of prolactin secretion which occurs in patients on some hypotensive drugs, notably methyldopa and reserpine. This is explained by the known ability of these drugs to deplete hypothalamic PIF. If prolactin can elevate blood pressure it is possible that the prolactin stimulating effect interferes with the hypotensive effect and that if the former could be eliminated much better control of arterial pressure might be achieved with much lower doses of the drugs. That this may be true is suggested by recent work which has shown that L-dopa treatment may lead to a substantial lowering of pressure in response to a dose of methyl dopa which had little or no hypotensive effect in the absence of L-dopa. Of course, L-dopa could have acted in many different ways but its suppression of prolactin secretion should be considered. If this does prove to be important it offers the possibility of much more effective blood pressure control using low doses of methyldopa in conjunction with the apparently safe and well-tolerated specific prolactin suppressor, 2-bromo-α-ergokryptine.

(Biglieri, Schambelan, Slaton, Stockigt, 1970: Bryant, Douglas, Ashburn, 1971: Calne, Reid, 1973: Fisch, Freedman, Myatt, 1972: Gibberd, Small, 1973: Harris, 1969: Kriss, Futcher, 1949: Laragh, 1970: Manku, 1973: Miall, 1959: Mulrow, Boyd, 1972: Ndeti, Horrobin, Burstyn, Hopcraft, 1972: Rado, Szende, Borbely, Banos, Tako, Fischer, 1970: Robinson, 1958: Sasaki, Nowaczynski, Kuchel, Chavez, Ledoux, Gauthier, Genest, 1972: Soffer, Gabrilove, Jacobs, 1949: Soffer, Lesnick, Sorkin, Sobotka, Jacobs, 1944: Watanabe, Parks, Kopin, Weise, 1971: Weir, Briggs, Browning, Mack, Naismith, Taylor, Wilson, 1971: Woods, 1967.)

Chapter 24

MIGRAINE

There is again no direct evidence relating prolactin with migraine but the indirect evidence is perhaps stronger than most of the other cases discussed in this section of the book.

The first part of the evidence relates to the epidemiology of migraine which indicates that it is liable to occur in situations in which prolactin secretion is likely to be elevated. Migraine may occur at times of stress, after prolonged sleep at a period when stress has been removed (e.g. weekends), in the premenstrual period, in individuals on estrogen therapy and in women on oral contraceptives. The evidence that these are all times when prolactin secretion may be elevated has been presented elsewhere in this book.

The second line of evidence relates to the studies of fluid and electrolyte balance which have been carried out in patients with migraine. Obviously only a very small proportion of migraine sufferers has been studied at all vigorously in this way. However those who have been studied have been shown to retain sodium and potassium and water immediately before and during a migraine attack. Termination of the attack appears to be signalled by a rise in the excretion of sodium, potassium and water.

The third line of evidence is that all the effective drugs which are used in the treatment or prevention of migraine probably suppress prolactin secretion. This has been specifically shown to be the case with ergot derivatives and clonidine. I am not aware of any direct work on methysergide and prolactin secretion but the drug is a serotonin antagonist and serotonin is a known stimulator of prolactin secretion.

Thus three quite separated types of evidence points to a possible role for prolactin in migraine. I should like to make it quite clear that I am not saying that prolactin causes migraine in the sense that all or even most people exposed to a given level of prolactin will develop migraine. I am suggesting that the relationship is much more like the one between smoking and lung cancer, namely that of a population exposed to a given level of prolactin some, because of their constitution, will develop a typical migaine attack. Prolactin can therefore cause migraine and a lowering of prolactin levels may perhaps be able to prevent migraine.

Migraine will, however, occur only in those whose constitution predisposes them to migraine attacks: in this sense prolactin may be said not to cause migraine but merely to provide the background conditions in which a migraine attack may develop. (Dalessio, 1972: Dalton, 1964: Fluckiger, 1972: Grant, 1968: HOrrobin, (Dalessio, 1972: Dalton, 1964: Fluckiger, 1972: Grant, 1968: Horrobin, 1973: Mears, Grant, 1962: Pendl, 1973: Philips, 1968.)

Chapter 25

ASTHMA

In this chapter I should like to suggest that the relationship between prolactin and asthma may be similar to the possible relationship between prolactin and migraine. This is not that prolactin is a cause of asthma but that a given level of prolactin may be required as a permissive factor before an attack of asthma can develop. If the prolactin level is below this then an attack may not occur in the presence of the normal predisposing factors. On the other hand elevating prolactin levels may provoke attacks in those susceptible to asthma but not in normal individuals.

A possible mechanism for prolactin-permitted bronchospasm might be a movement of potassium from the smooth muscle cells leading to a state of hyperexcitability (chapter 19). In this situation stimuli which were normally unable to provoke smooth muscle contraction might lead to bronchospasm.

The clues which suggest that prolactin might in some way be related to asthmatic attacks are as follows:

1. Attacks may be induced by stressful situations or by exercise. Prolactin secretion is elevated in both situations (chapter 5).

2. Some women regularly experience premenstrual asthma. Prolactin levels may be elevated at this time (chapter 18).

3. Steroid therapy is almost always effective in preventing attacks provided that the dose is sufficient. Prolactin secretion is suppressed by high doses of steroids (chapter 6, 12.)

Chapter 26

RHEUMATOID ARTHRITIS AND
COLLAGEN DISEASES

The most striking evidence relating prolactin to rheumatoid arthritis was provided by Jasmin and Bois in rats. In a complex series of experiments on hypophysectomised or adrenalectomised animals they showed that in the presence of some adrenal deficiency prolactin injections could consistently and reliably produce a highly specific arthritic syndrome within 10-20 days. Some growth hormone was essential for the response to develop. Growth hormone itself or other foreign protein injections could produce a very inconsistent syndrome in only a proportion of animals after many weeks of injection. The prolactin syndrome was quite different in being highly specific and consistent and in occurring in virtually all the animals.

The characteristics of the syndrome were edema and inflammation of the periarticular tissues with white cell infiltration, particularly by mononuclear phagocytes. The synovial membranes were grossly affected and often protruded into the joint cavity. Most striking of all, however, was the distribution of the affected joints. While any joint could be attacked, the small joints of the paws were the ones invariably damaged in all animals.

As far as human rheumatoid arthritis is concerned, the main clues which might suggest prolactin involvement are as follows:

1. The relief afforded by steroid therapy.

2. The characteristic early morning stiffness which occurs when prolactin levels are at their peak.

3. The fact that many patients with rheumatoid arthritis show increased cutaneous capillary fragility. This is similar to the increased fragility seen in diabetics with retinopathy and in normal women at or just before the time of menstruation. It

may be caused by increased prolactin levels. (chapter 27)

4. The possible precipitation of the disease by stress, admission to hospital, illness or surgery. It has, of course, been shown that the incidence of stressful episodes preceding the development of rheumatoid arthritis was not different from that in a control population who did not develop the disease. From this the conclusion has frequently been drawn that stressful episodes are not important in initiating the disease. While this may be true, it is most certainly not a logical conclusion from the study. It ignores the possibility that a stressful episode may initiate the disease in someone who is susceptible to rheumatoid arthritis but not in someone who is not susceptible.

5. The monthly premenstrual exacerbation shown by a few patients.

6. In a very preliminary study we have shown that three patients with rheumatoid arthritis who were on steroid therapy and who therefore should have had suppressed prolactin levels in fact had prolactin levels above the normal range. This work is being extended and it will clearly be necessary to attempt to control in some way for the effect of stress since patients with the disease are obviously stressed and this alone may elevate prolactin levels.

I suggest therefore that the hypothesis that rheumatoid arthritis may, in those susceptible to the disease, be precipitated and maintained by rises in prolactin secretion is at least worth consideration. First it offers a completely new approach to the condition and second if correct it offers the hope of rational therapy since a safe drug for the suppression of prolactin secretion is now available.

Using completely the opposite approach Ingvarsson attempted to treat patients with rheumatoid arthritis by means of prolactin injections, the rationale being that these might increase adrenal steroid output. He showed that it might be possible for prolactin to restore adrenal responsiveness to ACTH and claimed that prolactin injections produced improvement in some cases. However placebo effects were not excluded and some of the good results attributed to prolactin occurred after completion of the treatment course. Some patients became worse and one went on to develop systemic lupus erythematosus.

Apart from the single patient just mentioned evidence relating prolactin to the so-called collagen diseases is completely indirect and mainly relates to individuals on some form of estrogen therapy. There are several reports of rheumatic symptoms with anti-nuclear antibodies and LE cells developing in patients taking oral contraceptives. Usually the situation improved or reversed completely on stopping the pill. Most of the women involved seem to have been taking a mestranol-containing pill.

In rats a syndrome very similar to polyarteritis nodosa develops in about 10% of old animals which, of course tend to have high circulating prolactin levels. The syndrome can be induced in young animals by estrogen treatment. Again of course this is no evidence for any involvement of prolactin but is merely a possible clue pointing in that direction.

(Bole, Friedlander, Smith, 1969: Cutts, 1966: Ingvarsson, 1969a, 1969b: Jasmin, bois, 1959a, 1959b: Mund, Simson, Rothfield, 1963: Pimstone, 1968: Potter, Duthie 1961: Potter, Wigzell, 1957: Schleicher, 1968.)

Chapter 27

DIABETES MELLITUS

Because the metabolic actions of prolactin are similar in some ways to those of growth hormone this seems a good reason for considering the possibility that prolactin may be involved in some forms of diabetes mellitus. Many years ago Houssay and his colleagues studied the diabetognic actions of pituitary hormones in hypophysectomised, partially pancreatectomised animals. By "diabetogenic" they meant an ability to elevate blood sugar and to promote ketone body formation. Growth hormone was the most potent, ACTH the least potent, with prolactin in the middle.

Most of the metabolic evidence has been reviewed in chapter 4. It is unfortunately sparse. In normal humans and animals and in juvenile diabetics prolactin given for short periods and in moderate dosage produces nothing more than a slight elevation in blood glucose and/or reduction in glucose tolerance. The effects are much more marked in hypophysectomised juvenile diabetics and in hypopituitary dwarfs. In both groups there are wide individual variations and it is clear that the effect of prolactin depends very much on the consitution of and the hormonal environment in the individual into whom the prolactin is being injected. There have, of course, been no studies of the effects of very prolonged courses of prolactin treatment.

Some of the most interesting evidence relating prolactin to diabetes mellitus comes from menstrual cycle studies. From the time of ovulation to menstruation there is a small but clear cut rise in basal plasma glucose concentration paralleled by a similar fall in glucose tolerance. Cramer in 1942 analysed a very extensive Canadian experience of emergency diabetic admissions. He found that far more women were admitted in diabetic coma during the few days before onset of menstruation and the one or two days afterwards than could be accounted for on the basis of a random distribution of risk throughout the menstrul cycle. This phenomenon has continued to be described in the literature and recently there was reported a case of a women who went into diabetic coma at or just before menstruation with every cycle until she was stabilised by being placed on oral contraceptive therapy. There is no doubt that in a proportion of women there is a clear luteal phase elevation of prolactin levels, with a probable premenstrual peak in at least some and the possibility that this may be involved in the cyclic changes seen in some female diabetics is obviously worth exploration.

Prolactin may also be involved in the deterioration of glucose tolerance which may take place at the time of stress, particularly surgery. There is now excellent evidence that prolactin secretion is consistently elevated in surgical patients even pre-operatively and that surgery itself produces a very sharp rise in plasma levels (chapter 5).

More evidence comes from the study of cutaneous capillary fragility as indicated by the timed application of a vacum by means of a capsule on the skin surface. It has been known for many years that entirely normal women may consistently show a peak of increased fragility at or just before the onset of every menstrual period. It has also been known for some time that some diabetics consistently show such increased fragility but it has only recently been demonstrated that there is a remarkably consistent relationship between such cutaneous fragility and a liability to develop diabetic retinopathy. This strongly suggests that the skin capillaries may be used as indicators of a generalised capillary disorder and also that there are two relatively clear-cut types of diabetics, those who have small vessel disease and those who do not. An obvious possibility to be explored is that prolactin may be particularly involved in those with the vascular type of disease.

One problem which must be taken note of by anyone investigating any relationship between prolactin and diabetes is that prolactin appears to have extensive actions on potassium metabolism. Changes in potassium balance can, of course, by themselves alter glucose tolerance.

One slightly bizarre possible relationship between prolactin and diabetes concerns the oral antidiabetic agents. Both tolbutamide and chlorpropamide are known to be of value in patients with diabetes insipidus provided that this is not of the nephrogenic type. They exert this action partly by increasing residual ADH secretion and partly by increasing the sensitivity of the kidneys to ADH. Prolactin can both stimulate ADH secretion and increase renal sensivity to ADH and at the least it is a plausible hypothesis to suggest that the drugs act by stimulating prolactin secretion. If prolactin has a diabetogenic effect and the oral drugs have antidiabetogenic effects, then if prolactin is under some form of feedback control relating to some aspects of carbohydrate metabolism it makes sense that its secretion should be increased by antidiabetic drugs.

(Brewer, 1938: British Medical Journal, 1970: Cramer, 1942: Hunter, Bloom, Kelsey, Porter, 1971: Moses, Numan, Miller, 1973: Weissman, Shenkman, Gregerman, 1971.)

Chapter 28

EPILEPSY

The effect of prolactin on potassium metabolism provides a logical basis for considering its possible role in epilepsy (chapter 19). At the renal level mineralocorticoids and prolactin have directly opposing actions on potassium, the former promoting potassium loss and the latter potassium retention. If the two also have opposing actions at the cellular level then mineralocorticoids will tend to promote the movement of potassium into cells while prolactin will tend to promote its extrusion. The loss of potassium from cells which can occur in the "sick cell syndrome" supports this concept since this syndrome frequently occurs in situations in which prolactin levels are known to be elevated.

When potassium moves out from nerve and muscle cells they tend to be depolarised, first becoming hyperexcitable and then inexcitable. At least during the hyperexcitable phase of the process they would presumably be more likely to take part in an epileptic attack, either apparently spontaneous or in response to some form of epileptogenic focus or stimulus. In individuals not constitutionally liable to develop epilepsy no epileptic attack would occur but in ones liable to do so, an attack would develop. Prolactin has been shown first to excite and then to inhibit human uterine smooth muscle (fig 2): other systems have not as yet been tested but if a similar series of events occurs with nervous tissue then prolactin could be epileptogenic.

The clinical evidence is at the moment scanty but does indicate that this lead may be worth following up.

1. Chlorpromazine injections are now one of the standard techniques used by electroencephalograph (electrocorticograph) experts in order to trigger epileptiform discharges in those under investigation for epilepsy. Endocrinologists are now beginning to use chlorpromazine injections as a test of how well the hypothalamic-pituitary axis can respond to a powerful stimulus to prolactin secretion. It is worth

considering the possibility that part of the chlorpromazine effect may be mediated via prolactin. Imipramine, amitryptyline, tolbutamide, reserpine and haloperidol are all probable stimulators of prolactin secretion and all are known potentiators of epileptiform discharges.

2. Some women consistently experience epileptic attacks in the premenstrual period and at no other time. Prolactin levels are probably elevated at this time.

3. There seems to be a greater risk of epileptic attacks at night or in the very early morning than at any other times. Prolactin levels are elevated during these periods.

4. There is a greatly increased risk of epileptic attacks in pregnancy toxemia.

As with migraine and asthma I suggest that prolactin will precipitate epilepsy only in those consitutionally predisposed to it. "Normal" individuals with similar levels will not develop epilepsy but as prolactin levels are elevated the proportion of people in the population who will show epileptiform discharges will steadily rise.

(Betts, Kalra, Cooper, Jeavons, 1968: Davison, 1965: Kiloh, Davison, Osselton, 1961: Kiloh, McComas, Osselton, 1972.)

Chapter 29

NATURAL AND DRUG-INDUCED
PARKINSONISM

Natural Parkinsonism is associated with a deficiency of cerebral serotonin and dopamine. In the hypothalamus the dopamine deficiency leads among other things, to a failure of PIF secretion with a consequent elevation of prolactin secretion. Parkinsonism may be induced by a number of drugs, among them phenothiazines, methyldopa and reserpine, all of which may also lead to a deficiency of PIF with an elevation of prolactin secretion. Treatment with L-dopa tends to restore hypothalamic dopamine and to suppress prolactin secretion. Similar changes probably occur in hypothalamic MIF and pituitary MSH secretion.

Parkinsonism is usually attributed to the dopamine deficiency and this is presumably the initial cause. However there is no evidence that the dopamine deficiency itself, as distinct from some consequence of it, is the actual cause of the neuromuscular disorder. On the basis of the evidence outlined in the first paragraph, MIF/PIF deficiency or prolactin/MSH excess or both could be the basis of the neuromuscular problems.

I should like to suggest that it is possible that the hypothalamic content of the releasing and inhibiting factors themsleves may be crucial to the development of neuromuscular abnormalities, with an overall deficiency leading to a Parkinson-like state and an overall excess to a dyskinetic state. The main evidence is:

1. MIF may improve Parkinson-like states even in the absence of the pituitary gland. It must therefore have an action which is independent of MSH.

2. MSH may worsen Parkinsonism, possibly by reducing MIF secretion.

3. TRH may improve Parkinsonism, even in the absenc e of the pituitary so again it cannot be acting via TSH.

4. L-dopa, amphetamines and tricyclic anti-depressants may all produce dyskinetic states. They can all elevate the hypothalamic levels of releasing and/or inhibiting facto

Again the evidence in favour of the hypothesis is at best indirect, but it is worth putting forward as it could suggest alternative therapeutic approaches to Parkinsonism.

(Coppen, Metcalfe, Carroll, Morris, 1972: Cotzias, Van Woert, Schiffer, 1967: Gibber(Small, 1973: Kamberi, Mical, Porter, 1969: Kastin, 1967: Kastin, Barbeau, 1972: Plot Kastin, Anderson, Schally, 1971: Plotnikoff, Prange, Breese, Anderson, Wilson, 1972: Robins, 1973: Sandler, Goodwin, Leask, Ruthven, 1973: Schneider, McCann, 1970: S Burton, Thody, Plummer, Goolamali, Bates, 1973.)

Chapter 30

MYOCARDIAL INFARCTION AND
THROMBO-EMBOLIC DISEASES

Again, of course, there is no direct evidence relating myocardial infarction and other forms of thrombo-embolic disease to prolactin. However, it is obvious that a number of situations which are known to be associated with high prolactin levels are also associated with a high risk of myocardial infarction

Myocardial infarction is relatively common in surgical patients. Perhaps surprisingly it is almost as common or may even be more common pre-operatively as post-operatively. Prolactin levels are elevated pre-operatively presumably because of the stress associated with waiting for a surgical operation and there is a further very sharp rise during the operation itself (chapter 5).

Oral contraceptives can produce galactorrhea and at least those with a relatively high estrogen content probably produce moderate elevations of prolactin secretion in women. The relationship between oral contraceptives and an increased risk of myocardial infarction and thromboembolic disease has been well documented. In particular the greater part of the risk seems to be related to the estrogen content of the pills and it is the estrogen component which would be responsible for any stimulation of prolactin secretion. Prolactin levels are also elevated during pregnancy and the puerperium and myocardial infarction at these times seems more likely to occur than in non-pregnant and non-lactating women of similar age.

Estrogen therapy in males also seems to predispose to the development of myocardial infarction and thromboembolic disease. In one controlled trial with about seventy patients in each group, 20 men on estrogen therapy developed a myocardial infarction or cerebrovascular accident within six months whereas none of the control group did. In another uncontrolled trial, of 57 patients on estrogen, 17 developed a myocardial infarction or cerebro-vascular accident. Excess water retention often complicated the therapy suggesting that stimulation of prolactin secretion had occurred. In the Veterans Administration trial of estrogen therapy in prostatic cancer, the improved results as far as the cancer was concerned were more than counterbalanced by a substantial increase in death from cardiovascular causes. Interestingly enough the best cancer and worst cardiovascular results were obtained with a small group of 47 patients who received estrogen plus reserpine, a particularly potent combination as far as stimulation of prolactin secretion is concerned.

Drug-associated myocardial infarction is also interesting. Tricyclic anti-depressants appear to be able to precipitate myocardial infarction in some patients and a similar thing is true of reserpine. Evidence has been presented elsewhere (chapters 19 and 27) which suggests that the oral antidiabetic drugs may perhaps stimulate prolactin secretion. There is of course, a considerable controversy surrounding the suggestion that the oral antidiabetic drugs may be associated with myocardial infarction. However in a recent 6-year prospective study 19.7% of 71 patients treated with oral drugs developed ischemic heart disease but only 9.5% of 115 patients treated by diet alone did so. This does not exclude the possibility that those treated with the oral drugs were more difficult to control and therefore more liable to develop myocardial infarction.

Myocardial infarction may occur during sudden severe exercise in those unaccustomed to it or may be associated with a period of stress. In both situations prolactin levels are likely to be elevated.

There is a well-known relationship between increasing hardness of water and a reduced incidence of cardiovascular death. In the United States it has been shown that this seems to correlate more closely with the lithium content of the water than with any other parameter. Lithium may suppress prolactin secretion and those on a relatively high lithium intake would be expected to have lower levels of circulating prolactin.

One possible site at which prolactin might act is the platelet. Platelet adhesiveness may be enhanced by surgery or by therapy with synthetic estrogens. There is some evidence in man that the synthetic estrogens may be more potent stimulators of prolactin secretion than the natural ones.

Apart from the possible action of prolactin in promoting myocardial infarction its role in the various pathophysiological states which may occur in the post-infarction state should also be considered, particularly with regard to its effects on potassium metabolism. Anyone who has suffered a myocardial infarction is likely to be in a severely stressed state with a substantial elevation of prolactin secretion. This would tend to cause renal sodium, potassium and water retention but would also tend to cause a movement of potassium out from cells (chapter 19). This outward movement would cause a tendency to depolarisation with a consequent increased risk of the development of cardiac arrhythmias which are, of course, so common after myocardial infarction. The various treatments which have been proposed for post-infarction arrhythmias, notably potassium, glucose and insulin therapy and cortisol, are believed to operate by increasing the movements of potassium into cells. The cortisol certainly and the GKI therapy probably would also suppress prolactin secretion and might promote an inward movement of potassium this way. In view of the post-infarction problems which are posed by fluid and electrolyte retention and cardiac arrhythmias a trial of a drug such as 2-bromo-α-ergokryptine in myocardial infarction would appear to be justified.

(Bagshawe, Curtis, Garnett, 1965: Blachly, 1969: Bolton, Hampton, Mitchell, 1968: Boyle, Bhatia, Hadden, Montgomery, Weaver, 1972: British Medical Journal, 1969: Canning, Green, Mulcahy, 1969: Clark, Ray, Paredes, Ragland, Costiloe, Smith, Wolf, 1967: Committee on Safety of Drugs, 1970: Coull, Crooks, Dingwall-Fordyce, Scott, Weir, 1970: Daniel, Campbell, Turnbull, 1967: Datey, Nanda, 1967: Dear, Jones, 1971 Ginz, 1970: Goldstein, 1969: Gunther, Kohorn, 1968: Hadden, Montgomery, Weaver, 1972: Hampton, Gorlin, 1972: Heefner, 1973: Hunter, 1968: Husaini, 1971: Irey, Manion, Taylor, 1970: L'Hermite, Delvoye, Nokin, Vekemans, Robyn, 1972: McDowel Louis, McDevitt, 1967: Mittra, 1965, 1966: Newball, Byar, 1972: Oliver, 1970: Poller, Thomson, Tabiowo, Priest, 1969: Robinson, Higano, Cohen, 1963: Rosen, Mushin, Kilpatrick, Campbell, Davies, Harrison, 1966: Salonen, 1968: Saunders, Carey, Hewitt, Jones, 1971: Stitt, Clayton, Crawford, Morris, 1973: Vessey, Doll, 1969: Veterans, Administration Cooperative Urological Research Group, 1967: Voors, 1969, 1970: Waxler, Kimbiris, Van den Broeck, Segal, Likoff, 1971: Weiss, 1972: Wright, 1942.)

Chapter 31

MENTAL ILLNESS

As far as I am aware, it has never previously been suggested that prolactin is in any way involved in mental illness. Yet virtually every drug which is used in psychiatry, including TRH, either stimulates or suppresses prolactin secretion. Prolactin is bound to cerebral tissue, can alter the activity of hypothalamic neurons and has effects on electrolyte metabolism in general, and potassium metabolism in particular, which depending on their degree might produce neuronal excitation or depression. There are therefore excellent a priori reasons for considering that prolactin may in some way be intimately involved in the regulation of behaviour.

In order to understand what follows it is essential to be conversant with fig. 8 which shows what is now known of the regulation of prolactin secretion. There appear to be three hypothalamic regulating factors. TRH is of course the same substance which stimulates TSH output and which has been reported to produce very rapid relief of depression. PRF has not yet been isolated but there is evidence that it and TRH may be under the control of neurons which release noradrenaline or serotonin as transmitters. Both noradrenaline and serotonin can stimulate prolactin secretion but they have no direct action on the pituitary, nor do they act via PIF. PIF is an inhibitory factor which can block the release of prolactin: it appears to be secreted continuously and a fall in its rate of secretion leads to an elevation of prolactin secretion. The production of PIF is regulated by neurons which employ dopamine as a transmitter. The secretion of prolactin by the pituitary can act back on the hypothalamus by means of the so-called "short feedback loops". Elevated levels of prolactin have been shown definitely to elevate hypothalamic PIF and they almost certainly also depress hypothalamic TRH and PRF secretion.

Of the drugs used in psychiatry, the main ones which alter prolactin secretion and their probable modes of action are as follows:

1. The phenothiazines deplete hypothalamic PIF and elevate prolactin secretion.

As a consequence of the short feedback loops the elevated prolactin levels may suppress hypothalamic TRH and PRF secretion.

2. The monoamine oxidase inhibitors elevate hypothalamic PIF and suppress prolactin secretion. They may directly elevate PRF but this is unable to overcome the PIF. inhibition.

3. The actions of the tricyclic antidepressants and of amphetamines are uncertain but they both stimulate prolactin secretion, possibly by stimulating PRF secretion.

4. Lithium probably suppresses prolactin secretion but this has not definitely been established. The mode of action is unknown.

Biological bases of behavior

This chapter attempts to set out some precise and readily testable hypotheses which suggest that prolactin and the hypothalamic factors which regulate its secretion are at the heart of the problem of the biological bases of behavior. The hypotheses are not necessarily inconsistent with any of the other biological hypotheses so far proposed which largely refer to amines and transmitter substances. It is possible that the end-point of these other systems may be their interaction with the prolactin-regulating mechanism. The main advantage of the hypotheses I am proposing is that they are readily testable now in human patients using techniques which are simple and require only blood sampling. There is therefore no need to enter into long discussions about the validity of this or that type of animal model to this or that type of depression or schizophrenia. I freely admit that it is unlikely that my hypotheses are true. However, as Popper has pointed out, provided that a hypothesis genuinely is testable, improbability, perhaps surprisingly, is a virtue. A testable hypothesis will stimulate research and lead to advances in knowledge even if it is not true. An improbable hypothesis which turns out to be true will lead to advances in knowledge much more dramatic than those which occur when a probable hypothesis turns out to be true.

The hypothesis starts from the assumption that the immediate basis of all behavior is neuronal activity in particular neural circuits. The microanatomy and basic connections of these circuits are likely to be determined by genetic factors and early environmental experience. However, which functional inter-connections are made may depend on the biochemical environment of the brain. In particular I suggest that the particular connections which determine the pattern of normal or abnormal behavior are concentrated in the hypothalamic region and that is the biochemical environment there which will govern the switches.

Although obviously there is room for much argument I should like to suggest as a somewhat rough and ready starting point that there may be considered to be five basic types of behavior, normal, neurotic, depressive, manic and schizophrenic. Obviously dividing lines are blurred, the divisions are arbitrary. Their purpose is simply to provide a basis for discussion. One of the striking things about these groups is that it is now possible by the use of drugs to produce in apparently "normal" individuals behavior patterns characteristic of the other four states. This strongly suggests that even entirely normal brains contain the basic neuronal circuits required to produce neurosis, depression, mania and schizophrenia and that the expression or otherwise of these circuits depends on biochemical factors.

I suggest that basic genetic and early environmental factors will lay down the fundamental microcircuitry and determine the susceptibility of an individual to the abnormal behavior groups. Some individuals, for example, may have a basic anatomical circuitry which is such that even large changes in biochemistry will be insufficient to push them into one or other of the abnormal groups. Other individuals may have circuits which are such that even in the presence of a normal biochemical environment they become depressed. Other intermediate individuals may become depressed only in the presence of the appropriate biochemical changes which may, of course, originate in environmental events. Similar things will be true of the other abnormal categories.

Further I suggest that there is a strictly limited number of patterns of biochemical abnormality and that the variety of actual behavior comes from the interaction of each pattern with the microcircuitry of the individual. In other words the detailed pattern of the illness will depend on the patient's genetic and environmental history but the basic nature of the illness, whether it be depression or schizophrenia and so on, will depend on the basic biochemistry.

The hypothesis suggests, of course, that mental illness is of the smoking and lung cancer type of disease pattern rather than the plague type (chapter 12). By this I mean that the expression of the disease will depend not on the biochemistry alone but on the interaction of that biochemistry with the constitution of the individual. A numerical example may help. Suppose that there is a biochemical pattern which leads to depression and that this pattern may be arbitrarily divided into grades from 0 (normality) to 3 (very severe abnormality). The incidences of depression in populations with biochemical characteristics of the same type might then be as follows:

Grade	
0	6%
1	32%
2	51%
3	60%

Some people with normal biochemistry might have such unfortunate neuronal circuitry that they were depressed. The incidence of depression would rise as the biochemistry became more and more abnormal. Two consequences are, however, clear: some people who were depressed would have no biochemical abnormalities and some people with severe biochemical abnormalities would not be depressed. In spite of these facts comparison of the groups would leave no doubt about the relationship between the biochemical abnormality and the disease. It is very important both for those who are proposing biochemical hypotheses and those who are criticizing them to appreciate that the findings of "normal" biochemistry in some diseased persons and of "abnormal" biochemistry in some apparently normal persons in no way provide evidence against the biochemical concept.

One of the interesting things about psychiatry is that it is very widely accepted that diseases as destructive in their impact as the major psychoses must have some biological basis. Many, but of course not all, feel that such shattering phenomena cannot be explained on the basis of the influence of environmental factors. In contrast, there is an almost equally wide acceptance of the concept that the neuroses have "psychological" rather than biological bases although rarely, if ever, is the precise meaning of the word "psychological" spelled out. There often appears to be a sensation of hopelessness with regard to those who suffer from "neuroses" or from an "inadequate personality". It seems to be frequently felt that while some such people may be helped by drugs and others by intensive psychotherapy, the problem is too overwhelming and too rooted in environmental problems for psychiatry to have more than a marginal impact.

The hypothesis proposed in this chapter, in contrast, suggests that the neuroses as well as the psychoses may have a biological basis. Again as with depression, some individuals will have neurotic nervous systems even in the presence of normal biochemistry while others will function normally even in the presence of an abnormal "neurotic" biochemistry. The majority, however, will exhibit normal behaviour with normal biochemistry but with an increasing risk of becoming overtly neurotic as the biochemistry becomes more abnormal. This concept is unlikely to be readily accepted by most investigators yet almost all will regularly experience an example of it even though they may not have thought of it in this light. I refer, of course, to the mood changes which occur during the menstrual cycle in a large number of women. There can be no doubt that these mood changes occur and that in many women they are of a pattern which most psychiatrists would classify as neurotic. There is also no doubt that they are consistently associated with the endocrine and metabolic changes which take place in the luteal phase of the cycle and that they can be modified by changing the endocrine environment. The fact that even during the follicular phase psychological testing may indicate that women who suffer from the premenstrual syndrome are "neurotic" in no way detracts from the biological concept. It confirms the idea that these women have neurotic tendencies which may be suppressed in one biochemical environment but may be allowed to flourish in another.

I propose that the key factors in the hypothalamic environment which determine psychiatric state are TRH, PRF, PIF and prolactin and it is the balance between these which will decide whether an individual will reveal neurotic, manic, depressive or schizophrenic tendencies. As I have said it is unlikely that this hypothesis in its basic form will prove true but it does have the virtue of being immediately and precisely testable in human beings and if it is so tested progress is inevitable. Each situation will be discussed in detail later in the chapter but the basic propositions are outlined here.

1. Neurotic behaviour will occur in susceptible individuals when prolactin secretion is moderately stimulated by simultaneous but relatively small rises in TRH and PRF and by a similar fall in PIF. There are the changes which probably take place during the luteal phase of the menstrual cycle in some women and during the stimulation of prolactin secretion by stress.

2. The depressed state depends on the hypothalamic concentrations of TRH and PRF: when these are below normal, depression will be likely to occur. This fall

in TRH/PRF could occur because of a primary reduction in the activity of the neurones controlling their secretion or because of a fall in PIF secretion or more likely because of both. A fall in PIF secretion will lead to a rise in prolactin secretion which by the short feedback loop mechanism would suppress TRH/PRF secretion.

3. Mania will be likely to occur in individuals with low PIF, elevated prolactin and low TRH/PRF levels who for some reason begin to secrete large amounts of PRF. They will thus have low PIF, high PRF, very high prolactin and very low TRH levels. Thus as far as PRF and overt mood are concerned mania and depression will form a bipolar disease with mania at one extreme, depression at the other and normality in the middle. But as far as prolactin is concerned mania and depression will form a monopolar illness with depressives one stage removed from normality and manics a further stage away from normality along the same path.

4. Schizophrenia will occur when there is a primary elevation of PRF or TRH, possibly due to stimulation by serotonin or by noradrenaline, or a primary elevation of PIF. PRF or TRH elevation will elevate prolactin levels and by the short feedback loop also lead to PIF elevation. PIF elevation will suppress prolactin secretion and by the feedback mechanism lead to elevation of TRH and PRF. The crucial factor will be the simultaneous elevation of PRF/TRH and PIF.

Neuroses

The basic hypothesis is that during the luteal phase of the menstrual cycle and during situations of stress, prolactin secretion is elevated by a rise in PRF and a fall in PIF. The change in prolactin secretion itself may be important as in humans prolactin injections may cause irritability and lethargy. Unfortunately, with the exception of the premenstrual syndrome there are no satisfactory studies of biological changes in neuroses. The idea that prolactin is important gains support from the relief from the neurotic features of the syndrome which may be obtained by treatment with progesterone or lithium, both of which may suppress prolactin secretion. The electrolyte changes which occur in the syndrome could be accounted for by increased prolactin secretion. (Chapter 18).

Depression

The hypothesis suggests that depression will tend to occur whenever the sum of TRH + PRF falls. This end result could be achieved in three distinct ways:

1. By a primary fall in TRH secretion.

2. By a primary fall in PRF secretion.

3. By a primary fall in PIF secretion. This will allow prolactin secretion rates to rise and this in turn by the short feedback loops will suppress TRH and PRF secretion.

TRH and PRF secretion are probably determined primarily by activation of nora-drenaline and serotonin-containing neurons. PIF is regulated primarily by dopamine containing neurons. My own feeling is that the third mechanism is likelty to be more often important than the other two, mainly because of the relationships between electrolyte balance and thyroid function in depression.

The hypothesis is consistent with the following findings:

1. Depression may frequently be produced in normal individuals by treatment with α-methyldopa or reserpine. Both drugs increase prolactin secretion by depleting the hypothalamus of PIF.

2. Monoamine oxidase inhibitors which elevate hypothalamic PIF secretion and reduce prolactin secretion may relieve depression.

3. Amphetamines and tricyclic antidepressants which elevate prolactin secretion probably primarily by elevating PRF secretion may relieve depression.

4. TRH which elevates prolactin secretion may relieve depression.

5. There is some evidence that depression may be associated with depression of cerebral noradrenaline or serotonin activity which in turn would be associated with hypothalamic PRF and TRH depletion.

6. L-dopa therapy which elevates hypothalamic PIF content may relieve depression in some patients.

7.   Feeding of tryptophan would be expected to elevate hypothalamic TRH and PRF activity and has been reported to relieve depression in some patients. Conversely, diversion of tryptophan from the serotonin to the kynurenine pathway as in patients with pyridoxine deficiency and/or on oral contraceptives may be associated with depression. Correction of the defect with pyridoxine may relieve the depression.

8.   Oral contraceptives which elevate prolactin secretion by depressing PIF secretion would be expected to cause depression.

9.   The sodium retention which has been reported in depressive illness could be accounted for by excess prolactin secretion.

10. The reduced carbohydrate tolerance which is so frequently a feature of depressive illness could be explained by elevated prolactin secretion.

11. The recent demonstration of reduced thyroxine plasma levels in depression could be accounted for partly by prolactin suppression of TRH secretion and partly by prolactin interference with the action of TSH on the thyroid.

12. The elevated cortisol levels and reduced suppression by dexamethasone are probably in part a response to the stress of a depressive illness. However they might in part be brought about by a prolactin-induced increase in the sensitivity of the adrenal cortex to ACTH.

13. The elevation of blood pressure which has been reported in depression might be explained by elevated prolactin secretion.

Mania

The hypothesis suggests that mania arises from a situation in which there is a lowering of hypothalamic PIF, an elevation of prolactin secretion and a consequent lowering of hypothalamic TRH and PRF. In susceptible subjects these changes will lead to depression but in those not susceptible the changes could be present without overt depression. I suggest that there is then superimposed on this situation a rise in PRF secretion brought about by over-activity of neurons releasing either serotonin or noradrenaline or both. This high PRF coupled with a low PIF will lead to very high rates of prolactin secretion coupled with severe suppression of hypothalamic TRH. Thus in comparison with depression, PIF levels will be similar but both TRH and prolactin levels will become even more abnormal than in depression, but with the abnormality in the same direction from normal. The PRF levels will however be abnormal in a direction directly opposite to that seen in depression. I suggest that PRF rather than TRH is primarily involved in mania because the manic features which may be produce by amphetamines are associated with elevation of prolactin but not of TSH secretion. The hypothesis can explain the following findings;

1. There is some evidence which suggests that manic-depression is a bipolar disease but other evidence that it is a unipolar disease with mania further removed from normality than depression. The hypothesis incorporates both these concepts without strain suggesting that the disease is bipolar as far as PRF is concerned but unipolar as far as TRH and prolactin are concerned.

2. The greater degree of sodium retention which has been reported in mania as compared to depression could be explained by higher prolactin levels in the former.

3. The greater reduction of plasma thyroxine levels which has been reported in mania as compared to depression could also be explained by higher prolactin levels which would produce a greater suppression of TRH secretion and possibly a greater interference with the action of TSH on the thyroid.

4. The production of manic features by amphetamine or tricyclic antidepressant treatment in susceptible patients may be explained by their effects on PRF.

5. The reported worsening of mania in some patients by feeding with serotonin precursors and the improvement supposedly brought about by methysergide might be explained.

6. Mania may be treated by phenothiazines or haloperidol which deplete hypothalamic PIF and would be expected to elevate prolactin levels still further. This elevation would help to suppress hypothalamic PRF by means of the short feedback loop. Interestingly it has often been reported that relief of the mania may coincide with the development of drug-induced Parkinsonism. If as suggested in chapter 29 Parkinsonism is associated with low levels of hypothalamic releasing factors, the simultaneous relief of mania and appearance

of Parkinsonism would be neatly explained.

Schizophrenia

The hypothesis suggests that schizophrenia will be likely to occur in those individuals who are susceptible whenever a primary elevation takes place in PRF, TRH or PIF levels. A primary elevation in the releasing factors will lead to an elevation of prolactin secretion: the short feedback loop will attempt to return this to normal by elevating PIF. A primary elevation in PIF will lead to suppression of prolactin secretion followed by an attempt to return it to normal by elevation of the releasing factors. In one case there may be some suppression of prolactin secretion and in the other some elevation but in both there will be a simultaneous elevation of the hypothalamic levels of both releasing and inhibiting factors: it is this simultaneous elevation which I suggest may be crucial. Different forms of schizophrenia might be brought about by differences between the three primary changes interacting with individuals of different constitutions.

The hypothesis could explain the following features:

1. The success of treatments involving phenothiazines which are known to deplete hypothalamic PIF and which will secondarily reduce TRH and PRF levels.

2. The precipitation in susceptible individuals of schizophrenic features by L-dopa, amphetamines, tricyclic antidepressants, LSD and MAO inhibitors, all of which are capable of elevating hypothalamic PRF, TRH or PIF.

3. The effect of disulfiram in precipitating schizophrenic features in susceptible individuals. This drug inhibits the conversion of dopamine to other catecholamines and might therefore be expected to cause accumulation of dopamine which is the stimulator of PIF secretion.

4. The syndrome of periodic catatonia might be specifically accounted for by cyclic surges of TRH release. PBI and BMR tend to be elevated during the catatonic periods and at this time there is reduced water and sodium excretion. These effects could be accounted for by stimulation of TSH and prolactin secretion. Thyroxine prevents the psychotic episodes in most cases and would, of course, be expected to suppress TRH secretion.

Testing the hypothesis

One of the problems with all the biochemical models of psychiatric disease proposed so far is the impossibility of measuring in cerebral tissue in humans the concentrations and turnover rates of the various substances thought to be vitally involved. As a result it has been necessary to resort to two rather unsatisfactory ruses, the development of animal models and the study of metabolites of the key substances which may appear in various body fluids. While each approach has its enthusiasts I think it is not unfair to say that outside this enthusiastic circle the results are felt to be unconvincing. There is no doubt that animal models have proved very valuable in screening compounds with possible activity on the brain and in studying in detail the metabolism of these and of naturally occurring compounds. But unfortunately one cannot ask an animal how it feels and this imposes clear limitations on how far the results of animal experiments can be applied to man.

On the whole biochemical studies of human patients have, however, proved rather less satisfactory than the animal studies. Results have been contradictory and confusing and a particularly disappointing but recurrent feature has been the failure of groups of research workers to be able to repeat work which they themselves had reported. Much of the trouble arises from a failure to appreciate the need for study under metabolically controlled conditions and without the influence of drugs. This latter problem is becoming almost insuperable since many drugs have effects which persist for weeks after cessation of therapy and it is clearly unethical in most cases to withdraw an effective drug for the purposes of a research project.

One of the major advantages of the hypothesis proposed in this chapter is that it can in large measure be tested by using techniques which are already available (chapter 15). Basal plasma TSH and prolactin estimations can give an idea of the balance between factors promoting and inhibiting secretion. Chlorpromazine testing gives a good indication of the degree of inhibition being exerted by PIF while TRH testing indicates the responsiveness of the pituitary cells. The tests are simple to perform, are reliable and raise no ethical problems.

As I have repeatedly stated it is not likely that the ideas presented in this chapter are correct. However they do seem to explain in a relatively satisfactory way the clinical features of the various types of mental illness and their responsiveness to particular types of drugs. The most important feature is their testability and if patients with various types of psychiatric disorder were systematically tested by means of TRH and chlorpromazine it seems very likely that our knowledge of the biological basis of psychiatry would advance substantially.

(Adams, Wynn, Rose, Seed, Folkard, Strong, 1973: Angst, 1956: Braithwaite, Goulding, Theano, Bailey, Coppen, 1972: Carranza-Acevedo, 1967: Carroll, Frazer, Schless, Mendels, 1973: Coppen, Metcalfe, Carroll, Morris, 1972: Coppen, Prange, Whybrow, Noguera, 1972: Coppen, Shaw, 1963: Coppen, Shaw, Farrell, 1963: Davies, Carroll, Mowbray, 1972: Gibbons, 1960: Heine, Sainsbury, Chynoweth, 1969: Janowsky, El-Yousef, Dans, Hubbard, Sekerke, 1972: Kastin, Ehrensing, Schalch, Anderson, 1972: Lancet, 1968: Lapin, Oxenkrug, 1969: Lewis, 1971:.Medical Research Council, 1972: Mellerup, Plenge, Vendsborg, Rafaelsen, Kjeldsen, Agerback, 1972: Prnage, Wilson, Lara, Alltop, Breese, 1972: Price, Thornton, Mueller, 1967: Russell, 1960: Rybakowski, Sowinski, 1973: Sachar, 1973: Schildkraut, 1965: Schottstaedt, Grace, Wolff, 1956: Simpson, Waal-Manning, 1971: Van der Velde, Gordon, 1969: Weil-Malherbe, Szara, 1971: Winston, 1969.)

Chapter 32

CANCER

The experimental and clinical evidence relating prolactin to cancer was reviewed in chapter 11. References quoted there will not normally be quoted again here. In summary the data demonstrates quite clearly that mammary cancers in rodents may be prolactin-dependent and that suppression of prolactin secretion by one means or another will inhibit tumor growth while stimulation of prolactin secretion will accelerate it. There is suggestive evidence in humans that some breast cancers may be prolactin-dependent. This is shown by favorable responses to hypopjysectc and to L-Dopa treatment and also by the in vitro demonstration that in cultures of some tumors the activity of the pentose shunt pathway can be shown to depend on prolactin. It has been suggested that prostatic carcinoma may be prolactin-depender although here both the animal and human evidence is as yet negligible.

A more interesting, because possibly more generally applicable, finding is that stimulation of prolactin secretion may be associated with a blocking of tumor induc tion and a slowing down or abolition of tumor growth. A whole series of treatment: which have in common the fact that they stimulate prolactin secretion may greatly reduce the number of animals which develop tumors and the number of tumors per animal in response to treatment with 3MC or DMBA: once the tumors are established, however, these same treatments enhance their growth. It would be most interesting to carry out similarly extensive experiments on tumors arising in tissues which are not apparently target organs for prolactin. The crucial question to be answered is whether prolactin can inhibit - and also stimulate - rat mammary tumors because the mammary gland is a prolactin target organ or whether the stimulation is a specific target organ effect while the inhibition is a more general phenomenon which might be applied to the prevention and elimination of tumors anywhere in the body.

There are a number of reports of inhibition of growth of other animal tumors by chlorpromazine and reserpine both of which are powerful stimulators of prolactin secretion. They also both have many other effects any one of which might be involved in the tumor inhibition. Tumors reported to be inhibited include leukemia, mastocytoma, sarcoma and melanoma in mice.

In man there is also some evidence that prolactin may perhaps be involved in defence against tumors, although again the evidence is indirect. Pituitary stalk section and estrogen treatment may both produce remission of breast cancer in some women, as may pregnancy. In man estrogen therapy of prostatic cancer has been relatively successful and although this is usually attributed to the local action of the estrogen on prostatic tissue, a more general action operating via prolactin has been neither looked for nor excluded. Interestingly in the large Veterans Administration trial, the best results as far as the cancer was concerned were obtained in a group of 47 patients who received both estrogen and reserpine. It seems unlikely that the reserpine had any local effect on the tumors. The combination of estrogen and reserpine is, however, a very powerful stimulus to prolactin secretion.

One interesting recent finding is that in long stay mental patients (i.e. those whose tumors, if any, would have arisen during their time in hospital rather than before admission) the incidence of cancer seems to be lower than that in the general population. The difference was particularly evident with lung, gut, prostate and bladder tumors and with leukaemia. There was no difference in breast cancer incidence. Clearly there are a thousand possible explanations for this finding, but it may not be irrelevant that most long stay mental patients are on some form of phenothiazine therapy.

There are other fascinating findings which could have many explanations but which could perhaps also be accounted for on the basis of the idea that prolactin offers some form of defence against malignancy. There seems to be a small but definite reduced risk of cancer in patients with diabetes: there is some evidence that some diabetics may have raised prolactin levels. An increased risk of cancer has been reported in men whose risk of developing cardiovascular disease has been reduced by taking a diet high in polyunsaturated fat: other trials failed to demonstrate this but it is a niggling fact that in three different situations, diabetes, estrogen treatment of prostatic cancer and dietary therapy with unsaturated fats there have been reports of an inverse relationship between the risk of cancer and the risk of myocardial infarction.. Patients with asthma (chapter 25) and other forms of allergy have been reported to have a reduced risk of developing cancer. Survival rate has been reported better in those surgically treated lung cancer patients who develop severe infections. In asthma and infections prolactin levels may be

elevated. All of these rather surprising findings are open to criticism on statistical and other grounds and all have many other explanations apart from the one of an involvement of prolactin. At this stage they are nothing more than ideas as to areas which might be worth investigating. A certain interest is added to them, however, by the fact that if prolactin should prove capable of stimulating defence mechanisms against cancer, then drugs to stimulate its secretion are readily available and could be immediately used as adjuncts to therapy.

One relationship which requires investigation is that between plasma prolactin levels and various types of cancer. It has been reported for both breast cancer and prostatic cancer that the more advanced the disease the more elevated are plasma prolactin levels. There are clearly several possible explanations for this:

1. The prolactin is causing the disease and those individuals with more prolactin have more severe disease. This does not seem very likely as the evidence seems to indicate that the prolactin levels rise as the disease progresses although hard evidence from serial studies in the same patient is non-existent.

2. The elevated prolactin levels are a response to bony involvement. The relation between prolactin and calcium metabolism is not known. Prolactin does however promote urinary calcium excretion and if calcium were entering the blood from osteolytic lesions it would make sense to elevate prolactin secretion in order to help eliminate it. If this were true then prolactin elevation would be related to bony involvement and calcium metabolism rather than to tumor type or any other aspect of progression.

3. The elevated prolactin levels are part of the body's response to malignant disease of any type. If this were true then it should be found that prolactin levels are elevated not only in prostatic and mammary cancer but in any form of malignant disease.
(Belkin, Hardy, 1957: Cohen, 1972: Csatary, 1972: Ederer, Leren, Turpeinen, Frantz 1971: Goldin, Burton, Humphreys, Venditte, 1957: Gottlieb, Hazel, Broitman, Zamc Katz, Kunofsky, Patton, Allaway, 1967: Kessler, 1970: Levij, Polliack, 1970: Meers, Papioannou, 1972: Pearce, Dayton, 1971: Van Woert, Palmer, 1969.)

Chapter 33

OTHER ASPECTS

The possible roles of prolactin in physiology and disease have not yet even been outlined, let alone explored in detail. Some of the possible new areas of investigation are briefly mentioned in this chapter.

It has been reported that some women with glaucoma may experience regular premenstrual exacerbations. It would not be surprising if prolactin had some action on the secretion of aqueous humor in view of its effects on fluid and electrolyte movements at other sites. Interestingly, the intra-ocular pressure tends to be highest in the early morning when prolactin levels are at a peak and then it falls off during the day. (Dalton, 1964: Davson, 1969.)

Nothing is known about the potentially important actions of prolactin on the gut. Again because of its effects on fluid and electrolyte balance it would not be surprising if prolactin interacted with other nerves and hormones in the regulation of gut secretions. The increased gastric secretion and peptic ulceration brought about by reserpine have not been fully explained as yet. (Jarvik, 1970.)

The possible inter-relationships between prolactin and calcium metabolism have been mentioned elsewhere in the book. Prolactin certainly causes increased urinary calcium excretion but other aspects have not yet been explored. In sarcoidosis, and in metastatic prostatic and mammary cancers when calcium disturbances may be severe, prolactin levels are often elevated but whether this is simply an association or whether one is causing the other is quite unknown.

The effects of prolactin on cholesterol metabolism are probably also well worth investigation. Patients treated with phenothiazines tend to develop elevated plasma cholesterol levels. The reasons for the cholesterol elevations seen in myxedema and the nephrotic syndrome are quite unknown although in both cases prolactin levels are probably elevated. (Clark, Ray, Paredes, Ragland, Costiloe, Smith, Wolf, 1967.)

Finally it has been suggested that prolactin may be involved in increasing sensitivity to pain. If pain endings are sensitive to potassium and if prolactin causes extrusion of potassium from cells with consequent increased sensitivity of nerve endings, this would make sense. (Skutsch, 1972.)

Section C: Hypothesis

Chapter 34

THE ROLE OF PROLACTIN IN HUMAN PHYSIOLOGY AND DISEASE

In the last five years our knowledge of human prolactin has expanded dramatically. Five years ago it seemed to be a hormone which although at one time vital for human survival was destined to become a vestigial hormone, killed by a bottle ! Now it is apparent that its roles in the body are many, with lactation being only one, and perhaps not the most important.

The outstanding feature of prolactin physiology - and this may well turn out to be true of other hormones as well - is that it never acts alone. It always functions in conjunction with at least one and often several other hormones. Pure and classical methods of endocrinology which attempt to look at the effect of one hormone in isolation will not in their strict purist form give much apart from negatives where prolactin is concerned. Prolactin will yield up its secrets only to the alchemist who is prepared to throw at least one other hormone into the soup!

Physiological actions of prolactin

As yet the basic actions of prolactin on protein, carbohydrate, lipid and other metabolic pathways have been barely studied. When they are it may well be found that prolactin is a hormone whose importance is on a level with that of insulin, growth hormone or cortisol and that many of the anomalies which are at present only too obvious may become more amenable when prolactin is added to the brew.

As far as actions on specific target organs are concerned, the best established ones seem to be those on the mammary gland, the kidney, the steroid-synthesising glands and the male accessory glands. Less well studied are effects on the uterus, the hematopoietic system and on the brain. There are reasons for believing that prolactin may in some way be involved in the body's defence system. The best documented is its rapid secretion in response to stressful stimuli of almost any kind. Much less well documented is the possibility that a particular role may be in the elimination of certain forms of infection and of small groups of neoplastic cells.

With all these physiological actions of prolactin there are two outstanding points to be noted:

1. The effects of prolactin consistently depend on interactions with other hormones and those of other hormones depend on interactions with prolactin. Frequently prolactin seems to be in the position of amplifying or even of changing the direction of the effect of another hormone on a target tissue. This has been most clearly shown in the case of the interaction between prolactin, aldosterone and ADH at renal level.

2. The effects of prolactin may often be partially or completely imitated by other hormones. Again this has been particularly clearly shown in the case of the kidney where oxytocin has actions which in some respects are very similar to those of prolactin.

Since prolactin can in many ways be imitated and since patients with an isolated prolactin deficiency or an isolated excess due to a prolactin-secreting tumor rarely show any serious disabilities or abnormalities, it may well be asked whether the multifarious actions of prolactin are of much significance. The question can only be answered in the context of an endocrine system composed of many interlocking components which has been shaped by hundreds of millions of years of evolution. In such a system it is probable that there are several semi-independent ways of tackling any problem which is of genuinely vital significance. It is also probable that destruction of any one of these will leave the overall system working near normally. But this is very far from saying that the system destroyed is of no significance even though the overall mechanism still functions. The principle is very close to the fail-safe or redundancy principle so familiar to designers of all types of modern electronic control equipment. The point of this is that vital circuits may be independently duplicated or even triplicated so that if one or two of the circuits cease to function, the machinery as a whole will not fail. In a spacecraft, for example, there may be three independent circuits controlling temperature. Two of these can fail and the spacecraft temperature will remain normal. But try telling the spacemen that the two destroyed circuits were therefore of no significance! Yet this form of reasoning is all too frequently applied by physiologists working on control systems which are almost certainly considerably more complicated than those of a spacecraft.

The fact that the overall system can work near normally in the presence of an excess or a deficiency of a hormone is therefore no good reason for denying the hormone a role in the system. What role then does prolactin play? It seems to me that the most likely possibility is that its primary function is to amplify or to attenuate when appropriate, the actions of hormones which by themselves might be functioning either inadequately or excessively. Thus in the presence of a partial deficiency of aldosterone, when the aldosterone secreted would be insufficient by itself to produce adequate renal sodium retention, the action of the available aldosterone could be dramatically elevated by a rise in prolactin secretion. In the presence of an aldosterone-secreting tumor the effect of the excess aldosterone on renal function may be mitigated by reducing prolactin secretion and so effectively abolishing the powerful sodium-retaining effects of the steroid. Excess cortisol secretion may diminish prolactin secretion and so reduce the effect on ACTH on the adrenal: diminished cortisol secretion may have the opposite effect.

Thus a deficiency or an excess of almost any of the hormones with which prolactin interacts may be at least partially compensated for by changes in prolactin levels. The change in prolactin levels will of course attenuate or amplify the actions of all the other normally working hormones: the homeostatic mechanisms will then produce appropriate changes in the levels of these hormones and the end result will be that the functioning of the whole system has been slightly modified in order to compensate for the one malfunctioning unit. A primary and sustained deficiency or excess of prolactin itself will have little apparent effect provided that all the other hormonal mechanisms are working adequately. They will simply adjust levels up or down in order to compensate for the abnormal attenuation or amplification of their action. On the other hand rapid changes in prolactin levels will be much more difficult to cope with. The endocrine system may be thrown into something approaching chaos as it attempts to compensate for rapid alterations in the tissue effectiveness of a given hormone secretion rate.

Apart from the situation of rapid change, hormonal regulation in the steady state will break down if a hormone deficiency or excess is too extreme to be compensated by changes in prolactin levels. Prolactin, for example, may be able to amplify the action of small amounts of ACTH by increasing precursor supply but it cannot compensate for a total lack of ACTH. In the presence of a small excess of ADH and water retention prolactin may compensate by a falling level which will reduce the effect of the ADH on the kidneys. This will also reduce the effect of aldosterone whose secretion rate will tend to rise in compensation. But if the excess of ADH is such that prolactin falls to a level where mineralocorticoids have little or no renal action, then salt loss will ensue.

The other situation when hormonal regulation will break down is when two or more hormonal defects are present simultaneously. The prolactin mechanism may compensate for one but unless the other requires a prolactin shift of the same magnitude and in the same direction it cannot compensate for the second simultaneously. Sometimes in compensating for one hormonal problem another, not apparent in the uncompensated state, may be revealed. A possible example of this may occur during chlorpropamide therapy for diabetes mellitus. Evidence has been presented to suggest that this may stimulate prolactin secretion. This would be expected to amplify the effect of ADH, among other hormones, and to lead to water retention. Most people, however, presumably with a normally flexible control of ADH secretion do not run into any difficulty and seem able to reduce their ADH secretion appropriately. About 4% of individuals do not and may run into difficulties because of excess water retention. The chlorpropamide in these individuals exposes an endocrine defect which would not normally have become apparent.

Are there any actions which are carried out by prolactin alone and which cannot by duplicated by other hormones? It seems probable that the action on the mammary gland comes into this category. Two women with apparent prolactin deficiency as shown by sensitive bioassay were identified initially because of a failure to lactate. Another possible effect which may be specific to prolactin alone is the potassium-rataining action. The body may be able to compensate for the retaining action of high prolactin levels by means of the kaliuretic action of the mineralocorticoids: it may not be able to compensate for the reverse disturbance in potassium metabolism occurring in the absence of prolactin. The two women with prolactin deficiency both suffered from recurrent muscular weakness which can be a feature of disturbances in potassium metabolism.

The action of prolactin on potassium therefore deserves intensive exploration. Mineralocorticoids at the kidney cause potassium loss and they stimulate the movements of potassium into cells. Prolactin at the kidney causes potassium retention: if its cellular action is also opposite to that of mineralocorticoids it should cause potassium to move out of cells. The overall effect might therefore be expected to be reduction of intracellular potassium, increase of extracellular potassium and reduction of potassium excretion. The last two effects might interact in a complicated way as a result of increased delivery of potassium to the renal tubules. It is interesting to speculate on the possibility that the intracellular potassium loss occuring in the "sick cell syndrome" which not infrequently develops in those with, for example, congestive cardiac or hepatic failure, may be partly attributed to the elevated prolactin levels which are probably present in these conditions.

It is possible that these effects of prolactin may have profound consequences on neuromuscular function. An elevation of extracellular and diminution of intracellular potassium concentrations would tend to depolarise nerve fibres making them themselves more easily excited but also able to release smaller amounts of transmitter. The overall effect on the central nervous system might well be a depression of activity coupled with an increased susceptibility to the development of epileptic attacks. This of course is typical of the situation seen during phenothiazine therapy when prolactin levels are high.

Equally interesting are the possible effects in muscle, particularly heart muscle. The depletion of intracellular potassium would in the initial stages make heart muscle more excitable and more likely to develop arrhythmias but later would tend to produce a complete loss of excitability. Again the possibility that such changes may be important in arrhythmias occurring during anesthesia and surgery should not be overlooked. Particularly striking is the fact that every one of the cases of hypoaldosteronism so far reported has been accompanied by some form of cardiac arrhythmia, usually heart block. Here the unopposed actions of prolactin, probably present in high concentration in compensation for the lack of aldosterone, would be expected to produce particularly serious effects on potassium metabolism.

Some of the effects of prolactin on smooth muscle might also be explained on this sort of basis. Again prolactin would be expected to produce first an increase in excitability with depolarisation and then a loss of all activity. We have noticed that very frequently prolactin causes a flurry of increased activity on initially adding it to a bath containing a uterine strip but that very soon this dies away and a prolonged inhibition of activity develops. (figure 2)

The relationships between oxytocin and prolactin are interesting because at three separate end organs there is some evidence that they may imitate one another or compete for similar receptor sites. At the kidney under conditions when aldosterone causes sodium excretion and ADH causes water excretion either prolactin or oxytocin may restore the sodium-retaining effect of aldosterone and the water-retaining effect of ADH. This presumably indicates that prolactin and oxytocin can occupy similar renal receptor sites. In contrast in more normal situat oxytocin may have a natriuretic action: this might possibly be explained if it is inherently a less effective molecule than prolactin and competes with prolactin for receptor sites.

The other examples of prolactin-oxytocin interaction are less direct and clear-cut. In the mammary gland oxytocin may slow down or prevent the involution which normally takes place after prolactin withdrawal. It was this effect which was similar enough to a prolactin action which led to Benson and Folley's probably mistaken conclusion that oxytocin injections could promote prolactin secretion: at that time they did not believe that oxytocin could have such a prolactin-like effect on the mammary gland. In the uterus too there is some evidence of an interaction since prolactin may inhibit oxytocin-induced contractions though that in itself is no evidence whatsoever of an interaction at receptor level.

If prolactin and oxytocin can indeed occupy the same receptor sites then this indicates that at least for some types of activity most of the constituents of the prolactin molecule may be redundant. This seems most nearly true of the kidney where the effects of the two hormones in animals treated with cortisol or a high salt intake are virtually identical apart from the fact that the action of a single dose of prolactin seems much more prolonged than that of a single dose of oxytocin. The prolonged action suggests the possibility that one of the functions of the larger molecular size may be in some way to stabilise the binding of the hormone to its receptor site. Oxytocin would then be a short-acting and prolactin a long-acting hormone.

Prolactin and disease

Prolactin may be involved in disease in several different ways. First, as with other hormones there could be a primary deficit or excess of the hormone. A prolactin deficit is likely to have only limited effects since many of the actions of prolactin on target organs may be imitated and compensated for by other hormones. Provided that the other endocrine control mechanisms are functioning normally the only consequences of a prolactin deficiency are likely to be disturbances in potassium metabolism and a failure of lactation. The lack of prolactin might be likely to lead to renal potassium loss and an excess of intracellular potassium.

An isolated excess of prolactin would be likely to have even less effect than an isolated deficiency provided that other parts of the endocrine system were functioning normally. An excess of prolactin can be compensated for by appropriate secretion or suppression of all the hormones with which prolactin interacts.

Despite this apparent lack of pathophysiological consequences prolactin may be important in disease in a number of ways. First of all in situations where there is another hormonal abnormality, an excess or deficiency of prolactin secretion may lead to pathological situations which are obviously extensions of normal physiology. Some examples of this are as follows:

1. In the presence of an isolated excess of ADH, the consequent water retention may lead to suppression of prolactin secretion with failure of the normal interaction between prolactin and aldosterone. Excessive salt loss will then occur.

2. An isolated aldosterone deficiency will lead to an excess of prolactin secretion in an attempt to compensate for the sodium loss. This will lead to excessive potassium retention.

3. An excess of aldosterone secretion will lead to sodium retention, suppression of prolactin secretion and a loss of the normal sodium-retaining effect of mineralocorticoids. The suppression of prolactin secretion will lead to excessive potassium loss.

4. In any situation when there is a combined elevation of prolactin secretion with that of ADH and/or aldosterone there will be abnormal renal retention of fluid

and electrolytes with the development of edema.

5. An excess of adrenal glucocorticoid secretion may lead to a suppression of prolactin secretion with potassium loss and a failure of the normal sodium-retaining effect of mineralocorticoids.

6. A failure of adrenal steroid secretion will lead to an excess of prolactin secretion which may lead to potassium retention and a failure of normal water excretion.

7. Primary hypothyroidism may lead to elevated prolactin secretion as a result of excess TRH secretion. This may lead to increased water retention.

8. In any situation in which prolactin levels are elevated, provided that the other endocrine conditions are correct, galactorrhea may occur.

It is conceivable that in the future a number of other pathophysiological problems caused by prolactin in conjunction with other hormones may be demonstrated. The most likely area for this to happen may be in the field of carbohydrate metabolism where some forms of diabetes may perhaps be caused by excess prolactin secretion.

The effects of prolactin so far discussed will probably occur in all individuals, irrespective of constitution, who are exposed to the appropriate levels of prolactin and other hormones. It seems possible that there may be a whole range of other diseases which may be precipitated by a given level of prolactin in those individuals who are constitutionally susceptible. At the same level of prolactin, most other people who are not constitutionally susceptible to the disease will not develop it. In these diseases the relationship between prolactin and the appearance of the disease is not a simple and conventional causal one. It is much more akin to the relationship between smoking and lung cancer or to that between use of a relatively safe drug and the appearance of untoward side effects in a small proportion of users. In the sense that smoking causes lung cancer and drugs cause side effects, prolactin may be said to cause these diseases. But this does not mean that in any given population prolactin levels will necessarily be higher in those who develop the diseases. What it does mean is that if prolactin is involved, lowering the prolactin level, even though that level may not appear to be particularly elevated, should prevent or alleviate the disease process. With this type of disease a simple study of the relationship between prolactin levels and the disease can never hope to give definitive results because prolactin levels may be the same in those with and without the disease yet in spite of this prolactin will be responsible for the appearance of the disease in susceptible persons. The only definitive way to get an answer is to manipulate deliberately the prolactin levels in a diseased population and to look for changes in the disease process. If prolactin is involved, a lowering of prolactin levels will in some of the diseased individuals produce objective improvement: this may occur even if prolactin levels in the diseased population are apparently normal before treatment. It is very likely that with this type of pathological process, end organ sensitivity is more important than plasma levels of the hormone.

The diseases which may be of this type are many. They include migraine, asthma, epilepsy, rheumatoid arthritis, collagen diseases, some forms of mental illness, myocardial infarction and other forms of thrombo-embolic diseases. The striking thing about this is that it is almost a definitive list of those illnesses where very little progress has been made in recent years in spite of a colossal expenditure of money on research. For this reason alone it might be thought worthwhile to investigate a radically new concept, namely that these diseases may all be precipitated by prolactin acting in individuals who are constitutionally susceptible. A further reason for looking at the idea is that if it is correct, a method of treatment is already available in the form of 2-bromo-α-ergokryptine which seems to be a specific suppressor of prolactin secretion.

I fully admit that the hypothesis is somewhat wild and very unlikely to be true. However, Popper has pointed out that provided that a hypothesis is testable, improbability is actually a virtue. If a probable hypothesis turns out to be true the advance made is inevitably relatively small. If an improbable hypothesis turns out to be true, the resultant complete revolution in thought leads to dramatic advances. I sometimes feel that grant-giving bodies should set some money aside for the support of ideas which, although highly improbable would if true lead to tremendous advances. Clearly I have a vested interest here, but the prolactin hypothesis is immediately testable and if it proves true will lead to immediate and dramatic advances in therapy in a whole range of diseases in which morale of both patients and doctors tends to be low because of the relative lack of progress. I hope therefore that many scientists will be stimulated to start work in this area.

Finally I should like to raise the question of what prolactin is doing when its secretion rate rises in response to virtually any form of stress. To take a strictly teleological approach, it would be surprising if it were not doing something and I should like to suggest that it may be doing at least three different things, mobilising metabolic resources to cope with the situation, preventing loss of fluid and electrolytes, and also in some way stimulating the mechanisms which help to eliminate viruses, foreign cells and malignant cells from the body. It is interesting that there appear to be a number of situations where prolactin secretion may be elevated and where there is a reduced incidence of cancer. The proposition that prolactin may be involved in stimulating the body's defences against cancer should also be relatively easy to test since drugs like chlorpromazine which are powerful stimulators of prolactin secretion are readily available. It should be possible for example to test the effectiveness of radiotherapy plus chlorpromazine treatment against radiotherapy plus placebo or to test the effect of giving chlorpromazine for two months post-operatively to those undergoing surgery for malignant disease. Again the hypothesis is highly improbable but again it is readily testable and could immediately lead to advances in therapy.

REFERENCES

Adamopoulos, D.A., Loraine, J.A., Lunn, S.F., Coppen, A.J., Daly, R.J. Endocrine profiles in premenstrual tension. Clinical Endocr., 1, 283-92, 1972.

Adams, P.W., Wynn, V., Rose, D.P., Seed, M., Folkard, J., Strong, R. Effect of pyridoxine hydrochloride (vitamin B6) upon depression associated with oral contraception. Lancet 1, 897-904, 1973.

Ahmad, A.B.J., George, B.C., Gonzalez-Auvert, C., Dingman, J.F. Increased plasma arginine-vasopressin in clinical adrenocortical insufficiency and its inhibition by glucosteroids. J. Clin. Invest., 46, 111, 1967.

Ahmad, N., Lyons, W.R. Lactation in pituitary autografted rats. Endocrinology, 78, 837-44, 1966.

Ahmad, N., Lyons, W.R. Effects of sibling and non-sibling pituitary grafts and ovine luteotrophic hormone in Long-Evans female rats. Proc. Soc. Exp. Biol. Med., 140, 765-9, 1972.

Ahmad, N., Lyons, W.R., Ellis, S. Luteotrophic activity of rat hypophysial mammotrophin. Endocrinology, 85, 378-80, 1969.

Ajika, K., Kalra, S.P., Fawcett, C.P., Krulich, L., McCann, S.M. The effect of stress and nembutal on plasma levels of gonadotropins and prolactin in ovariectomised rats. Endocrinology, 90, 707-15, 1972.

Ajika, K., Krulich, L., Fawcett, C.P., McCann, S.M. Effects of estrogen on plasma and pituitary gonadotropins and prolactin and on hypothalamic releasing and inhibiting factors. Neuroendocrinology, 9, 304-15, 1972.

Akikusa, Y. Effect of starvation on synthesis and release of growth hormone and prolactin in the rat anterior pituitary. Endocrinol. Jap., 18, 411-16, 1971.

Alexander, D.P., Britton, H.G., Buttle, H.L., Nixon, D.A. Prolactin in the sheep foetus. Res. Vet. Sci., 13, 188-9, 1972.

Amenomori, Y., Chen, C.L., Meites, J. Serum prolactin levels in rats during different reproductive states. Endocrinology, 86, 506-10, 1970.

Amenomori, Y., Meites, J. Effects of a hypothalamic extract on serum prolactin levels during the estrus cycle and lactation. Proc. Soc. Exp. Biol. Med., 134, 492-5, 1970.

Anderson, L.L., Peters, J.B., Melampy, R.M., Cox, D.F. Changes in adenohypophysial cells and levels of somatotrophin and prolactin at different reproductive stages in the pig. J. Reprod. Fertil., 28, 55-65, 1972.

Anderson, M.S., Bowers, C.Y., Kastin, A.J., Schalch, D.S.,Schally, A.V., Snyder, P.J., Utiger, R.D., Wilber, J.F., Wise, A.J. Synthetic thyrotropin releasing hormone: a potent stimulator of thyrotropin secretion in man. New Eng. J. Med., 285, 1279-83, 1971.

Angrist, B.M., Gershon, S., Levitan, S.J., Blumberg, A.G. Lithium-induced diabetes insipidus-like syndrome. Compr. Psychiat., 11, 141, 1970.

Angst, J. Zur frage der psychosen bei behandlung mit disulfiram. Schweiz. Med. Wschr. 86, 1304-6, 1956.

Antliff, H.R., Prasad, M.R., Meyer, R.K. Action of prolactin on seminal vesicles of guinea pig. Proc. Soc. Exp. Biol. Med., **103**, 77-80, 1960.

Apostolakis, M. Prolactin. Vitam. Horm. **26**, 197, 1968.

Apostolakis, M., Kapetanakis, S., Lazos, G., Madena-Pyrgaki, A. Plasma prolactin activity in patients with galactorrhea after treatment with psychotropic drugs. pp. 349-354 in Lactogenic Hormones, ed. G.E.W. Wolstenholme and J. Knight, Churchill Livingstone, 1972

Arai, Y., Lee, T.H. A double antibody radioimmunoassay procedure for ovine pituitary prolactin Endocrinology, **81**, 1041-6, 1967.

Arai, Y., Suzuki, Y. Biphasic lactogenic response of male rat mammary glands after a single injection of reserpine. J. Endocrinol., **50**, 697-8, 1971.

Arai, Y., Suzuki, Y., Masuda, S. Effects of ergocornine on reserpine-induced lactogenic response of male rat mammary glands. Endocrinol. Jap. **19**, 111-4, 1972.

Argonz, J., Del Castillo, E.B. A syndrome characterised by estrogenic insufficiency, galactorrhea and decreased urinary gonadotropin. J. Clin. Endocr., **13**, 79-87, 1953.

Arimura, A., Dunn, J.D., Schally, A.V. Effect of infusion of hypothalamic extracts on serum prolactin levels in rats treated with nembutal, CNS depressants or bearing hypothalamic lesions. Endocrinology, **90**, 378-83, 1972.

Arimura, A., Saito, T., Muller, E.E., Bowers, C.Y., Sawano, S., Schally, A.V. Absence of prolactin-release inhibiting activity in highly purified LH-releasing factor. Endocrinology, **80**, 972-4, 1967.

Armstrong, D.T., Greep, R.O. Effect of gonadotrophic hormones on glucose metabolism by luteinized rat ovaries. Endocrinology, **70**, 701-10, 1962.

Armstrong, D.T., King, E.R. Uterine progesterone metabolism and progestational response: effects of estrogen and prolactin. Endocrinology, **89**, 191-7, 1971.

Armstrong, D.T., Knudsen, K.A., Miller, L.S. Effects of prolactin upon cholesterol metabolism and progesterone biosynthesis in corpera lutea of rats hypophysectemised during pregnancy. Endocrinology, **86**, 634-41, 1970.

Armstrong, D.T. Miller, L.S., Knudsen, K.A. Regulation of lipid metabolism and progesterone production in rat corpera lutea and ovarian interstitial elements by prolactin and luteinizing hormone. Endocrinology, **85**, 393-401, 1969.

Aron, M., Marescaux, J. Hypothalamic control of the secretion of prolactin in the guinea pig. C.R. Soc. Biol. (Paris), **156**, 1916-18, 1962.

Arroyo, H., Aubert, L. Hypersecretion of prolactin in hypothyroidism. Presse. Med. **79**, 146, 1971.

Asano, M. Studies on urinary prolactin with special reference to carcinoma of the prostate. Jap. J. Urol., **53**, 901-18, 1962.

Asano, M. Basic experimental studies of the pituitary prolactin-prostate inter-relationship. J. Urol., **93**, 87-93, 1965.

Asano, M., Kanzaki, S., Sekiguchi, E., Tasaka, T. Inhibition of prostatic growth in rabbits with anti-ovine prolactin serum. J. Urol. **106**, 248-52, 1971.

Astarabadi, T. The effect of growth and lactogenic hormones on renal compensatory hypertrophy in hypophysectomised rats. Quent. J. Exp. Physiol., **48**, 85-92, 1963.

Atkins, H.J.B., Bulbrook, R.D., Falconer, M.A., Hayward, T.L., Maclean, K.S., Schurr, P.H. Ten years experience of steroid assays in the management of breast cancer. Lancet, **ii**, 1255-60, 1968.

Atkins, H.J.B., Bulbrook, R.D., Falconer, M.A., Hayward, J.L., Maclean, K.S., Schurr, P.H. Usefulness of discriminant functions. Lancet, **ii**, 1260-63, 1968.

Aubry, R.H., Nankin, H.R., Moses, A.M., Streeten, D.H.P. Measurement of osmotic threshold for vasopressin release in human subjects and its modification by cortisol. J. Clin. Endocr., **25**, 1481, 1965.

August, J.T., Nelson, D.H., Thorn, G.W. Response of normal subjects to large amounts of aldosterone. J. Clin. Invest., **37**, 1549-1555, 1958.

Averill, R.L. Failure of luteotrophic function due to pituitary grafts in the rat hypothalamus. Neuroendocrinology, **5**, 121-31, 1969.

Baird, D.T. Effect of luteinising hormone, follicle stimulating hormone and prolactin on steroid secretion by the autotransplanted ovary of the ewe. J. Endocr., **43**, xviii-xix, 1969

Baer, L., Platman, S.R., Fieve, R.R. The role of electrolytes in affective disorders. Arch. Gen. Psychiat., **22**, 108-113, 1970.

Bagshawe, K.D., Curtis, J.R., Garnett, E.S. Effect of prolonged hydrocortisone administration on potassium metabolism. Lancet **1**, 18-21, 1965.

Baldwin, R.L., Martin, R.J. Protein and nucleic acid synthesis in rat mammary gland during early lactation. Endocrinology, **82**, 1209-16, 1968.

Barger, A.C., Berlin, R.D., Tulenko, J.F. Infusion of aldosterone, 9-α-fluorohydrocortisone into the renal artery of normal and adrenalectomized dogs: effect on electrolyte and water excretion. Endocrinol., **62**, 804-15, 1958.

Barker, J.R., Richmond, C. Breast carcinoma culture. A reliable method and study of hormonal effects. Br. J. Surg., **58**, 302, 1971a.

Barker, J.R., Richmond, C. Human breast carcinoma culture: the effects of hormones. Br. J. Surg., **58**, 732-4, 1971b.

Barnawell, E.B. Analysis of the direct action of prolactin and steroids on mammary tissue of the dog in organ culture. Endocrinology, **80**, 1083-9, 1967.

Bartke, A. Influence of prolactin on male fertility in dwarf mice. J. Endocr., **35**, 419-20, 1966.

Bartke, A. Influence of pituitary homografts on the weight of seminal vesicles in castrated mice. J. Endocr., **38**, 195-6, 1967.

Bartke, A. Effects of prolactin and luteinizing hormone on the cholesterol stores in the mouse testis. J. Endocr., **49**, 317-24, 1971a.

Bartke, A. The maintenance of gestation and initiation of lactation in the mouse in the absence of pituitary prolactin. J. Reprod. Fertil., **27**, 121-4, 1971b.

Bartke, A. Effects of prolactin on spermatogenesis in hypophysectomised mice. J. Endocr., **49**, 311-6, 1971c.

Bartke, A., Lloyd, C.W. Influence of prolactin and pituitary isografts on spermatogenesis in dwarf mice and hypophysectomised rats. J. Endocr., **46**, 321-9, 1970.

Bartosik, D., Romanoff, E.G., Watson, D.J., Scricco, E. Luteotrophic effects of prolactin in the bovine ovary. Endocrinology, **81**, 186-94, 1967.

Bast, J.D., Melampy, R.M. Luteinizing hormone, prolactin and ovarian 20 α-hydroxysteroid dehydrogenose levels during pregnancy and pseudopregnancy in the rat. Endocrinology, **91**, 1499, 1972.

Bates, R.W. Species difference in hormonal control of intestinal weight and food intake of rats and pigeons. Proc. Soc. Exp. Biol. Med., **120**, 721-4, 1965.

Bates, R.W. Delay of hormonally induced diabetes by amino-glutethimide and metyrapone in partially pancreatectomized rats having transplantable pituitary tumours. Concomitant failure to prevent splanchnomegaly. Endocrinology, **86**, 107-19, 1970.

Bates, R.W., Milkovic, S.M.S., Garrison, M.M. Concentration of prolactin, growth hormone and ACTH in blood and tumor of rats with transplantable mammotropic pituitary tumors. Endocrinology, **71**, 943-8, 1962.

Bates, R.W., Milkovic, S.M.S., Garrison, M.M. Effects of prolactin, growth hormone and ACTH alone and in combination upon organ weights and adrenal function in normal rats. Endocrinology, **74**, 714-723, 1964.

Bates, R.W., Scow, R.O., Lacy, P.E. Induction of permanent diabetes in rats by pituitary hormones from a transplantable mammotropic tumour, changes in organ weights and the effect of adrenalectomy. Endocrinology, **78**, 826-36, 1966.

Bayle, T.D. Hypothalamic regulation of the secretion of prolactin in birds. Arch. Anat. Micr. Morph. Exp., **58**, 375-86, 1969.

Bayliss, P.F.C., Van't Hoff, W. Amenorrhea and galactorrhea associated with hypothyroidism. Lancet, ii, 1399-1400, 1969.

Beck, J.C., Gonda, A., Hamid, M.A., Morgen, R.O., Rubinstein, D., McGarry, E.E. Some metabolic changes induced by primate growth hormone and purified ovine prolactin. Metabolism, **13**, 1108-34, 1964.

Behrman, H.R., Orczyk, G.P., Macdonald, G.J., Greep, R.O. Prolactin induction of enzymes controlling luteal cholesterol ester turnover. Endocrinology, **87**, 1251-6, 1970.

Belanger, C., Shome, B., Friesen, H., Myers, R. Studies of the secretion of monkey placental lactogen. J. Clin. Invest., **50**, 2660-7, 1971.

Belkin, M., Hardy, W.G. Effect of reserpine and chlorpromazine on sarcoma 37, Science, **125**, 233-4, 1957.

Ben-David, M., Danon, A., Benveniste, R., Weller, C.P., Sulman, F.G. Results of radio-immunoassay of rat pituitary and serum prolactin after adrenalectomy and perphenazine treatment in rats, J. Endocr., **50**, 599-606, 1971.

Ben-David, M., Danon, A., Sulman, F.G. Acute changes in blood and pituitary prolactin after a single injection of perphenazine, Neuroendocrinology, **6**, 336-42, 1970.

Ben-David, M., Danon, A., Sulman, F.G. Evidence for antagonism between prolactin and gonadotrophin secretion: effect of methalibure on perphenazine-induced prolactin secretion in ovariectomised rats. J. Endocr. **51**, 719-25, 1971.

Ben-David, M., Dikstein, S., Sulman, F.G. Effect of different steroids on prolactin secretion in pituitary-hypothalamus organ co-culture, Proc. Soc. Exp. Biol. Med., **117**, 511-3, 1964.

Ben-David, M., Dikstein, S., Sulman, F.G. Production of lactation by non-sedative pheno-thiazine derivatives. Proc. Soc. Exp. Biol. Med., **118**, 265-70, 1965.

Ben-David, M., Heston, W.E., Rodbard, D. Mammary tumour potentiation of endogenous prolactin effect on mammary gland differentiation, J. Nat. Cancer Inst., **42**, 207-18, 1969.

Bengmark, S., Hesselsjo, R. The combined effect of prolactin and androsterone on the growth of rat seminal vesicle tissue in vitro. Urol. Intern., **16**, 387-90, 1963.

Bengmark, S., Hesselsjo, R. Endocrine dependence of rat seminal vesicle tissue in vitro. Urol. Intern., 17, 84-92, 1964.

Benson, G.K., Folley, S.J. Oxytocin as stimulator for the release of prolactin from the anterior pituitary. Nature, 177, 700, 1956.

Bergenstal, D.M., Lipsett, M.B. The anabolic effect of sheep prolactin in man. J. Clin. Invest., **37**, 877, 1958.

Berle, P., Apostolakis, M. Prolactin in human plasma during pregnancy and puerperium. Acta Endocrinol., (Kbh), **67**, 63-72, 1971.

Berle, P., Apostolakis, M. Prolactin concentrations under physiological and pathological conditions. Arch. Gynaekol., **211**, 220-1, 1971.

Berle, P., Apostolakis, M., Link, A. Lactotropic activity in human plasma during the menstrual cycle. Arch Gynaekol., **210**, 124-30, 1971.

Berle, P., Voigt, K.D. Plasma prolactin concentrations in women with breast cancer. Acta Endocr. (Kbh), Suppl., **159**, 38, 1972.

Bern, H.A., Nicoll, C.S. The comparative endocrinology of prolactin. Recet. Progr. Horm, Res., **24**, 681-720, 1968.

Berswordt-Wallrabe, I. von., Herlyn, U., Flaskamp, D., Hellige, G. Bioassay of the lactotropic hormone and its applicability in man. Arch. Gynaekol, **209**, 380-95, 1971.

Berswordt-Wallrabe, I. von., Herlyn, U., Jantzen, K. A modification of the pigeon crop sac assay for determination of lactogenic hormone in human serum. Acta Endocrinol (Kbh) Suppl., **100**, 169, 1965.

Berswordt-Wallrabe, I. von., Jantzen, K. Prolactin content of the blood serum before and after ovulation as measured by the pigeon crop test. Arch. Gynaekol., **202**, 238-9, 1965.

Berswordt-Wallrabe, R. von., Scheuer, A., Dahnke, H.G., Mosebach, K.O. Influence of prolactin and progesterone on nucleic acid metabolism in the prostate, vesicular gland and ductus deferens of juvenile hypophysectomised rats and orchidectomised rats. Acta Endocrinol. (Suppl) (Kbh), **152**, 7, 1971.

Besser, G.M., Edwards, C.R.W. Galactorrhoea..Brit. Med. J., **2**, 280-2, 1972.

Besser, G.M., Parke, L., Edwards, C.R.W., Forsyth, I.A., McNeilly, A.S. Galactorrhoea: successful treatment with reduction of plasma prolactin levels by bromo-ergocryptine. Brit. Med. J., **3**, 669-72, 1972.

Betts, T.A., Kalra, P.L., Cooper, R., Jeavons, P.M. Epileptic fits as a side effect of amitriptyline. Lancet **1**, 390-2, 1968.

Bewley, T.A., Li, C.H. Primary Structures of human pituitary growth hormone and sheep pituitary lactogenic hormone compared. Science, **168**, 1361-2, 1970.

Bewley, T.A., Li, C.H. Sequence comparison of human pituitary growth hormone, human chorionic somatomammotropin and ovine pituitary lactogenic hormone. Experientia, **27**, 1368-71, 1971.

Bewley, T.A., Li, C.H. Circular dichroism studies on human pituitary growth hormone and ovine pituitary lactogenic hormone. Biochem., **11**, 884-8, 1972.

Biglieri, E.G., Schambelan, M., Slaton, P.E., Stockigt, J.R. The intercurrent hypertension of primary aldosteronism. Circ. Res. **26-27**, Suppl. I, 195-202, 1970.

Billeter, E., Fluckiger, E. Evidence for a luteolytic function of prolactin in the intact cyclic rat using 2-Br- α -ergokryptine (CB 154), Experientia, **27**, 464-5, 1971.

Birge, C.A., Jacobs, L.S., Hammer, C.T., Daughaday, W.H. Catecholamine inhibition of prolactin secretion by isolated rat adenohypophyses. Endocrinology, **86**, 120-130, 1970.

Birkinshaw, M., Falconer, I.R. The localization of prolactin labelled with radioactive iodine in rabbit mammary tissue. J. Endocr., **55**, 323-334, 1972.

Bishop, W., Fawcett, C.P., Krulich, L., McCann, S.M. Acute and chronic effects of hypothalamic lesion on release of FSH, LH and prolactin in intact and castrated rats. Endocrinology, **91**, 643-56, 1972.

Bishop, W., Kalra, P.S., Fawcett, C.P., Krulich, L., McCann, S.M. The effects of hypothalamic lesions on the release of gonadotropins and prolactin in response to estrogen and progesterone treatment in female rats. Endocrinology, **91**, 1404-10, 1972.

Bishop, W., Orias, R., Fawcett, C.P., Krulich, L., McCann, S.M. Plasma gonadotropins and prolactin in pseudopregnancy in the rat. Proc. Soc. Exp. Biol. Med., **137**, 1411-4, 1971.

Blachly, P.H. Lithium content of drinking water and ischaemic heart disease. New Eng. J. Med. **281**, 682, 1969.

Black, D.A.K. Potassium metabolism. In *Clinical Disorders of Fluid and Electrolyte Metabolism*, pp. 121-149, ed. M.H. Maxwell, C.R. Kleeman, McGraw Hill, New York, 1972.

Blair-West, J.R., Coghlan, J.P., Denton, D.A., Funder, J.W., Nelson, J., Scoggins, B.A., Wright, R.D..Sodium homeostasis, salt appetite and hypertension. Circulation Res., **27**, Suppl. II, 251-266, 1970.

Blake, C.A., Sawyer, C.H. Nicotine blocks the suckling-induced rise in circulating prolactin in lactating rats. Science, **177**, 619-21, 1972.

Blake, C.A., Weiner, R.I., Sawyer, C.H. Pituitary prolactin secretion in female rats made persistently estrous or diestrous by hypothalamic deafferentation. Endocrinology, **90**, 862-71, 1972.

Blizzard, R.M., Drash, A.L., Jenkins, M.E., Spaudling, J.S., Glick, A., Weldon, V., Powell, G.F., Raiti, S. Comparative effects of animal prolactins and human growth hormone in hypopituitary children. J. Clin. Endocr. **26**, 852-8, 1966.

Boeskor, A., Gabbiani, G. Influence of hypophysectomy and pituitary hormones on dextran edema in rats. Endokrinologie, **53**, 217-21, 1968.

Bohr, H.H. The influence of different hormones on bone formation in rats. Acta Endocr., (Kbh), **58**, 116-22, 1968.

Bole, G.G., Friedlander, M.H., Smith, C.K. Rheumatic symptoms and serological abnormalities induced by oral contraceptives. Lancet **1**, 323, 1969.

Boler, J., Enzman, F., Folkers, K., Bowers, C.Y., Schally, A.V. The identity of chemical and hormonal properties of the thyrotropin releasing hormone and pyroglutamyl-histidyl-proline amide. Biochem. Biophys. Res. Commun., **37**, 705-10, 1969.

Bolton, C.E. Effect of prolactin and corticosterone on lipid synthesis by rabbit mammary gland explants. J. Endocr., **51**, xxi-ii, 1971.

Bolton, C.H., Hampton, J.R., Mitchell, J.R.A. Effect of oral contraceptive agents on platelets and phospholipids. Lancet **2**, 1336-41, 1968.

Bonnyns, M., Pasteels, J-L., Herlant, M., Van Haelst, L., Bastenie, P.A. Comparison between thyrotropin concentration and cell morphology of anterior pituitary in asymptomatic atrophic thyroiditis. J. Clin. Endocr., **35**, 722-28, 1972.

Boot, L.M. Prolactin and mammary gland carcinogenesis. The problem of human prolactin. Intern. J. Cancer, **5**, 167, 1970.

Bourdel, G., Champigny, O., Jacquot, R. Nutritional role of prolactin, progesterone and estradiol benzoate administered alone or in combination to castrated rats. Study of body composition. C.R. Acad. Sci. (Paris), **255**, 778-80, 1962.

Bowers, C.Y., Studies on the role of cyclic AMP in the release of anterior pituitary hormones. Ann. N Y Acad. Sci., **185**, 263-90, 1971.

Bowers, C.Y., Friesen, H.G., Folkers, K., On the mechanism of TRH-induced prolactin release. Clin. Res., **20**, 71, 1972.

Bowers, C.Y., Friesen, H.G., Hwang, P., Guyda, H.J., Folkers, K. Prolactin and thyrotropin release in man by synthetic pyroglutamyl-histidyl-prolinamide. Biochem. Biophys. Res. Commun., **45**, 1033-41, 1971.

Bowers, C.Y., Schally, A.V., Enzmann, F., Boler, J., Folkers, I.K. Porcine thyrotropin releasing hormone is (pyro) Glu-His-Pro (NH_2). Endocrinology, **86**, 1143-53, 1970.

Boyd, A.E., Lebovitz, H.E., Pfeiffer, J.B. Stimulation of human growth hormone secretion by L-Dopa. New Engl. J. Med., **283**, 1425-9, 1970.

Boyle, D., Bhatia, S.K., Hadden, D.R., Montgomery, D.A.D., Weaver, J.A. Ischaemic heart disease in diabetics. A prospective study. Lancet, **i**, 338-9, 1972.

Boyns, A.R., Cole, E.N., Golder, M.P., Danutra, V., Harper, M.E., Brownsey, B., Cowley, T., Jones, G.E., Griffiths, K..Prolactin studies with the prostate. In *Prolactin and Carcinogenesis. 4th Tenovus Workshop.* ed. A.R. Boyns and K. Griffiths. Alpha Omega Alpha Publishing Limited, Cardiff, 1972.

Boyns, A.R., Griffiths, K., eds. *Prolactin and Carcinogenesis. 4th Tenovus Workshop,* Alpha Omega Alpha Publishing Limited, Cardiff, 1972.

Braithwaite, R.A., Goulding, R., Theano, G., Bailey, J., Coppen, A. Clinical significance of plasma levels of tricyclic antidepressant drugs in the treatment of depression. Lancet **1**, 556-7, 1972.

Brauman, J., Brauman, H., Pasteels, J.L. Immunoassay of growth hormone in cultures of human hypophysis by the method of complement fixation: comparison of the growth hormone secretion and the prolactin activity. Nature (London), **202**, 1116-18, 1964.

Brenner, B.M., Berliner, R.W. Relationships between extracellular volume and fluid re-absorption by the rat nephron. Amer. J. Physiol., **217**, 6-12, 1969.

Brewer, J.I. Rhythmic changes in the skin capillaries and their relation to menstruation. Amer. J. Obstet. Gynec. **36**, 597-610, 1938.

British Medical Journal. Diabetes and menstruation. Brit. Med. J., **4**, 699, 1970.

British Medical Journal. Strokes and the pill. Brit. Med. J., **1**, 733, 1969.

Browning, H.G., Brown, A.L., Crisp, T.E., Gibbs, W.E. Response of ovarian isografts to purified FSH, LH and LTH in partially and completely hypophysectomized mice. Texas Rep. Biol. Med., **23**, 715-28, 1965.

Browning, H.C., Guzman, R. Intraocular ovarian isografts in female rats and their response to gonadotropins and to pituitary isografts. Endocrinology, **81**, 1311-8, 1967.

Bruce, J., Russell, G.F.M. Premenstrual tension: a study of weight changes and balances of water, sodium and potassium. Lancet, **ii**, 267, 1962.

Brumby, H.I., Forsyth, I.A. Bioassay of prolactin un the blood of goats at parturition. J. Endocr., **43**, xxiii-iv, 1969.

Bruni, J.E., Montemurro, D.G. Effect of hypothalmic lesions on the genesis of spontaneous mammary gland tumours in the mouse. Cancer Res., **31**, 854-60, 1971.

Bryant, G.D., Connan, R.M., Greenwood, F.C. Changes in plasma prolactin induced by acepromazine in sheep. J. Endocr., **41**, 613-4, 1968.

Bryant, E.E., Douglas, B.H., Ashburn, A.D. The effect of prolactin on blood pressure, blood volume and angiotensin response. J.Lab. Clin. Med., **78**, 795-6, 1971.

Bryant, G.D., Greenwood, F.C. Radioimmunoassay for ovine, caprine and bovine prolactin in plasma and tissue extracts. Biochem. J., **109**, 831-40, 1968.

Bryant, G.D., Greenwood, F.C. The concentrations of human prolactin in plasma measured by radioimmunoassay: experimental and physiological modifications; pp. 197-206, in *Lactogenic Hormones,* ed. G.E.W. Wolstenholme and J. Knight, Churchill Livingstone, 1972.

Bryant, G.D., Greenwood, F.C., Kann, G., Martinet, J., Denamur, R. Plasma prolactin in the oestrous cycle of the ewe: effect of pituitary stalk section. J.Endocr., **51**, 405-6, 1971.

Bryant, G.D., Greenwood, F.C., Linzell, J.L. Plasma prolactin levels in the goat: physiological and experimental modification. J. Endocr., **40**, iv-v, 1968.

Bryant, G.D., Linzell, J.L., Greenwood, F.C. Plasma prolactin in goats measured by radioimmunoassay: the effects of teat stimulation, mating behaviour, stress, fasting and of oxytocin, insulin and glucose injections. Hormones, **1**, 26-35, 1970.

Bryant, G.D., Siler, T.M., Greenwood, F.C., Pasteels, J.L., Robyn, C., Hubinont, P.O. Radioimmunoassay of a human pituitary prolactin in plasma. Hormones, **2**, 139-152, 1971.

Bulbrook, R.D., Hayward, J.L., Spicer, C.C. Relation between urinary androgen and corticoid excretion and subsequent breast cancer. Lancet, **ii**, 395-8, 1971.

Bulbrook, R.D., Wang, D.Y., Swain, M.C. Prolactin and breast cancer. In *Prolactin and Carcinogenesis. 4th Tenovus Workshop.* ed. A.R. Boyns and K. Griffith, Alpha Omega Alpha Publishing Limited, Cardiff, 1972.

Burstyn, P.G., Horrobin; D.F., Manku, M.S. Saluretic action of aldosterone in the presense of increased salt intake and restoration of normal action by prolactin or by oxytocin. J. Endocr., **55**, 369-76, 1972.

Butcher, R.L., Fugo, N.W., Collins, W.E. Semicircadian rhythm in plasma levels of prolactin during early gestation in the rat. Endocrinology, **90**, 1125-7, 1972.

Butler, T., Pearson, O.H. Regression of prolactin-dependent rat mammary carcenoma in response to anti-hormone treatment. Cancer Res., **31**, 817-20, 1971.

Butler, W.R., Malven, P.V., Willett, L.B., Bolt, D.J. Patterns of pituitary release and cranial output of LH and prolactin in ovariectomised ewes. Endocrinology, **91**, 793-801, 1972.

Buttle, H.L., Forsyth, I.A. Prolactin concentration and lactogenic activity in the plasma of lactating and pregnant goats. J. Endocr., **51**, xxxiii-iv, 1971.

Buttle, H.L., Forsyth, I.A., Knaggs, G.S. Plasma prolactin measured by radioimmunoassay and bioassay in pregnant and lactating goats and the occurrence of a placental lactogen. J. Endocr., **53**, 483-91, 1972.

Calne, D.B., Reid, J.L. Action of levodopa on the blood pressure of conscious rabbits. Medical Res. Soc. Proc. no. 18, Feb. 1973.

Cameron, E.H.D., Griffiths, K., Gleave, E.N., Stewart, H.J., Forrest, A.P.M., Campbell, H. Benig and malignant breast disease in South Wales: a study of urinary steroids. Brit. Med. J., **4**, 768-71, 1970.

Canfield, C.J., Bates, R.W. Nonpuerperal galactorrhea. New Eng. J. Med., **273**, 897-902, 1965.

Canning, B.S., Green, A.T., Mulcahy, R. Coronary heart disease in the puerperium. J. Obstet. Gynaec. Brit. Comm., **76**, 1018-20, 1969.

Carlsson, A., Dahlstrom, A., Fuxe, K., Hillard, N.A. Failure of reserpine to deplete noradrenaline neurons of α-methylnoradrenaline formed from α-methyl DOPA. Acta Pharmacol. Toxicol., **22**, 270-6, 1965.

Carlsson, S., Kullander, S., Muller, E.R.A. The distribution of ^{125}I-marked bovine prolactin and human chlorionic gonadotrophin in rats with experimental ovarian tumours. Acta Obstet. Gynecol. Scand., **51**, 175-82, 1972.

Carranza-Acevedo, J. Oral contraceptives and depression. Lancet **2**, 104, 1967.

Carroll, B.J., Frazer, A., Schless, A., Mendels, J. Cholinergic reversal of manic symptoms. Lancet **1**, 427-8, 1973.

Cassell, E.E., Meites, J,, Welsch, C.W. Effects of ergocornine and ergocryptine on growth of 7, 12-dimethyl-benzanthracene-induced mammary tumours in rats. Cancer Res., **31**, 1051-53, 1971.

Cehovic, G., Dettbarn, W-D., Welsch, F. Paraoxon: effects on rat brain cholinesterase and on growth hormone and prolactin of pituitary. Science, **175**, 1256-8, 1972.

Cehovic, G., Lewis, U.J., Van der Laan, W.P. Study of the action of some new analogues of cyclic AMP on the release of growth hormone and prolactin in vitro. C.R. Acad. Sci. D. (Paris), **271**, 1399-401, 1970.

Cehovic, G., Lewis, U.J., Van der Laan, W.P. Study of the action of adenosine-cyclic-3'-5'-monophosphate acid on release of growth hormone and prolactin in vitro. C.R. Acad. Sci. D. (Paris), **270**, 3119-22, 1970.

Celis, M.E., Taleisnik, S., Walter, R. Regulation of formation and proposed structure of the factor inhibiting the release of melanocyte-stimulating hormone. Proc. Nat. Acad. Sci. U.S.A., **68**, 1428-33, 1971.

Challis, J.R.G. Sharp increase in the circulating oestrogen immediately before parturition in sheep. Nature (Lond.), **229**, 208, 1971.

Champigny, O., Bourdel, G., Jacquot, R. Energy and nitrogen values in the rat during pregnancy and under the effect of prolactin. C.R. Acad. Sci. (Paris), **251**, 1664-5, 1960.

Chan, W.Y., Sawyer, W.H. Saluretic actions of neurohypophysial peptides in conscious dogs. Amer. J. Physiol., **201**, 799-803, 1961.

Channing, C.P., Taylor, M., Knobil, E , Nicoll, C.S., Nichols, C.W. Secretion of prolactin and growth hormone by cultures of adult simian pituitaries. Proc. Soc. Exp. Biol. Med., **135**, 540-2, 1970.

Chapman, V.M., Desjardins, C., Whitten, W.K. Pregnancy block in mice: changes in pituitary LH and LTH and plasma progestin levels. J. Reprod. Fertil., **21**, 333-7, 1970.

Chase, M.D., Geschwin, I.I., Bern, H.A. Synergistic role of prolactin in response of male rat sex accessories to androgen. Proc. Soc. Exp. Biol. Med., **94**, 680-3, 1957.

Chazov, E.I. Biosynthesis of hypophysis under different physiological conditions. Vopr. Med. Khim., **17**, 594-8, 1971.

Chazov, E.I. Biosynthesis of hypophysial hormones. Growth hormone and prolactin synthesis in the rat hypophysis under different physiological conditions. Vopr. Med. Khim., **17**, 594-8, 1971.

Cheever, E.V., Seavey, B.K., Lewis, U.J. Prolactin of normal and dwarf mice. Endocrinology, **85**, 698-703, 1969.

Chen, C.L., Amenomori, Y., Lu, K.H., Voogt, J.L., Meites, J. Serum prolactin levels in rats with pituitary transplants or hypothalamic lesions. Neuroendocrinology, **6**, 220-7, 1970.

Chen, C.L., Meites, J. Effects of thyroxine and thiouracil on hypothalamic PIF and pituitary prolactin levels. Proc. Soc. Exp. Biol. Med., **131**, 576-8, 1969.

Chen, C.L., Meites, J. Effects of estrogen and progesterone on serum and pituitary prolactin levels in ovariectomised rats. Endocrinology, **86**, 503-5, 1970.

Chen, C.L., Minaguchi, H., Meites, J. Effects of transplanted pituitary tumours on host pituitary prolactin secretion. Proc. Soc. Exp. Biol. Med., **126**, 317-20, 1967.

Chen, C.L., Voogt, J.L., Meites, J. Effect of median eminence implants of FSH, LH or prolactin on luteal function in the rat. Endocrinology, **83**, 1273-7, 1968.

Chesley, L.C. Water, electrolyte and acid-base disorders in pregnancy, pp. 995-1022, in *Clinical Disorders of Fluid and Electrolyte Metabolism*. ed. M.H. Maxwell, C.R. Kleeman, McGraw Hill, New York, 1972.

Chinn, M.A. Oestrogen therapy and migraine. Brit. Med. J., **2**, 699, 1968.

Choudary, J.B., Greenwald, G.S. Effect of an ectopic pituitary gland on luteal maintenance in the hamster. Endocrinology, **81**, 542-52, 1967.

Chrambach, A., Bridson, W.E., Turkington, R.W. Human prolactin: identification and physical characterization of the biologically active hormone by polyacrylamide gel electrophoresis. Biochem. Biophys. Res. Comm., **43**, 1296-1303, 1971.

Cirksena, W.J., Dirks, J.H., Berliner, R.B. Effect of caval ligation on response of proximal tubular sodium reabsorption to saline infusion. J. Clin. Invest., **44**, 1035, 1965.

Clark, D.H. Peptic ulcer in women. Brit. Med. J., **1**, 1254-5, 1953.

Clark, M.L., Ray, T.S., Paredes, A., Ragland, R.E., Costiloe, J.P., Smith, C.W., Wolf, S. Chlorpromazine in women with chronic schizophrenia: the effect on cholesterol levels and cholesterol-behaviour relationships. Psychosom. Med., **29**, 634-42, 1967.

Clark, R.H., Baker, B.L. Circadian periodicity in the concentration of prolactin in the rat hypophysis. Science, 143, 375-6, 1964.

Clark, S.W. Effects of suppressed prolactin levels during proestrus or estrus on induction and duration of pseudopregnancy. Biol. Reprod., 7, 138, 1972.

Clemens, J.A., Gallo, R.V., Whitmoyer, D.I., Sawyer, C.H. Prolactin responsive neurons in the rabbit hypothalamus. Brain Res., **25**, 371-9, 1971.

Clemens, J.A., Meites, J. Neuro-endocrine status of old constant-estrous rats. Neuroendocrinology **7**, 249-56, 1971.

Clemens, J.A., Minaguchi, H., Storey, R., Voogt, J.L., Meites, J. Induction of precocious puberty in female rats by prolactin. Neuroendocrinology, **4**, 150-6, 1969.

Clemens, J.A., Sar, M., Meites, J. Termination of pregnancy in rats by a prolactin implant in median eminence. Proc. Soc. Exp. Biol. Med., **130**, 628-30, 1969.

Clemens, J.A., Sar, M., Meites, J. Inhibition of lactation and luteal function in post-partum rats by hypothalamic implantation of prolactin. Endocrinology, **84**, 868-72, 1969.

Clemens, J.A., Shaar, C.J. Inhibition by ergocornine of initiation and growth of 7, 12-dimethylbenzanthracene-induced mammary tumours in rats: effect of tumour size. Proc. Soc. Exp. Biol. Med., **139**, 659-62, 1972.

Clemens, J.A., Shaar, C.J., Kleber, J.W., Tandy, W.A. Reciprocal control by the pre-optic area of LH and prolactin. Exper. Brain Res., **12**, 250-3, 1971.

Clemens, J.A., Shaar, C.J., Tandy, W.A., Roush, M.E. Effects of hypothalamic stimulation on prolactin secretion in steroid-treated rats. Endocrinology, **89**, 1317-20, 1971.

Clemens, J.A., Meites, J. Inhibition of hypothalamic prolactin implants of prolactin secretion, mammary growth and luteal function. Endocrinology, **82**, 878-81, 1968.

Clemens, J.A., Welsch, C.W., Meites, J. Effects of hypothalamic lesions on incidence and growth of mammary tumors in carcinogen-treated rats. Proc. Soc. Exp. Biol. Med., **127**, 969-72, 1968.

Cochrane, R. High blood pressure as a psychosomatic disorder: a selective review. Brit. J. Soc. Clin. Psychol., **10**, 61-72, 1971.

Cohen, M.H. Enhancement of the antitumor effect of bis-chloroethyl nitrosourea by psychotropic drugs and caffeine. Proc. Am. Ass. Cancer Res., **13**, 45, 1972.

Cole, R.D., Hopkins, T.R. Maintenance of the mammary gland in hypophysectomised-oöphorectomised rats by injections of prolactin. Endocrinology, **71**, 395-8, 1962.

Convey, E.M. Personal communication, quoted in Meites, Clemens, 1972.

Convey, E.M., Bretschneider, E., Hafs, H.D., Oxender, W.D. Serum levels of LH, prolactin and growth hormone after ejaculation in bulls. Biol. Reprod., **5**, 20-4, 1971.

Convey, E.M., Reece, R.P. Restoration of pituitary lactogen released in response to suckling. Proc. Soc. Exp. Biol. Med., **131**, 543-6, 1969.

Convey, E.M. Tucker, H.A., Smith, V.G., Zolman, J.J. Anim. Sci., **35**, 258, 1972.

Cook, B., Kaltenbach, C.C., Niswender, G.D., Norton, H.W., Nalbandov, A.V. Short term ovarian responses to some pituitary hormones infused in vivo in pigs and sheep. J. Anim. Sci., **29**, 711-8, 1969.

Cook, B., Nalbandov, A.V. The effect of some pituitary hormones on progesterone synthesis in vitro by the luteinized ovary of the common opossum. J. Reprod. Fertil., **15**, 267-75, 1968.

Coppen, A. The biochemistry of affective disorders. Brit. J. Psychiat. **113**, 1237-64, 1967.

Coppen, A., Metcalfe, M., Carroll, J.D., Morris, J.G.L., Levodopa and L-tryptophan therapy in Parkinsonism. Lancet 1, 654-8, 1972.

Coppen, A., Prange, A.J., Whybrow, P.C., Noguera, R. Abnormalities of indoleamines in affective disorders. Arch. Gen. Psychiat. **26**, 474-8, 1972.

Coppen, A.J., Shaw, D.M. Mineral metabolism in melancholia. Brit. Med. J. **2**, 1439-44, 1963.

Coppen, A.J., Shaw, D.M. Mineral metabolism in mania. Brit. Med. J. **1**, 71-5, 1966.

Coppen, A.J., Shaw, D.M. The distribution of electrolytes and water in patients after taking lithium carbonate. Lancet **2**, 805-6, 1967.

194

Coppen, A.J., Shaw, D.M., Farrell, J.P. Potentiation of the antidepressive effect of a mono-amine oxidase inhibitor by tryptophan. Lancet 1, 79, 1963.

Coppen, A.J., Shaw, D.M., Mangoni, A. Total exchangeable sodium in depressive illness. Brit. Med. J. 2, 295-8, 1962.

Costom, B.H., Grumbach, M.M., Kaplan, S.L. Effect of thyrotropin-releasing factor on serum thyroid-stimulating hormone. J. Clin. Invest., 50, 2219-25, 1971.

Cotes, P.M. Discussion, pp. 111-113. Prolactin and Carcinogenesis, 4th Tenovus Workshop. Ed. A.R. Boyns and K. Griffiths, Alpha Omega Alpha, Cardiff, 1972.

Cotzias, G.C., Van Woert, M.A., Schiffer, L.M. Aromatic amino acids and modification of Parkinsonism. New Eng. J. Med. 276, 374-9, 1967.

Coull, D.C., Crooks, J., Dingwall-Fordyce, I., Scott, A.M., Weir, R.D. Amitriptyline and cardiac disease. Lancet, 2, 590-1, 1970.

Cowie, A.T. Complete restoration of lactation in the goat after hypophysectomy. J. Endocr., 28, 267-79, 1964.

Cowie, A.T. Variations in the yield and composition of milk during lactation in the rabbit and the galactopoietic effect of prolactin. J. Endocr., 44, 437-50, 1969.

Cowie, A.T., Daniel, P.M., Knaggs, G.S. Lactation in the goat after section of the pituitáry stalk. J. Endocr., 28, 253-65, 1964.

Cowie, A.T., Hartmann, P.E., Turvey, A. The maintenance of lactation in the rabbit after hypophysectomy. J. Endocr., 43, 651-2, 1969.

Cowie, A.T., Tindal, J.S. The Physiology of Lactation. Edward Arnold, London, 1971.

Cowie, A.T., Tindal, J.S., Yokoyama, A. The induction of mammary growth in the hypophysectomised goat. J. Endocr., 34, 185-95, 1966.

Cramer, H.I. The influence of menstruation on carbohydrate tolerance in diabetes mellitus. Canad. Med. Ass. J. 47, 51-5, 1942.

Crosbie, W.A., Snowden, S., Parsons, V. Changes in lung capillary permeability in renal failure. Brit. Med. J. 4, 388-90, 1972.

Csatary, L.K. Chlorpromazines and cancer. Lancet, ii, 338-9, 1972.

Cumming, I.A., Brown, J.M., Goding, J.R., Bryant, G.D., Greenwood, F.C. Secretion of pro-lactin and luteinising hormone at oestrus in the ewe. J. Endocr., 54, 207-13, 1972.

Cutts, J.H. Vascular lesions resembling polyarteritis nodosa in rats undergoing prolonged stimulation with oestrogens. Brit. J. Exp. Path., 47, 401-4, 1966.

Dalessio, D.J. Wolff's Headache and other Head Pain, Oxford University Press, New York, 3rd ed. 1972.

Dalton, K. The Premenstrual Syndrome. Heinemann Medical Publications, London, 1964.

Daniel, D.G., Campbell, H., Turnbull, A.C. Puerperal thromboembolism and suppression of lactation. Lancet 2, 287, 1967.

Danon, A., Dikstein, S., Sulman, F.G. In-vivo assay for hypothalamic prolactin-inhibiting factor. J. Endocr., 46, 237-41, 1970.

Danon, A., Sulman, F.G. Storage of prolactin-inhibiting factor in the hypothalamus of perphenazine-treated rats. Neuroendocrinology, 6, 295-300, 1970.

Dao, T.L. Studies on mechanism of carcinogenesis in the mammary gland. Progr. Exp. Tumour Res., 11, 235-61, 1968.

Dao, T.L. Inhibition of tumor induction in chemical carcinogenesis in the mammary gland. Prog. Exp. Tumour Res., 14, 59-88, 1971.

Dao, T.L., Sinha, D. Oestrogen and prolactin in mammary carcinogenesis: in vivo and in vitro studies. pp. 189-194 in Prolactin and Carcinogenesis, 4th Tenovus Workshop. ed. A.R. Boyns and K. Griffiths, Alpha Omega Alpha, Cardiff, 1972.

Datey, K.K., Nanda, N.C. Hyperglycemia after acute myocardial infarction: its relation to diabetes mellitus. New Eng. J. Med., 276, 262-5, 1967.

Davey, M.J., Lockett, M.F. Actions and interactions of aldosterone monoacetate and neuro-hypophysial hormones on the isolated cat kidney. J. Physiol., 152, 206-19, 1960.

David, R.R., Asnis, M., Drucker, W.D. Disturbance of cortisol production in congenital aldosterone deficiency. J. Clin. Endocr., 35, 604-608, 1972.

Davies, B., Carroll, B.J., Mowbray, R.M. Depressive illness. Some research studies. Charles C. Thomas, Springfield, 1972.

Davies, J., Bull, G.M. Stimulation of synthesis of foetal haemoglobin in adult hamsters. Trans. Roy. Soc. Trop. Med. Hyg., 65, 78-81, 1971.

Davies, M.H. Is high blood pressure a psychosomatic disorder? A critical review of the evidence. J. Chronic Dis., 24, 239-58, 1971.

Davis, J.O. Editorial. Two important frontiers in renal physiology. Circulation, 30, 1-6, 1964.

Davis, J.O., Holman, J.E., Carpenter, C.C.J., Urquhart, J., Higgins, J.T. An extra-adrenal factor essential for chronic renal sodium retention in presence of increased sodium-retaining hormone. Circulation Res., 14, 17-31, 1964.

Davis, J.O., Howell, D.S., Hyatt, R.E. Sodium excretion in adrenalectomised dogs with chronic failure induced by pulmonary artery constriction. Amer. J. Physiol., 183, 263, 1955.

Davis, J.W., Liu, T.M.Y. The adrenal gland and lactogenesis. Endocrinology, 85, 155-60, 1969.

Davis, S.L. Plasma levels of prolactin, growth hormone and insulin in sheep following the infusion of arginine, leucine and phenylalanine. Endocrinology, 91, 549-555, 1972.

Davis, S.L. Reichart, L.E., Niswender, G.D. Serum levels of prolactin in sheep as measured by radioimmunoassay. Biol. Reprod., 4, 145-53, 1971.

Davison, K. EEG activation after intravenous amitriptyline. Electroenceph. Clin. Neurophysiol. 19, 298-300, 1965.

Davson, H. The intraocular pressure. pp 187-272 in The Eye, vol. 1, ed. H. Davson, Academic Press, New York, 2nd ed. 1969.

Dear, H.D., Jones, W.B. Myocardial infarction associated with the use of oral contraceptives. Ann. Intern. Med. 74, 236-9, 1971.

Debeljuk, L., Arimura, A., Sandow, J.K., Schally, A.V. Effects of cis-clomiphene on serum LH and prolactin levels and on the response to LH-RH in the ewe. J. Anim. Sci., 34, 294-6, 1972.

Debeljuk, L., Arimura, A., Schally, A.V. Lack of prolactin release-inhibiting activity in synthetic LH-releasing hormone. J. Clin. Endocr., 35, 918-920, 1972.

Delouis, C., Denamur, R. Induction of lactose synthesis by prolactin in rabbit mammary gland extracts. J. Endocr., 52, 311-19, 1972.

Del Pozo, E., Brun Del Re, R., Varga, L., Friesen, H. The inhibition of prolactin secretion in man by CB 154 (2-Br-α-ergokryptine). J. Clin. Endocr., 35, 768-70, 1972.

Demers, R., Henniger, G., Pretibial edema and sodium retention during lithium carbonate treatment. J. Amer. Med. Ass., 214, 1845-8, 1970.

Denamur, R., Delouis, C. Effects of progesterone and prolactin on the secretory activity and the nucleic acid content of the mammary gland of pregnant rabbits. Acta Endocr. (Kbh), 70, 603-18, 1972.

De Prospo, N.D. The role of adenohypophysial hormones and their target glands in isoquinoline dye hepatocarcinogenesis. J. Endocr., 37, 227-8, 1967.

De Voe, W.F., Ramirez, V.D., McCann, S.M. Induction of mammary secretion by hypothalamic lesions in male rats. Endocrinology, 78, 158-64, 1966.

De Wardener, H.E. Control of sodium reabsorption[1]. Brit. Med. J., 3, 611-6, 1969a.

De Wardener, H.E. Control of sodium reabsorption[2]. Brit. Med. J., 3, 676-83, 1969b.

De Wardener, H.E., Mills, I.H., Clapham, W.F., Hayter, C.J. Studies on the efferent mechanism of the sodium diuresis which follows the administration of intravenous saline in the dog. Clin. Sci., 21, 249-258, 1961.

Dewhurst, W.G. Nature, Lond., 218, 1130, 1968.

De Wied, D. Chlorpromazine and endocrine function. Pharmacol. Rev., 19, 251-88, 1967.

Dickerman, S., Clark, J., Dickerman, E., Meites, J. Effects of haloperidol on serum and pituitary prolactin and on hypothalamic PIF in rats. Neuroendocrinology, 9, 332-40, 1972.

Dieterle, P. Asymptomatic diabetes mellitus in hypertensive patients of renal weight, glucose tolerance and serum levels of insulin and nonesterified fatty acids in essential hypertension. German Med. Mon., 13, 478-83, 1968.

Dilley, D.A. Evaluation of immunoassay methods for prolactin in body fluids. U.S. Air Force Aerospace Med. Res. Lab., 1-24, 1966.

Dilley, W.G. Morphogenic and mitogenic effects of prolactin on rat mammary gland. Endocrinology, 88, 514-7, 1971.

Dilley, W.G., Nandi, S. Rat mammary gland differentiation in vitro in the absence of steroids. Science, 161, 59-60, 1968.

Dirks, J.H., Cirksena, W.J., Berliner, R.W. Effect of saline infusion on sodium reabsorption by the proximal tubule of the dog. J. Clin. Invest., 44, 1160-1170, 1965.

Djojosoebagio, S., Turner, C.W. Effect of a combincation of lactogenic, thyroid and parathyroid hormones on lactation in rats. Proc. Soc. Exp. Biol. Med., 116, 213-5, 1964.

Doerr-Schott, J., Stoeckel, M-E., Porte A., Reville, P. Ultrastructural modifications of pituitary prolactin cells in hypothyroid rats. C.R. Acad. Sci. D (Paris), 274, 2995-7, 1972.

Domanski, E., Skrzeczkowski, L., Stupnicka, E., Fitko, R., Dobrowolski, W. Effect of gonadotrophins on the secretion of progesterone and oestrogen by the sheep ovary perfused in situ. J. Reprod. Fertil., 14, 365-72, 1967.

Dominic, C.J. Observations on the reproductive phenomena of mice. Neuroendocrine mechanisms involved in the olfactory block to pregnancy. J. Reprod. Fertil., 11, 415-21, 1966.

Dominic, C.J. Effect of exogenous prolactin on olfactory block to pregnancy in mice exposed to urine of alien males. Indian J. Exp. Biol., 5, 47-8, 1967.

Donofrio, R.J., Reiter, R.J. Depressed pituitary prolactin levels in blinded anosmic female rats: role of the pineal gland. J. Reprod. Fertil., 31, 159-62, 1972.

Donoso, A.O., Bishop, W., Fawcett, C.D., Krulich, L., McCann, S.M. Effects of drugs that modify brain monoamine concentrations on plasma gonadotropin and prolactin levels in the rat. Endocrinology, 89, 774-84, 1971.

Donovan, B.T., Van der Werff Ten Bosch, J.J. The hypothalamus and lactation in the rabbit. J. Physiol (Lond.), 137, 410-20, 1957.

Dowd, A.J., Bartke, A. Serum levels of prolactin, LH and FSH and testis cholesterol content in rats from one to ten weeks of age. Biol. Reprod., 7, 115, 1972.

Dunn, J.D., Arimura, A., Scheving, L.E. Effect of stress on circadian periodicity in serum LH and prolactin concentrations. Endocrinology, 90, 29-33, 1972.

Earley, L.E. Sodium metabolism. pp. 95-120 in Clinical Disorders of Fluid and Electrolyte Metabolism. ed. M.H. Maxwell and C.R. Kleeman, McGraw Hill, New York, 1972.

Ebringer, A. Rheumatoid factor, vascular damage and hypertension. Brit. Med. J., 3, 110, 1970.

Ebringer, A., Doyle, A.E. Raised serum lgG levels in hypertension. Brit. Med. J., 2, 146-8, 1970.

Ectors, F., Danguy, A., Pasteels, J.L. Ultrastructure of organ cultures of rat hypophyses exposed to ergocornine. J. Endocr., 52, 211-12, 1972.

Ederer, F., Leren, P., Turpeinen, O., Frantz, I.D. Cancer among men on cholesterol lowering diets. Lancet, **2**, 203-6, 1971.

Edwards, C.R.W., Forsyth, I.A., Besser, G.M. Amenorrhoea, galactorrhoea and primary hypothyroidism with high circulating levels of prolactin. Brit. Med. J. **3**, 462-4, 1971.

Ehni, G., Eckles, N.E. Interruption of the pituitary stalk in the patient with mammary cancer. J. Neurosurg., **16**, 628-51, 1959.

Elghamry, M.I., Grunert, E. The effect of estrogen and progesterone on the glycogenetic response to prolactin in ovariectomised mice. Zbl Veterinaermed., **16**, 41-5, 1969.

Elghamry, M.I., Said, A., Elmougy, S.A. The effect of lactogenic hormone on liver glycogen and blood glucose in ovariectomised mice. Naturwissenschaften, **53**, 530, 1966.

Elsair, J., Denine, R. Action of sheep prolactin on plasma free fatty acid levels and blood sugar in the normal fasting child. Rev. Eur. Etud. Clin. Biol.,**15**, 899-905, 1970.

Emerson, C.H., Utiger, R.D. New Eng. J. Med. **287**, 328, 1972.

Ensor, D.M., Edmondson, M.R., Phillips, J.G. Prolactin and dehydration in rats. J. Endocr., **53**, 1:x-1x, 1972.

Evans, A.J. The in vitro effect of prolactin on β-glucuronidase in the testis of the rat. J. Endocr., **24**, 233-44, 1962.

Evered, D., Horrobin, D.F., Nassar, B. Fluid and electrolyte changes in a woman with severe premenstrual syndrome. Unpublished, 1973.

Everett, J.W. Luteotrophic function of autografts of the rat hypophysis. Endocrinology **54**, 685-90, 1954.

Falconer, I.R. The distribution of ^{131}I or ^{125}I-labelled prolactin in rabbit mammary tissue after intravenous or intraductal injection. J. Endocrinol., **53**, viii-ix, 1972.

Falconer, I.R., Fiddler, T.J. Effects of intraductal administration of prolactin, actinomycin D and cycloheximide on lipoprotein lipase activity in the mammary glands of pseudopregnant rabbits. Biochim. Biophys. Acta, **218**, 508-14, 1970.

Farnsworth, W.E. Prolactin and the prostate. pp 217-225 in *Prolactin and Carcinogenesis. 4th Tenovus Workshop*, ed. A.R. Boyns and K. Griffiths, Alpha Omega Alpha, Cardiff, 1972.

Farooq, A., Denenberg, V.H., Ross, S., Sawin, P.B., Zarrow, M.X. Maternal behaviour in the rabbit: endocrine factors involved in hair loosening. Amer. J. Physiol., **204**, 271-4, 1963.

Faure, J., Friconneau, C. Influence of prolactin on the electroencephalogram in the rabbit. Rev. Neurol., **101**, 308-16, 1959.

Fell, L.R., Beck, C., Brown, J.M., Catt, K.J., Cumming, I.A., Goding, J.R. Solid phase radioimmunoassay of ovine prolactin in antibody-coated tubes. Prolactin secretion during estradiol treatment, at parturition and during milking. Endocrinol., **91**, 1329-42, 1972.

Fell, L.R., Beck, C., Brown, J.M., Cumming, I.A., Goding, J.R. Radioimmunoassay for ovine prolactin. The secretion of prolactin as affected by milking, oestradiol administration and onset of parturition. J. Reprod. Fertil., **28**, 133-4, 1972.

Fichman, M.P., Brooker, G. Deficient renal cyclic adenosine 3', 5'-monophosphate production in nephrogenic diabetes insipidus. J. Clin. Endocr., **35**, 35-47, 1972.

Finn, C.A., Martin, L. The onset of progesterone secretion during pregnancy in the mouse. J. Reprod. Fertil., **25**, 299-300, 1971.

Fiorindo, R.P., Nicoll, C.S. Inhibitory and stimulatory effects of rat median eminence extract on prolactin secretion in vitro by rat adenohypophysis. Fed. Proc., **28**, 437, 1969.

Fisch, I.R., Freedman, S.H., Myatt, A.V. Oral contraceptives, pregnancy and blood pressure. J. Am. Med. Ass., **222**, 1507-10, 1972.

Fisher, E.R., Fisher, B. Experimental studies of factors influencing hepatic metastases, XIV. Effect of prolactin. Cancer Res., **23**, 1532-8, 1963.

Fisher, E.R., Fisher, B. Antiprolactin and experimentally-induced hepatic metastases. Proc. Soc. Exp. Biol. Med., **123**, 364-7, 1966.

Fleischer, N., Bureus, R., Vale, W., Dunn, T., Guillemin, R. Preliminary observations on the effect of synthetic thyrotropin releasing factor on plasma thyrotropin levels in man. J. Clin. Endocr., **31**, 109-12, 1970.

Fluckiger, E. Drugs and the control of prolactin secretion, in *Prolactin and Carcinogenesis. 4th Tenovus Workshop*. ed. A.R. Boyns, and K. Griffiths, Alpha Omega Alpha Publishing, Cardiff, 1972.

Fluckiger, E., Lutterbeck, P.M., Wagner, H.R., Billeter, E., Antagonism of 2-Br-α-ergokryptine methanesulphonate (CB 154) to certain endocrine actions of centrally active drugs. Experientia, **28**, 924-5, 1972.

Fluckiger, E., Wagner, H.R. 2-Br-α-ergokryptine: beeinflussung von Fertilitat und Laktation bei der Ratte. Experientia, **24**, 1130-1, 1968.

Foley, T.P., Jacobs, L.S., Hoffman, W., Daughaday, W.H., Blizzard, R.M. Human prolactin and thyrotropin concentration in the serum of normal and hypopituitary children before and after the administration of synthetic thyrotropin releasing hormone. J. Clin. Invest., **51**, 2143-50, 1972.

Foley, T.P., Owings, J., Hayford, J.T., Blizzard, R.M. Serum thyrotropin responses to synthetic thyrotropin-releasing hormone in normal children and hypopituitary patients. J. Clin., Invest., **51**, 431-7, 1972.

Forbes, A.P., Henneman, P.H., Griswold, G.C., Albright, F. Syndrome characterised by galactorrhea, amenorrhea and low urinary FSH: comparison with acromegaly and normal lactation. J. Clin. Endocr., **14**, 265-71, 1954.

Forsyth, I.A. The detection of lactogenic activity in human blood by bioassay. J. Endocr., **46**, iv-v, 1970.

Forsyth, I.A. Use of a rabbit mammary gland organ culture system to detect lactogenic activity in blood. pp. 151-167 in *Lactogenic Hormones,* ed. G.E.W. Wolstenholme and J. Knight, Churchill Livingstone, 1972.

Forsyth, I.A., Besser, G.M., Edwards, C.R.W., Francis, L., Myres, R.P. Plasma prolactin activity in inappropriate lactation. Brit. Med. J., **3**, 225-7, 1971.

Forsyth, I.A., Edwards, C.R.W. Human prolactin, its isolation, assay and clinical applications. Clin. Endocr., **1**, 293-314, 1972.

Forsyth, I.A., Myres, R.P. Human prolactin. Evidence obtained by the bioassay of human plasma. J. Endocr., **51**, 157-68, 1971.

Frantz, A.G., Kleinberg, D.L. Prolactin: evidence that it is separate from growth hormone in human blood. Science, **170**, 745-6, 1970.

Frantz, A.G., Kleinberg, D.L., Noel, G.L. Physiological and pathological secretion of human prolactin studied by in vitro bioassay. pp. 137-150 in *Lactogenic Hormones.* ed. G.E.W. Wolstenholme and J. Knight, Churchill Livingstone, 1972a.

Frantz, A.G., Kleinberg, D.L., Noel, G.L. Studies on prolactin in man. Rec. Progr. Hormone Res., **28**, 527-90, 1972b.

Frantz, A.G., Rabkin, M.T. Human growth hormone: clinical measurement, response to hypoglycemia and suppression by corticosteroids. N. Eng. J. Med., **271**, 1375-81, 1964.

Frantz, A.G., Rabkin, M.T. Effects of estrogen and sex difference on secretion of human growth hormone. J. Clin. Endocr. **25**, 1470-80, 1965.

Frantz, W.L., Turkington, R.W. Formation of biologically active ^{125}I-prolactin by enzymatic radioiodination. Endocrinology, **91**, 1545-48, 1972.

Frazer, L.E., Spicer, C.C., Williams, P.C., Young, S. Detection and attempted assay of mammotrophic activity in women's blood and urine. Brit. J. Cancer, **15**, 243-51, 1961.

Freeman, M.E., Neill, J.D. The pattern of prolactin secretion during pseudopregnancy in the rat: a daily nocturnal surge. Endocrinology, **90**, 1292-4, 1972.

Freeman, M.E., Reichert, L.E., Neill, J.D. Regulation of the proestrus surge of prolactin secretion by gonadotropin and estrogens in the rat. Endocrinology, **90**, 232-8, 1972.

Friesen, H.G. Synthesis and secretion of placental lactogen and other proteins by the placenta. Recent Progr. Hormone Res., **25**, 161-205, 1969.

Friesen, H.G. Human placental lactogen and human pituitary prolactin. Clin. Obstet. Gynecol., **14**, 669-84, 1971.

Friesen, H.G. Discussion, pp. 115 in *Prolactin and Carcinogenesis. 4th Tenovus Workshop,* ed. A.R. Boyns and K. Griffiths, Alpha Omega Alpha Publishing, Cardiff, 1972.

Friesen, H.G. Discussion, p. 588 after paper by Frantz, Kleinberg, Noel, 1972b.

Friesen, H., Belanger, C., Guyda, H., Hwang, P. The synthesis and secretion of placental lactogen and pituitary prolactin. pp. 83-103 in *Lactogenic Hormones,* ed. G.E.W. Wolstenholme and J. Knight. Churchill Livingstone, 1972.

Friesen, H., Guyda, H. Biosynthesis of monkey growth hormone and prolactin in vitro. Endocrinology, **88**, 1353-62, 1971.

Friesen, H., Guyda, H., Hardy, J. The biosynthesis of human growth hormone and prolactin. J. Clin. Endocr., **31**, 611-24, 1970.

Friesen, H., Guyda, H., Hwang, P. Prolactin synthesis in primates. Nature (New Biol.), **232**, 19-20, 1971.

Friesen, H., Guyda, H., Hwang, P., Tyson, J.E., Barbeau, A. Functional elevation of prolactin secretion: a guide to therapy. J. Clin. Invest., **51**, 706-9, 1972.

Friesen, H., Hwang, P., Guyda, H., Tolis, G., Tyson, J., Myers, R. A radio-immunoassay for human prolactin in *Prolactin and Carcinogenesis. 4th Tenovus Workshop,* ed. A.R. Boyns and K. Griffiths. Alpha Omega Alpha Publishing, Cardiff, 1972.

Friesen, H., Webster, B.R., Hwang, P., Guyda, H., Munro, R.E., Read, L. Prolactin synthesis and secretion in a patient with the Forbes-Albright syndrome. J. Clin. Endocr., **34**, 192-9, 1972.

Fujii, K., Uruta, Y. On the urinary excretion of pituitary prolactin. Bull. Tokyo Med. Dent. Univ., **12**, 109-16, 1965.

Furth, J. Influence of host factors on the growth of neoplastic cells. Cancer Res., **23**, 21-34, 1963.

Furth, J. Pituitary cybernetics and neoplasia. Harvey Lectures, **63**, 47-72, 1969.

Furth, J. Prolactin and carcinogenesis, in *Prolactin and Carcinogenesis. 4th Tenovus Workshop,* ed. A.R. Boyns and K. Griffiths, Alpha Omega Alpha Publishing, Cardiff, 1972.

Furth, J., Clifton, K.H., Gadsden, E.L., Buffet, R.F. Dependent and autonomous mammotropic pituitary tumors in rats. Cancer Res., **16**, 608-616, 1956.

Gachev, E.P. The role of prolactin in the maintenance of the lactose level in milk. Zh. Obshch. Biol. **24**, 382-3, 1963.

Gachev, E.P. An attempt at stimulating prolactin secretion by means of synthetic oxytocin. Dokl. Bolg. Akad. Nauk. **20**, 1357-9, 1967.

Gachev, E.P. On the mechanism of blocking lactation through diuretics. Arzneimittelforschung, **18**, 738-40, 1968.

Gachev, E.P. Physiological conditions for the secretion of prolactin from the anterior pituitary. Endokrinologie **53**, 352-4, 1968.

Gachev, E.P. Lactose synthesis as a function of prolactin dosage. Dokl. Bolg. Akad. Nauk. **22**, 717-8, 1969.

Gachev, E.P. Certain particularities of prolactin secretion during the milk retention experiment. Endokrinologie **54**, 81-4, 1969.

Gala, R.R. Prolactin production by the human anterior pituitary cultured in vitro. J. Endocr. **50**, 637-42, 1971.

Gala, R.R., Janson, P.A., Kuo, E.Y. The influence of neural blocking agents injected into the third ventricle of the rat brain and hypothalamic electrical stimulation on serum prolactin. Proc. Soc. Exp. Biol. Med. **140**, 569-72, 1972.

Gala, R.R., Reece, R.P. Influence of neurohumors on anterior pituitary lactogen production in vitro. Proc. Soc. Exp. Biol. Med. **120**, 220-2, 1965.

Gambrell, R.D., Greenblatt, R.B., Mahesh, V.B. Post-pill and pill-related amenorrhea-galactorrhea. Amer. J. Obstet. Gynec. **110**, 838-47, 1971.

Gati, I., Doszpod, J., Preisz, J. LTH production and steroid excretion during the menstrual cycle. Acta Physiol. Acad. Sci. Hung. **32**, 115-22, 1967.

Gay, V.L., Midgley, A.R., Niswender, G.D. Patterns of gonadotrophin secretion associated with ovulation. Fed. Proc. **29**, 1880-7, 1970.

Geschwind, I.I. Introduction: prolactin and carcinogenesis, in *Prolactin and Carcinogenesis. 4th Tenovus Workshop.* ed. A.R. Boyns & K. Griffiths, Alpha Omega Alpha Publishing, Cardiff, 1972.

Gharib, H., Hodgson, S.F., Gastineau, C.F., Scholz, D.A., Smith, L.A. Reversible hypothyroidism in Addison's disease. Lancet **2**, 734-6, 1972.

Gibberd, F.B., Small, E. Interaction between levodopa and methyldopa. Brit. Med. J. **2**, 90-1, 1973.

Gibbons, J.L. Total body sodium and potassium in depressive illness. Clin. Sci. **19**, 133-8, 1960.

Ginz, B. Myocardial infarction in pregnancy. J. Obstet. Gynaec. Brit. Comm. **77**, 610-5, 1970.

Goldin, A., Burton, R.M., Humphreys, S.R., Venditti, J.M. Antileukemia action of reserpine. Science **125**, 156-7, 1957.

Goldstein, M., Battista, A.F., Nakatani, S., Anaghoste, B. Drug-induced relief of the tremor in monkeys with mesencephalic lesions. Nature **224**, 382-4, 1969.

Goldstein, R.L. Fatal myocardial infarction associated with sub-clinical doses of imipramine. Canad. Psychiat. Ass. J. **14**, 407-8, 1969.

Goluboff, L.G., Ezrin, C. Effect of pregnancy on the somatotroph and the prolactin cell of the human adenohypophysis. J. Clin. Endocr. **29**, 1533-8, 1969.

Gomez Dumm, C.L., Echave Lanos, J.M. Variations in the Golgi complex of mouse prolactin cells at different times in a circadian period. Experientia **26**, 1123, 1970.

Goodman, H.G., Grumbach, M.M., Kaplan, S.L. Growth and growth hormone. II. New Eng. J. Med. **278**, 57-68, 1968.

Gottlieb, L.S., Hazel, M., Broitman, S., Samchek, N. Effects of chlorpromazine on a transplantable mouse mastocytoma. Fed. Proc. **19**, 181, 1960.

Gourdji, D., Kerdelhue, B., Tixier-Vidal, A.C.R. Acad. Sci. (Paris) **274**, 437-40, 1972.

Grady, K.L., Greenwald, G.S. Gonadotropic induction of pseudopregnancy in the cyclic hamster. Endocrinology **83**, 1173-80, 1968.

Grandiston, L. Luteolytic action of prolactin during estrous cycle of the mouse. Proc. Soc. Exp. Biol. Med. **140**, 323-5, 1972.

Grant, E.C.G. Relation between headaches from oral contraceptives and development of endometrial arterioles. Brit. Med. J. **3**, 402-5, 1968.

Graybiel, A.L., Sode, J. Diuretics, potassium depletion and carbohydrate intolerance. Lancet **2**, 265, 1971.

Grayhack, J.T., Bunce, P.L., Kearns, J.W., Scott, W.W. Influence of pituitary on prostatic response to androgen in the rat. Bull. Johns Hopkins Hosp. **96**, 154-63, 1955.

Grayhack, J.T., Lebowitz, J.M. Effect of prolactin on the citric acid of the lateral lobe of the prostate of the Sprague-Dawley rat. Invest. Urol. **5**, 87-94, 1967.

Green, A.R., Curzon, G. Decrease of 5-hydroxytryptamine in the brain provoked by hydrocortisone and its prevention by allopurinol. Nature **220**, 1095-7, 1968.

Green, H.H., Harrington, A.R., Valtin, H. Impaired water diuresis in rats with hereditary hypothalamic diabetes insipidus after adrenalectomy. p202 in Proc. 3rd Int. Contgr. Nephrology, Washington. Hans Huber, Basel, 1967.

Green, M.R., Bunting, S.L., Peacock, A.C. Changes in labeling pattern of ribonucleic acid from mammary tissue as a result of hormone treatment. Biochemistry **10**, 2366-71, 1971.

Green, M.R., Topper, Y.J. Some effects of prolactin, insulin and hydrocortisone on RNA synthesis by mouse mammary gland in vitro. Biochim. Biophys. Acta **204**, 441-8, 1970.

Greene, R., Dalton, K. The premenstrual syndrome. Brit. Med. J. **1**, 1007-14, 1953.

Greenwald, G.S. Luteotrophic complex of the hamster. Endocrinology **80**, 118-30, 1967.

Greenwald, G.S., Johnson, D.C. Gonadotropic requirements for the maintenance of pregnancy in the hypophysectomised rat. Endocrinology **83**, 1052-64, 1968.

Greenwood, F.C. discussion on pp 174-5 in *Prolactin and Carcinogenesis. 4th Tenovus Workshop.* ed. A.R. Boyns & K. Griffiths, Alpha Omega Alpha Publishing, Cardiff, 1972.

Greenwood, F.C., Hunter, W.M., Glover, J.S. The preparation of ^{131}I-labelled human growth hormone of high specific radioactivity. Biochem. J. **89**, 114-23, 1963.

Greenwood, F.C., Siler, T.M., Bryant, G.D., Morgenstern, L.L. Radioimmunoassay of human plasma prolactin: applications and problems. in *Prolactin and Carcinogenesis. 4th Tenovus Workshop.* ed. A.R. Boyns & K. Griffiths. Alpha Omega Alpha Publishing, Cardiff, 1972.

Gropper, L., Shimkin, M.B., Combination therapy of 3-methylcholanthrene-induced mammary carcinoma in rats: effect of chemotherapy, ovariectomy and food restriction. Cancer Res. **27**, 26-32, 1967.

Grossman, S., Buchberg, A.S., Brecher, E., Hallinger, L.M. Idiopathic lactation following thoracoplasty. J. Clin. Endocr. **10**, 729-34, 1950.

Grosvenor, C.E. Evidence that exteroceptive stimuli can release prolactin from the pituitary gland of the lactating rat. Endocrinology **76**, 340-2, 1965a.

Grosvenor, C.E. Effect of nursing and stress upon prolactin-inhibiting activity of the rat hypothalamus. Endocrinology **77**, 1037-42, 1965b.

Grosvenor, C.E. Disappearance rate of exogenous prolactin from serum of female rats. Endocrinology **80**, 195-202, 1967.

Grosvenor, C.E., Krulich, L., McCann, S.M. Depletion of pituitary concentration of growth hormone as a result of suckling in the lactating rat. Endocrinology **82**, 617-9, 1968.

Grosvenor, C.E., McCann, S.M., Nallar, R. Inhibition of nursing-induced and stress-induced fall in pituitary prolactin concentration in lactating rats by injection of acid extracts of bovine hypothalamus. Endocrinology **76**, 883-9, 1965.

Grosvenor, C.E., Maiweg, H., Mena, F. Effect of non-suckling interval on ability of prolactin to stimulate milk secretion in rats. Amer. J. Physiol. **219**, 403-8, 1970.

Grosvenor, C.E., Mena, F. Effect of auditory, olfactory and optic stimuli upon milk ejection and suckling-induced release of prolactin in lactating rats. Endocrinology **80**, 840-6, 1967.

Grosvenor, C.E., Mena, F. Evidence for a refractory period in the neuroendocrine mechanism for release of prolactin. Endocrinology **88**, 355-8, 1971.

Grosvenor, C.E., Mena, F., Maiweg, H., Dhariwal, A.P.S., McCann, S.M. Effect of hypothalamic extracts and exogenous prolactin on reaccumulation of prolactin in the pituitary of the lactating rat after suckling. J. Endocr. **47**, 339-46, 1970.

Grosvenor, C.E., Mena, F., Schaefgen, D.A. Effect of non-suckling interval and duration of suckling on the suckling-induced fall in pituitary prolactin concentration in the rat. Endocrinology **81**, 449-53, 1967.

Guillemin, R. p518 of discussion after Meites, Lu, Wuttke, Welsch, Nagasawa, Quadri, 1972.

Gunn, S.A., Gould, T.C., Anderson, W.A.D. The effect of growth hormone and prolactin preparations on the control by interstitial cell stimulating hormone of uptake of ^{65}Zn by the rat dorsolateral prostate. J. Endocr. 32, 205-14, 1965.

Gunther, M., Kohorn, E.J. Oestrogens and puerperal thrombosis. Brit. Med. J. 4, 769, 1968.

Gupta, K.K. Syndrome of inappropriate secretion of antidiuretic hormone. Lancet 1, 866, 1971.

Guyda, H., Friesen, H. The separation of monkey prolactin from monkey growth hormone by affinity chromatography. Biochem. Biophys. Res. Comm. 42, 1068-75, 1971.

Guyda, H., Hwang, P., Friesen, H. Immunologic evidence for monkey and human prolactin. J. Clin. Endocr. 32, 120-3, 1971.

Hadden, D.R., Montgomery, D.A.D., Weaver, J.A. Myocardial infarction in maturity-onset diabetics. A retrospective study. Lancet 1, 335-8, 1972.

Hafiez, A.A., Bartke, A., Lloyd, C.W. The role of prolactin in the regulation of testis function: the synergistic effects of prolactin and luteinizing hormone on the incorporation of (1-^{14}C) acetate into testosterone and cholesterol by testes from hypophysectomised rats in vitro. J. Endocr. 53, 223-30, 1972.

Hafiez, A.A., Lloyd, C.W., Bartke, A. The role of prolactin in the regulation of testis function: the effects of prolactin and luteinizing hormone on the plasma levels of testosterone and androstenedione in hypophysectomised rats. J. Endocr. 52, 327-32, 1972.

Hafiez, A.A., Philpott, J.E., Bartke, A. The role of prolactin in the regulation of testicular function: the effect of prolactin and luteinizing hormone on 3β-hydroxysteroid dehydrogenase activity in the testes of mice and rats. J. Endocr. 50, 619-23, 1971.

Haigler, K.D., Pittman, J.A., Hershman, J.M., Baugh, C.M. Direct evaluation of pituitary prolactin reserve utilizing synthetic thyrotropin releasing hormone. J. Clin. Endocr. 33, 573-81, 1971.

Halbert, D.R., Christian, C.D. Amenorrhea following oral contraceptives. Obstet. Gynec. 34, 161-7, 1969.

Hall, R. Thyrotrophin releasing hormone and thyroid function. Proc. Roy Soc. Med. in press, 1973.

Hall, R., Ormston, B.J., Besser, G.M., Cryer, R.J., McKendrick, M. The thyrotrophin releasing hormone test in diseases of the pituitary and hypothalamus. Lancet 1, 759-64, 1972.

Hamid, M.A., Rubenstein, D., Ferguson, K.A., Beck, J.C. The effect of growth hormone and prolactin preparations on the intermediary metabolism of rat adipose tissue. Biochem. Biophys. Acta 100, 179-92, 1965.

Hampton, J.R., Gorlin, R. Platelet studies in patients with coronary artery disease and in their relatives. Brit. Heart. J. 34, 465-71, 1972.

Hanwell, A., Linzell, J.L. Evaluation of the effects on cardiac output in the rat by prolactin and growth hormone. J. Endocr. 53, lvii-iii, 1972.

Harrington, F.E., Eggert, R.G., Wilbur, R.D. Induction of ovulation in chlorpromazine-blocked rats. Endocrinology 81, 877-81, 1967.

Harris, P.W.R. Malignant hypertension associated with oral contraceptives. Lancet 2, 466-7, 1969.

Harrold, B.P. Diabetic retinopathy and hypertension. Brit. J. Ophthalmol. 55, 225-32, 1971.

Hart, I.C. A solid phase radioimmunoassay for ovine and caprine prolactin using sepharose 6B: its application to the measurement of circulating levels of prolactin before and during parturition in the goat. J. Endocr. 55, 51-62, 1972.

Hart, I.C. Levels of prolactin in the blood of the goat during milking, throughout lactation and over a 24-hour period. J. Endocr. 55, xxviii, 1972.

Hartmann, P.E., Cowie, A.T. The changes occurring in the mammary glands of lactating rabbits after hypophysectomy and hormone replacement therapy. J. Reprod. Fertil. **21**, 372-3, 1970.

Hartmann, P.E., Cowie, A.T., Hosking, Z.D. Changes in enzymatic activity, chemical composition and histology of the mammary glands and metabolites in the blood of lactating rabbits after hypophysectomy and replacement therapy with sheep prolactin, human growth hormone or bovine growth hormone. J. Endocr. **48**, 433-48, 1970.

Hartmann, G., Endroczi, E., Lissak, K. The effect of hypothalamic implantation of 17-beta-oestradiol and systemic administration of prolactin on sexual behaviour in male rabbits. Acta Physiol. Acad. Sci. Hung. **30**, 53-9, 1966.

Hashimoto, I., Wiest, W.G. Luteotrophic and luetolytic mechanisms in rat corpora lutea. Endocrinology **84**, 886-92, 1969.

Heap, R.B., Perry, J.S., Rowlands, I.N. Corpus luteum function in the guinea pig: arterial and luteal progesterone levels and the effects of hysterectomy and hypophysectomy. J. Reprod. Fertil. **13**, 537-53, 1967.

Heefner, W.A. Dissecting hematoma of the coronary artery. A possible complication of oral contraceptive therapy. J. Am. Med. Ass. **223**, 550-1, 1973.

Heine, B.E., Sainsbury, P., Chynoweth, R.C. Hypertension and emotional disturbances. J. Psychiat. Res. **7**, 119-30, 1969.

Heizmann, A., Klaus, D. Der einfluss von Lithiumchlorid auf die blutdruckwirkung von renin, angiotensin und noradrenalin bei ratten. Klin. Wschr. **45**, 659-60, 1967.

Herbert, D.C., Hayashida, T. Prolactin localization in the primate pituitary by immuno-fluorescence. Science **169**, 378-9, 1970.

Herd, J.A. Behavior and cardiovascular function. Physiologist **14**, 83-9, 1971.

Herlant, M., Pasteels, J.L. Histophysiology of the human anterior pituitary. Meth. Achiev. Exp. Path. **3**, 250-305, 1967.

Hessov, I.B. Hypertension during chlorimipramine therapy. Brit. Med. J. **1**, 406, 1971.

Heuson, J.C., Waelbroeck-van Gaver, C., Legros, N. Growth inhibition of rat mammary carcinoma and endocrine changes produced by 2-bromo-α-ergokryptine, a suppressor of lactation and nidation. Europ. J. Cancer **6**, 353-6, 1970.

Hibbs, R.E. Gynecomastia associated with vitamin deficiency disease. Amer. J. Med. Sci. **213**, 176-7, 1947.

Higgins, J.T. Escape from the sodium-retaining effects of deoxycorticosterone in hypotensive and hypertensive dogs. Proc. Soc. Exp. Biol. Med. **134**, 768-72, 1970.

Hilf, R. Milk-like fluid in a mammary adenocarcinoma: biochemical characterization. Science **155**, 826-7, 1967.

Hilf, R. Mammary tumour growth and biochemistry as influenced by prolactin. pp 181-8 in *Prolactin and Carcinogenesis. 4th Tenovus Workshop.* ed. A.R. Boyns & K. Griffiths. Alpha Omega Alpha Publishing, Cardiff, 1972.

Hilf, R., Goldenberg, H., Bell, C. Effect of actidione (cycloheximide) on estrogen-induced biochemical changes in R3230AC mammary tumors, uteri and mammary glands. Cancer Res. **27**, 1485-93, 1967.

Hilf, R. Bell, C., Goldenberg, H., Michel, I. Effect of fluphenazine HC1 on R3230AC mammary carcinoma and mammary glands of the rat. Cancer Res. **31**, 1111-7, 1971.

Hilf, R., Bell, C., Michel, I. Influence of the mammotropic tumor MtTF4 on the growth and biochemistry of the R3230AC mammary carcinoma and mammary glands. Cancer Res. **27**, 482-9, 1967.

Hilf, R., Goldenberg, H., Michel, I., Carrington, M.J., Bell, C., Gruenstein, M., Meranze, D.R., Shimkin, M.B. Biochemical characteristics of mammary glands and mammary tumors of rats induced by 3-methylcholanthrene and 7, 12-dimethyl-benz(a)anthracene. Cancer Res. 29, 977-88, 1969.

Hilf, R., Michel, I., Bell, C. Biochemical and morphological responses of normal and neoplastic mammary tissue to hormone treatment. Recent Progr. Hormone Res. 23, 229-90, 1967.

Hilf, R., Michel, I., Bell, C., Freeman, J.J., Borman, A. Biochemical and morphologic properties of a new lactating mammary tumor line in the rat. Cancer Res. 25, 286-99, 1965.

Hilf, R., Michel, I., Silverstein, G., Bell, C. Effect of actinomycin D on estrogen-induced changes in enzymes and nucleic acids of R3230AC mammary tumors, uteri and mammary glands. Cancer Res. 25, 1854-9, 1965.

Hillarp, N.A., Fuxe, K., Dahlstrom, A. Demonstration and mapping of central neurons containing dopamine, noradrenaline and 5-hydroxytryptamine and their reactions to psychopharmaca. Pharmacol. Rev. 18, 727-41, 1966.

Hilliard, J., Spies, H.G., Lucas, L., Sawyer, C.H. Effect of prolactin on progestin release and cholesterol storage by rabbit ovarian insterstitium. Endocrinology 82, 122-31, 1972.

Hixon, J.E., Armstrong, D.T. Inhibition of gonadotropin-induced ovulation by prolactin. Endocrinology 89, 584-90, 1971.

Hixon, J.E., Clegg, M.T. Influence of the pituitary on ovarian progesterone output in the ewe: effects of hypophysectomy and gonadotropic hormones. Endocrinology 84, 828-34, 1969.

Hohmann, P., Cole, R.D. Hormonal effects on amino acid incorporation into lysine-rich histones in the mouse mammary gland. J. Mol. Biol. 58, 533-40, 1971.

Hokfelt, T., Fuxe, K. Effects of prolactin and ergot alkaloids on the tubero-infundibular dopamine neurons. Neuroendocrinology 9, 100-22, 1972.

Hopkins, T.F., Meites, J. Effects of epsilon-amino-caproic acid on prolactin-inactivating and fibrinolytic activities of streptokinase-activated plasminogen. Proc. Soc. Exp. Biol. Med. 112, 830-2, 1963.

Hopkins, T.F., Meites, J., Ratner, A. Inactivation of prolactin by human blood serum and plasmin (fibrinolysin) Proc. Soc. Exp. Biol. Med. 106, 140-1, 1961.

Horrell, E., Kilpatrick, R., Major, P.W. A comparison of the effects of pituitary hormones and aminophylline on progestational hormone production by the rabbit ovary in vivo. J. Endocr. 55, 205-6, 1972.

Horrobin, D.F. Some effects of long-term progesterone treatment in rabbits and their relevance to pre-eclampsia. Lancet 1, 170-3, 1968.

Horrobin, D.F. Pathophysiology of pre-eclampsia and of eclampsia. East Afr. Med. J. 48, 163-175, 1971.

Horrobin, D.F. Prevention of migraine by reducing prolactin levels? Lancet 1, 777, 1973.

Horrobin, D.F., Lipton, A., Muiruri, K.L., Manku, M.S., Bramley, P.S., Burstyn, P.G. An inhibitory effect of prolactin on the response of rat myometrium to oxytocin. Experientia 29, 109-10, 1973.

Horrobin, D.F., Lloyd, I.J. Pre-eclamptic toxaemia: possible relevance of progesterone, salt and frusemide. J. Obstet. Gynaec. Brit. Comm. 77, 253-8, 1970.

Horrobin, D.F., Lloyd, I.J., Lipton, A., Burstyn, P.G., Durkin, N., Muiruri, K.L. Actions of prolactin on human renal function. Lancet 2, 352-4, 1971.

Horrobin, D.F., Manku, M.S., Burstyn, P.G. Effect of intravenous prolactin infusion on arterial blood pressure in rabbits. Cardiovasc. Res. in press, 1973.

Horrobin, D.F., Manku, M.S., Burstyn, P.G. Saluretic action of aldosterone in the presence of excess cortisol: restoration of salt-retaining action by prolactin. J. Endocr. 56, 343-4, 1973.

Horrobin, D.F., Manku, M.S., Muriuki, P.B., Burstyn, P.G. Saluretic action of deoxycorticosterone acetate in rabbits in the presence of excess cortisol: restoration of salt-retaining action by prolactin. Submitted for publication, 1973.

Horrobin, D.F., Manku, M.S., Robertshaw, D. Water-losing action of anti-diuretic hormone in the presence of excess cortisol. Restoration of normal action by prolactin or by oxytocin. J. Endocr. in press, 1973.

Houssay, B.A., Anderson, E., Bates, R.W., Li, C.H. Diabetogenic activity of prolactin. Endocrinology 57, 55-63, 1955.

Houssay, B.A., Penhos, J.C. Diabetogenic action of pituitary hormones on adrenalectomized, hypophysectomized dogs. Endocrinology 59, 637-41, 1956.

Huggins, C.B. Two principles in endocrine therapy of cancers: hormone deprival and hormone interference. Cancer Res. 25, 1163-7, 1965.

Huggins, C.B., Briziarelli, G., Sutton, H. Rapid induction of mammary carcinoma in the rat and the influence of hormones on the tumors. J. Exp. Med. 109, 25-41, 1959.

Huggins, C.B., Grand, L.C., Brillantes, F.P. Mammary cancer induced by a single feeding of polynuclear hydrocarbons and its suppression. Nature 189, 204-5, 1961.

Huggins, C.B., Russell, P.S. Quantitative effects of hypophysectomy on testis and prostate of dogs. Endocrinology 39, 1-7, 1946.

Hunter, P.R. Myocardial infarction following surgical operations. Brit. Med. J. 4, 725-8, 1968.

Hunter, P.R., Bloom, A., Kelsey, J.H., Porter, R. Cutaneous capillary resistance and retinal haemorrhage in diabetes. Diabetologia 7, 20-4, 1971.

Huntingford, P.J. The inter-relationship of pituitary hormones and the maintenance of lactation. J. Obstet. Gynaec. Brit. Comm. 70, 929-46, 1963.

Husaini, M.H. Myocardial infarction during pregnancy. Postgrad. Med. J. 47, 660-5, 1971.

Huseby, R.A., Thomas, L.B. Histological and histochemical alterations in the normal breast tissues of patients with advanced breast cancer being treated with estrogenic hormones. Cancer 7, 54-74, 1954.

Hwang, P., Friesen, H., Hardy, J., Wilensky, D. Biosynthesis of human growth hormone and prolactin by normal pituitary glands and pituitary adenomas. J. Clin. Endocr. 33, 1-7, 1971.

Hwang, P., Guyda, H., Friesen, H. A radioimmunoassay for human prolactin. Proc. Nat. Acad. Sci. USA 68, 1902-6, 1971.

Hwang, P., Guyda, H., Friesen, H. Purification of human prolactin. J. Biol. Chem. 247, 1955-8, 1972.

Ichinose, R.R., Nandi, S. Lobuloalveolar differentiation in mouse mammary tissue in vitro. Science 145, 496-7, 1964.

Ieiri, T. Effects of thyroidectomy and triiodothyronine on the synthesis and release of growth hormone and prolactin. Jap. J. Physiol. 21, 551-62, 1971.

Ieiri, T., Akikusa, Y., Yamamoto, K. Synthesis and release of prolactin and growth hormone in vitro during the estrous cycle of the rat. Endocrinology 89, 1533-7, 1971.

Ieiri, T., Nobunaga, T., Yamamoto, K. Fluctuations in the synthesis and release of prolactin by the anterior pituitary of the rat during the oestrous cycle. J. Endocr. 55, 451-2, 1972.

Illingworth, D.V., Perry, J.S. The effect of hypophysial stalk section on the corpus luteum of the guinea pig. J. Endocr. 50, 625-35, 1971.

Ingalls, W., Hafs, H.D., Oxender, W.D. Growth hormone, prolactin and luteinizing hormone in heifers before and after parturition. J. Dairy Sci. 54, 768, 1971.

Ingvarsson, C.G. Prolactin in rheumatoid arthritis (a therapeutic test). Acta Rheum. Scand. 15, 4-17, 1969.

Ingvarsson, C.G. The action of prolactin on the adrenocortical function. Acta Rheum. Scand. 15, 18-20, 1969.

Irey, N.S., Manion, W.C., Taylor, H.B. Vascular lesions in women taking oral contraceptives. Arch. Path. (Chicago) 89, 1-8, 1970.

Irvin, T.T., Modgill, V.K., Hayter, C.J., McDowall, D.G., Goligher, J.C. Plasma volume deficits and salt and water excretion after surgery. Lancet, 2, 11 59-61, 1972.

Ito, A., Martin, J.M., Grindeland, R.E., Takizawa, S., Furth, J. Mammotropic and somatotropic hormones in sera of normal rats and in rats bearing primary and grafted pituitary tumors. Int. J. Cancer 7, 416-29, 1971.

Ivanteeva, E.P. Determination of prolactin in the urine by the immunological method. Probl. Endokr. Gormonoter 9, 99-101, 1963.

Jackson, W.P.U. Post-thyroidectomy hypothyroidism, hypoparathyroidism, exophthalmos and galactorrhea with normal menstruation: metabolic response to probenecid. J. Clin. Endocr., 16, 1245-50, 1956.

Jacobs, E.C. Effects of starvation on sex hormones in the male. J. Clin. Endocr. 8, 227-32, 1948.

Jacobs, L.S., Bauman, J.E., Daughaday, W.H. Hypothalamic influences on prolactin secretion in man. J. Lab. Clin. Med., 78, 818, 1971.

Jacobs, L.S., Mariz, I.K., Daughaday, W.H. A mixed heterologous radioimmunoassay for human prolactin. J. Clin. Endocr. 34, 484-90, 1972.

Janowsky, D.S., El-Yousef, M.K., Dans, J.M., Hubbard, B., Sekerke, H.J. A cholinergic-adrenergic hypothesis of mania and depression. Lancet, 1, 1236, 1972.

Jarvik, M.E. Drugs used in the treatment of psychiatric disorders. pp. 151-203 in *Pharmacological Basis of Therapeutics*, ed. L.S. Goodman and A. Gilman, 4th ed. Macmillan, New York, 1970.

Jasmin, G., Bois, P. Development of an acute polyarthritis in rats treated with prolactin. Arthritis Rheum., 2, 460-4, 1959.

Jasmin, G., Bois, P. Polyarthritis produced in rats by treatment with prolactin and growth hormone. Endocrinology, 65, 494-9, 1959.

Jean, C. Action of prolactin and sematotropic hormone on the differentiation and embryonic development of the mammary gland of mice. Ann. Endocrinol. (Paris), 32, 629-37, 1971.

Jepson, J.H., Lowenstein, L. Effect of prolactin on erythropoiesis in the mouse. Blood, 24, 726-38, 1964.

Jepson, J.H., Lowenstein, L. Erythropoiesis during pregnancy and lactation. I. Effect of various hormones on erythropoiesis during lactation. Proc. Soc. Exp. Biol. Med., 120, 500-4, 1965.

Jepson, J.H., Lowenstein, L. The effect of testosterone, adrenal steroids and prolactin on erythropoiesis. Acta Haemat. (Basel), 38, 292-9, 1967.

Johnson, R.M., Meites, J. Effect of cortisone, hydrocortisone and ACTH on mammary growth and pituitary prolactin content of rats. Proc. Soc. Exp. Biol. Med., 89, 455-8, 1955.

Joke, T. Factors affecting the plasma prolactin level in the cow and the goat as determined by radioimmunoassay. Endocrinol. Jap., 17, 393-401, 1970.

Josimovich, T.B., Boccella, L., Levitt, M.J. Detection of a lactogenic antigen in serum by antibodies to a chemically modified human chorionic somatomammotropin. J. Clin. Endocr., 33, 77-86, 1971.

Josimovich, J.B., Wilson, E.L., Leff, A. Vaginal mucification induced by pituitary prolactin and placental lactogen in mice. Gynecol. Invest., 1, 210-21, 1970.

Kahn, R.H., Baker, B.L. Prolactin content of the rat hypophysis following treatment with norethynodrel. Acta. Endocr. (Kbh), 51, 411-4, 1966.

Kalkhoff, R.K., Richardson, B.L., Beck, P. Relative effects of pregnancy, human placental lactogen and prednisolone on carbohydrate tolerance in normal and subclinical diabetic subjects. Diabetes, 18, 153-63, 1969.

Kalra, S.P., Ajika, K., Krulich, L., Fawcett, C.P., Quijada, M., McCann, S.M. Effects of hypothalamic and preoptic electrochemical stimulation on gonadotropin and prolactin release in proestrus rats. Endocrinology, **88**, 1150-8, 1971.

Kaltenbach, C.C., Graber, J.W., Niswender, G.D., Nalbandov, A.V. Luteotrophic properties of some pituitary hormones in non-pregnant or pregnant hypophysectomised ewes. Endocrinology, **82**, 818-24, 1968.

Kamberi, I.A. p.520 in discussion of paper by Meites, Lu, Wuttke, Welsch, Nagasawa, Quandri, Rec. Progr. Horm. Res., **28**, 471-516, 1972.

Kamberi, I.A., Mical, R.S., Porter, J.C. Luteinizing hormone releasing activity in hypophysial stalk blood and elevation by dopamine. Science, **166**, 388-90, 1969.

Kamberi, I.A., Mical, R.S., Porter, J.C. Prolactin-inhibiting activity in hypophysial stalk blood and elevation by dopamine. Experientia, **26**, 1150-1, 1970.

Kamberi, I.A., Mical, R.S., Porter, J.C. Effect of anterior pituitary perfusion and intraventricular injection of catecholamines on prolactin release. Endocrinology, **88**, 1012-20, 1971a.

Kamberi, I.A., Mical, R.S., Porter, J.C. Effects of melatonin and serotonin on the release of FSH and prolactin. Endocrinology, **88**, 1288-93, 1971b.

Kamberi, I.A., Mical, R.S., Porter, J.C. Pituitary portal vessel infusion of hypothalamic extract and release of LH, FSH and prolactin. Endocrinology, **88**, 1294-99, 1971c.

Kamberi, I.A. Mical, R.S., Porter, J.C. Hypophysial portal vessel infusion: in vivo demonstration of LRF, FRF and PIF in pituitary stalk plasma. Endocrinology, **89**, 1942-46, 1971d.

Kanematsu, S., Hilliard, J., Sawyer, C.H. Effect of hypothalamic lesions on pituitary prolactin content in the rabbit. Endocrinology, **73**, 345-8, 1963.

Kanematsu, S., Hilliard, J., Sawyer, C.H. Effect of reserpine on pituitary prolactin content and its hypothalamic site of action in the rabbit. Acta Endocr. (Kbh), **44**, 467-74, 1963.

Kanematsu, S., Sawyer, C.H. Effects of intrahypothalamic and intrahypophysial estrogen implants on pituitary prolactin and lactation in the rabbit. Endocrinology, **72**, 243-52, 1963.

Kanematsu, S., Sawyer, C.H. Effect of intrahypothalamic implants of reserpine on lactation and pituitary prolactin content in the rabbit. Proc. Soc. Exp. Biol. Med., **113**, 967-9, 1963.

Kann, G. Changes of plasma concentrations of luteinizing hormone and prolactin during the estrous cycle of ewes. C.R. Acad. Sci. D. (Paris), **272**, 2934-7, 1971.

Kann, G. Radioimmunoassay of plasma prolactin in sheep. C.R. Acad. Sci. D. (Paris), **272**, 2808-11, 1971.

Kaplan, S.L., Grumbach, M.M., Friesen, H.G. Effect of thyrotropin releasing factor on release of human pituitary prolactin. Clin. Res., **20**, 254, 1972.

Kaplan, S.L., Grumbach, M.M., Friesen, H.G., Costom, B.H. Thyrotropin releasing factor effect on secretion of human pituitary prolactin and thyrotropin in children and in idiopathic hypopituitary dwarfism: further evidence of hypophysiotropic hormone deficiencies. J. Clin. Endocr., **35**, 825-30, 1972.

Karg, H., Schams, D., Reinhardt, V. Effects of 2-Br-α-ergokryptine on plasma prolactin level and milk yield in cows. Experientia, **28**, 574-6, 1972.

Karsch, F.J., Cook, B., Ellicott, A.R., Foster, D.L., Jackson, G.L., Nalbandov, A.V. Failure of infused prolactin to prolong the life span of the corpus luteum in the ewe. Endocrinology, **89**, 272-5, 1971.

Kastin, A.J. Modification of Parkinsonism. New Eng. J. Med., **276**, 1041, 1967.

Kastin, A.J., Barbeau, A. Can. Med. Ass. J., **107**, 1079, 1972.

Kastin, A.J., Ehrensing, R.H., Schalch, D.S., Anderson, M.S. Improvement in mental depression with decreased thyrotropin response after administration of thyrotropin-releasing hormone. Lancet, **2**, 740-2, 1972.

Katz, F.H., Romfh, P., Smith, J.A. Episodic secretion of aldosterone in supine man: relationship to cortisol. J. Clin. Endocr., **35**, 178-81, 1972.

Katz, J., Kunofsky, S., Patton, R.E., Allaway, N.C. Cancer mortality among patients in New York mental hospitals. Cancer, **20**, 2194-9, 1967.

Kawakami, M., Kimura, F., Wakabayashi, K. Electrical stimulation of the hippocampus under the chronic preparation and changes of LH, FSH and prolactin levels in serum and pituitary. Endocrinol. Jap., **19**, 85-96, 1972.

Keenan, T.W. Prolactin, the Golgi apparatus and milk secretion. J. Dairy Sci., **53**, 1349-52, 1970.

Kellett, J.M. Evolutionary theory for the dichotomy of the functional psychoses. Lancet, **i**, 860-3, 1973.

Kennedy, T.G., Armstrong, D.T., Extra-ovarian effect of prolactin on vaginal mucification in the rat. Endocrinology, **90**, 815-22, 1972.

Kennedy, T.G., Armstrong, D.T. Extra-ovarian action of prolactin in the regulation of uterine fluid accumulation in rats. Endocrinology, **90**, 1503-9, 1972.

Kessler, I.I. A genetic relationship between diabetes and cancer. Lancet, **1**, 218-20, 1970.

Khazan, N., Danon, A. Effect of progestogenic hormones on the endocrine system. Arch. Intern. Pharmacodyn., **141**, 261-286, 1962.

Kiloh, L.G., Davison, K., Osselton, J.W. An electroencephalographic study of the analeptic effects of imipramine. Electroenceph. Clin. Neurophysiol., **13**, 216, 1961.

Kiloh, L.G., McComas, A.J., Osselton, J.W. *Clinical Electroencephalography*, 3rd ed. Butterworth, London, 1972.

Kilpatrick, R., Armstrong, D.T., Greep, R.O. Maintenance of the corpus luteum by gonadotrophins in the hypophysectomised rabbit. Endocrinology, **74**, 453-61, 1964.

Kim, U. Pituitary function and hormonal therapy of experimental breast cancer. Cancer Res. **25**, 1146-56, 1965.

Kim, U., Furth, J. Relation of mammary tumours to mammotropes, I. Induction of mammary tumors in rats. Proc. Soc. Exp. Biol. Med., **103**, 640-2, 1960.

Kim, U., Furth, J. Relation of mammary tumours to mammotropes II. Hormone responsiveness of transplanted mammary tumours. Proc. Soc. Exp. Biol. Med., **103**, 643-5, 1960.

Kim, U., Furth, J., Clifton, K.H. Relation of mammary tumours to mammotropes. III. Hormone responsiveness of transplanted mammary tumours. Proc. Soc. Exp. Biol. Med., **103**, 646-50, 1960.

Kim, U., Furth, J., Yannopoulos, K. Observations on hormonal control of mammary cancer. Estrogen and mammotropes. J. Natl. Cancer Inst., **31**, 233-50, 1963.

Kinch, R.A.H., Plunkett, E.R., Devlin, M.C. Post-partum amenorrhea-galactorrhea of hypothyroidism. Amer. J. Obstet. Gynec., **105**, 766-72, 1969.

Kleeman, C.R. Water metabolism. pp. 215-295 in *Clinical Disorders of Fluid and Electrolyte Metabolism.* ed. M.H. Maxwell, C.R. Kleeman, McGraw Hill, New York, 1972.

Kleinberg, D.L., Frantz, A.G. Human prolactin: measurement in plasma by in vitro bioassay. J. Clin. Invest., **50**, 1557-68, 1971.

Kleinberg, D.L., Noel, G.L., Frantz, A.G. Chlorpromazine stimulation and L-dopa suppression of plasma prolactin in man. J. Clin. Endocr., **33**, 873-6, 1971.

Koch, Y., Chow, Y.F., Meites, J. Metabolic clearance and secretion rates of prolactin in the rat. Endocrinology, **89**, 1303-8, 1971.

Koch, Y., Lu, K-H., Meites, J. Biphasic effects of catecholamines on pituitary prolactin release in vitro. Endocrinology, **87**, 673-5, 1970.

Kohner, E.M., Dollery, C.T., Lowy, C., Schumer, B. Effect of diuretic therapy on glucose tolerance in hypertensive patients. Lancet, 1, 986-90, 1971.

Kohnlein, H.E., Bianchi, L., Biermann, F.J. Der Einfluss von Lactation hormone auf die ischamisierte Rattenniere. Arzneimittelforsch, 16, 480-87, 1966.

Kolodny, R.C., Jacobs, L.S., Daughaday, W.H. Mammary stimulation causes prolactin secretion in non-lactating women. Nature (London), 238, 284-6, 1972.

Kolodny, R.C., Jacobs, L.S., Masters, W.H., Toro, G., Daughaday, W.H. Plasma gonadotropins and prolactin in male homosexuals. Lancet, 2, 18-20, 1972.

Koprowski, J.A. Prolactin and growth hormone circadian periodicity in lactating cows Proc. Soc. Exp. Biol. Med., 140, 1012-4, 1972.

Koprowski, J.A., Tucker, H.A. Failure of oxytocin to initiate prolactin or luteinizing hormone release in lactating dairy cows. J. Dairy Sci., 54, 1675-80, 1971.

Kordon, C., Javoy, F., Vassent, G., Glowinski, J. Blockade of superovulation in the immature rat by increased brain serotonin. Europ. J. Pharmacol., 4, 169-74, 1968.

Kovaleva, I.G., Ryshka, F.Y., Dilman, V.M. Inhibition of lipolytic activity of human growth hormone with sheep prolactin derivative (anaprolactin). Acta Endocrinol. (Kbh), 69, 209-18, 1972.

Kowalski, E., Dabrowski, Z., Stepniewski, M. Prolactin activity in blood samples of women in the time of functional uterine bleedings. Ginek. Pol., 40, 125-31, 1969.

Koyama, H., Sinha, D., Dao, T.L. Effects of hormones and 7, 12, -dimethylbenzanthracene on rat mammary tissue grown in organ culture. J. Natl. Cancer Inst., 48, 1671-80, 1972.

Kragt, C.L., Meites, J. Dose-response relationships between hypothalamic PIF and prolactin release by rat pituitary tissue in vitro. Endocrinology, 80, 1170-3, 1967.

Kraicer, P.F., Strauss, J.F. Ovulation block produced by an inhibitor of luteotrophin, ergocornine. Acta Endocrinol., 65, 698-706, 1970.

Krant, M.J., Brandrup, C.S., Greene, R.S., Pochi, P.E., Strauss, T.S. Sebaceous gland activity in breast cancer. Nature, 217, 463-5, 1968.

Kriss, J.P., Futcher, P.H. Renal excretion and tubular reabsorption of salt in Cushing's syndrome after intravenous administration of hypertonic sodium chloride. J. Clin. Endocrinol., 9, 13. 1949.

Kuhn, N.J. Progesterone withdrawal as the lactogenic trigger in the rat. J. Endocr., 44, 39-54, 1969a.

Kuhn, N.J. Specificity of progesterone inhibition of lactogenesis. J. Endocr., 45, 615-6, 1969b.

Kumaresan, P., Anderson, R.R., Turner, C.W. Effect of graded levels of lactogenic hormone upon mammary gland growth and lactation in rats. Proc. Soc. Exp. Biol. Med., 123, 581-4, 1966.

Kuo, E.Y., Gala, R.R. Radioimmunoassay of rat prolactin comparing prolactin obtained from anterior pituitary organ culture with that distributed by the National Institute of Arthritis and Metabolic Diseases. Biochim. Biophys. Acta, 264, 462-71, 1972.

Kwa, H.G., Feltkamp, C.A., Van der Gugten, A.A., Verhofstad, F. The rate of elimination of prolactin as a determinant factor for plasma levels assayed in rats. J. Endocr., 48, 299-300, 1970.

Kwa, H.G., Van der Gugten, A.A., Sala, M., Verhofstad, F. Effect of pituitary tumours and grafts on plasma prolactin levels. Eur. J. Cancer, 8, 39-54, 1972.

Kwa, H.G., Van der Gugten, A.A., Verhofstad, F. Radioimmunoassay of rat prolactin. Europ. J. Cancer, 5, 571-9, 1969.

Kwa, H.G., Verhofstad, F. Radioimmunoassay of rat prolactin. Biochim. Biophys. Acta, 133, 186-8, 1967.

La Bella, F., Krass, M., Fritz, W., Vivian, S., Shin, S., Queen, G. Isolation of cytoplasmic granules containing growth hormone and prolactin from bovine pituitary. Endocrinology, **89**, 1094-102, 1971.

La Bella, F.S., Vivian, S.R. Effect of synthetic TRF on hormone release from bovine anterior pituitary in vitro. Endocrinology, **88**, 787-9, 1971.

Lal, H.B. Glucose tolerance in hypertension. Indian Heart J., **21**, 55-60, 1969.

Lamming, G.E., Moseley, S., McNeilly, J.R. Prolactin release in the ewe at parturition and first suckling. J. Endocr., **55**, xxvii, 1972.

Lancet. Amines, alerting and affect. Lancet, **1**, 1237-8, 1968.

Lange, K. Capillary permeability in myxedema. Amer. J. Med. Sci., **208**, 5, 1944.

Lapin, L.P., Oxenkrug, G.F. Intensification of the central serotoninergic processes as a possible determinant of thymoleptic effect. Lancet, **1**, 132, 1969.

Laragh, J.H. Oral contraceptives and hypertensive disease. Circulation, **42**, 983-5, 1970.

Lasnitzki, I. The effect of prolactin on rat prostate gland in organ culture. pp 200-6 in. *Prolactin and Carcinogenesis. 4th Tenovus Workshop.* ed. K. Griffiths and A.R. Boyns. Alpha Omega Alpha Publishing, Cardiff, 1972.

Lavoie, J. Lactation after surgery. Can. J. Surg., **11**, 464-5, 1968.

Lawrence, A.M., Landau, R.L. Impaired ventral prostate affinity for testosterone in hypophysectomised rats. Endocrinology, **77**, 1119-25, 1965.

Leaf, A., Bartter, F.C., Santos, R.F., Wrong, O. Evidence in man that urinary electrolyte loss induced by pitressin is a function of water retention. J. Clin. Invest., **32**, 868, 1953.

Léake, R.E., Mayne, R., Barry, J.M. Increase during lactation of RNA synthesis by isolated liver nuclei. Biochem. Biophys. Acta. **157**, 198-200, 1968.

Lee, R.V., Jampol, L.M., Brown, W.V. New Engl. J. Med., **284**, 93, 1971.

Lemay, A., Labrie, F. Calcium-dependent stimulation of prolactin release in rat anterior pituitary in vitro by N^6-monobutyryl adenosine $3'$, $5'$-monophosphate. FEBS Lett, **20**, 7-10, 1972.

Lemon, H.M. Oestriol and prevention of breast cancer. Lancet, **i**, 456-7, 1973.

Levij, I.S., Polliack, A. Inhibition of chemical carcinogenesis in the hamster cheek pouch by chlorpromazine. Nature, **228**, 1096-7, 1970.

Levinsky, N.G., Lalone, R.C. The mechanism of sodium diuresis after saline infusion in the dog. J. Clin. Invest., **42**, 1261, 1963.

Levinsky, N.G., Lalone, R.C. Sodium excretion during acute saline loading in dogs with vena caval constriction. J. Clin. Invest., **44**, 565, 1965.

Lewis, U.J., Singh, R.N.P., Seavey, B.K. Human prolactin: isolation and some properties. Biochem. Biophys. Res. Commun., **44**, 1169-76, 1971.

Lewis, U.J., Singh, R.N.P., Seavey, B.K. Problems in the purification of human prolactin in *Prolactin and Carcinogenesis. 4th Tenovus Workshop.* ed. A.R. Boyns and K. Griffiths, Alpha Omega Alpha Publishing, Cardiff, 1972.

Lewis, U.J., Singh, R.N.P., Sinha, Y.N., Vanderlaan, W.P. Electrophoretic evidence for human prolactin. J. Clin. Endocr., **33**, 153-6, 1971.

Lewis, W.H. Iatrogenic psychotic depressive reaction in hypertensive patients. Am. J. Psychiatry, **127**, 1416-7, 1971.

L'Hermite, M., Copinschi, G., Golstein, J., Vanhaelst, L., Leclercq, R., Bruno, O.D. Prolactin release after injection of thyrotrophin-releasing hormone in man. Lancet, **1**, 763-5, 1972.

L'Hermite, M., Delvoye, P., Nokin, J., Vekemans, M., Robyn, C. Human prolactin secretion as studied by radioimmunoassay in *Prolactin and Carcinogenesis. 4th Tenovus Workshop.* ed. A.R. Boyns and K. Griffiths, Alpha Omega Alpha Publishing, Cardiff, 1972.

L'Hermite, M., Stauric, V., Robyn, C. Human pituitary prolactin during pregnancy and post-partum as measured in serum by a radioimmunoassay. Acta Endocrinol. (Kbh) Suppl., **159**, 37, 1972.

Li, C.H. Comparative chemistry of lactogenic hormones. Gen. Comp. Endocrinol., Suppl., **2**, 1, 1969.

Li, C.H. Recent knowledge of the chemistry of lactogenic hormones. pp. 7-22, in *Lactogenic Hormones*. ed. G.E. Wolstenholme and J. Knight, Churchill Livingstone, 1972.

Li, C.H., Dixon, J.S., Chune, D. Primary structure of the human chorionic sematomammotropin (HCS) molecule. Science, **173**, 56-8, 1971.

Li, C.H., Dixon, J.S., Liu, W.K. Human pituitary growth hormone, XIX. The primary structure of the hormone. Arch Biochem. Biophys., **133**, 70-91, 1969.

Li, C.H., Dixon, J.S., Lo, T-B., Schmidt, K.D., Pankou, Y.A. Studies on pituitary lactogenic hormone. XXX. The primary structure of the sheep hormone. Arch. Biochem. Biophys., **141**, 705-37, 1970.

Li, C.H., Yamashiro, D. The synthesis of a protein possessing growth promoting and lactogenic activities. J. Amer. Chem. Soc., **92**, 7608-9, 1970.

Lindsay, D., Poulson, E., Robson, J.M. The effect of 5-hydroxytryptamine on pregnancy. J. Endocr., **26**, 85-96, 1963.

Linkie, D.M., Niswender, G.D. Serum levels of prolactin, luteinizing hormone and follicle stimulating hormone during pregnancy in the rat. Endocrinology, **90**, 632-7, 1972.

Lipsett, M.B., Bergenstal, D.M. Lack of effect of human growth hormone and ovine prolactin on cancer in man. Cancer Res., **20**, 1172-8, 1960.

Llerena, O., Llerena, L., Molina, A., Butler, T., Pearson, O.H. Prolactin-dependent rat mammary cancer: a model for man? Trans. Assoc. Amer. Phys., **82**, 225-38, 1969.

Locker, D., Superstine, E., Sulman, F.G. Endocrine effects of thalidomide and its analogues. Arch. Int. Pharmacodyn. Ther., **194**, 39-55, 1971.

Lockett, M.F. A comparison of the direct renal actions of pituitary growth and lactogenic hormones. J. Physiol. (London), **181**, 192-9, 1965.

Lockett, M.F., Nail, B. A comparative study of the renal actions of growth and lactogenic hormones in rats. J. Physiol. (London), **180**, 147-56, 1965.

Lockett, M.F., Roberts, C.N. Hormonal factors affecting sodium excretion in the rat. J. Physiol., **167**, 581-90, 1963.

Lockwood, D.H., Turkington, R.W., Topper, Y.J. Hormone-dependent development of milk protein synthesis in mammary gland in vitro. Biochim. Biophys. Acta, **130**, 493-501, 1966.

Loewenstein, J.E., Mariz, I.K., Peake, G.T., Daughaday, W.H. Prolactin bioassay by induction on n-acetyllactosamine synthetase in mouse mammary gland explants. J. Clin. Endocr., **33**, 217-24, 1971.

Lorscheider, F.L., Reineke, E.P. The influence of lactational intensity and exogenous prolactin on serum thyroxine levels in the rat. Proc. Soc. Exp. Biol. Med., **138**, 1116-8, 1971.

Lostroh, A.J., Li, C.H. Stimulation of the sex accessories of hypophysectomised male rats by non-gonadotrophic hormones of the pituitary gland. Acta Endocrinol. (Kbh), **25**, 1-16, 1957.

Lu, K-H., Amenomori, Y., Chen, C-L., Meites, J. Effects of centrally acting drugs on serum and pituitary prolactin levels in rats. Endocrinology, **87**, 667-72, 1970.

Lu, K-H., Koch, Y., Meites, J. Direct inhibition by ergocornine of pituitary prolactin release. Endocrinology, **89**, 229-33, 1971.

Lu, K-H., Meites, J. Inhibition by L-dopa and monoamine oxidase inhibitors of pituitary prolactin release: stimulation by methyldopa and D-amphetamine. Proc. Soc. Exp. Bio. Med., **137**, 480-3, 1971a.

Lu, K-H., Meites, J. Unpublished, quoted in Meites, Clemens, 1972. 1971b.

Lu, K-H., Meites, J. Effects of L-dopa on serum prolactin and PIF in intact and hypophysectomised, pituitary-grafted rats. Endocrinology, 91, 868-72, 1972.

Lu, K-H., Shaar, C.J., Kortright, K.H., Meites, J. Effects of synthetic TRH on in vitro and in vivo prolactin release in the rat. Endocrinology, 91, 1540-45, 1972.

Lunn, T., Cole, E., Boyns, A.R., Nassar, B., Horrobin, D.F. Studies of plasma prolactin levels in clinical disorders of fluid and electrolyte balance. Unpublished, 1973.

Lutterbeck, P.M., Pryor, J.S., Varga, L., Wenner, R. Treatment of non-puerperal galactorrhoea with an ergot alkaloid. Brit. Med. J., 3, 228-9, 1971.

Lyons, W.R. The hormonal basis for "witches' milk". Proc. Soc. Exp. Biol. Med., 37, 207-209, 1937.

Lyons, W.R., Page, E. Detection of mammotropin in the urine of lactating women. Proc. Soc. Exper. Biol. Med., 32, 1049, 1935.

McAttee, J.W., Trenkle, A. Effects of feeding, fasting, glucose or arginine on plasma prolactin levels in the bovine. Endocrinology, 89, 730-4, 1971.

McCalister, A., Welbourne, R.B. Stimulation of mammary cancer by prolactin and the clinical response to hypophysectomy. Brit. Med. J., 1, 1669-70, 1962.

McCormick, G.M., Moon, R.C. Hormones influencing post-partum growth of 7, 12-dimethylbenzanthracene-induced rat tumours. Cancer Res., 27, 626-31, 1967.

MacDonald, G.J. Ovarian function and progestin content in response to gonadotropin. J. Reprod. Fertil., 19, 299-308, 1969.

MacDonald, C.J., Yoshinaga, K., Greep, R.O. Maintenance of luteal function in rats by rat prolactin. Proc. Soc. Exp. Biol. Med., 136, 687-8, 1971.

McDowell, F., Louis, S., McDevitt, E. A clinical trial of Premarin in cerebrovascular disease. J. Chron. Dis., 20, 679-84, 1967.

McGarry, E.E., Beck, J.C. Some metabolic effects of ovine prolactin in man. Lancet, 2, 915-6, 1962.

McGarry, E.E., Beck, J.C. Biological effects of non-primate prolactin and human placental lactogen. pp. 361-83 in *Lactogenic Hormones*. ed. G.E.W. Wolstenholme and J. Knight, Churchill Livingstone, 1972.

MacLean, P. Effects of prolactin in vitro on the metabolism of glucose by rat mammary gland. Biochim. Biophys. Acta, 42, 166-7, 1960.

MacLeod, R.M. Influence of norepinephrine and catecholamine-depleting agents on the synthesis and release of prolactin and growth hormone. Endocrinology, 85, 916-23, 1969.

MacLeod, R.M. Inhibition of the in vitro synthesis of pituitary prolactin and growth hormone by mouse pituitary isografts. Proc. Soc. Exp. Biol. Med., 133, 339-41, 1970.

MacLeod, R.M., Abad, A. Thyroid inhibition of rats bearing transplantable hormone-producing pituitary tumours. Proc. Soc. Exp. Biol. Med., 128, 120-5, 1968.

MacLeod, R.M., Abad, A. On the control of prolactin and growth hormone synthesis in rat pituitary glands. Endocrinology, 83, 799-806, 1968.

MacLeod, R.M., Abad, A., Eidson, L.L. In vivo effect of sex hormones on the in vitro synthesis of prolactin and growth hormone in normal and pituitary tumor-bearing rats. Endocrinology, 84, 1475-83, 1969.

MacLeod, R.M., Bass, M.B., Hwang, S.C., Smith, M.C. Intermediary metabolism in the liver and adipose tissue of rats with hormone-secreting pituitary tumours. Endocrinology, 82, 253-65, 1968.

MacLeod, R.M., Fontham, E.H. Influence of ionic environment on the in vitro synthesis and release of pituitary hormones. Endocrinology, 86, 863-9, 1970.

MacLeod, R.M., Fontham, E.H., Lehmeyer, J.E. Prolactin and growth hormone production as influenced by catecholamines and agents that affect brain catecholamines. Neuroendocrinology, 6, 283-94, 1970.

MacLeod, R.M., Lehmeyer, J.E. Regulation of the synthesis and release of prolactin. pp. 53-76 in *Lactogenic Hormones*. ed. G.E.W. Wolstenholme and J. Knight, Churchill Livingstone, 1972.

McNeilly, J.R. A solid phase radioimmunoassay for ovine prolactin. J. Endocr. 49, 141-9, 1971.

McNeilly, J.R., Lamming, G.E. The effect of perphenazine on the level of prolactin in sheep blood. J. Endocr., 50, 359-60, 1971.

Majumder, G.C., Turkington, R.W. Adenosine 3′, 5′-monophosphate dependent and independen protein phosphokinase enzymes from mammary gland. J. Biol. Chem., 246, 2650-7, 1971a.

Majumder, G.C., Turkington, R.W. Hormonal regulation of protein kinase and adenosine 3′, 5′-monophosphate binding protein in developing mammary gland. J. Biol. Chem., 246, 5545-54, 1971b.

Malarkey, W.B., Daughaday, W.H. Divergent effects of medroxyprogesterone acetate on growth hormone and prolactin in the MSI-TW15 tumour bearing rat. Endocrinology, 90, 909-14, 1972.

Malarkey, W.B., Daughaday, W.H. The influence of levodopa and adrenergic blockade on growth hormone and prolactin secretion in the MSI-TW15 tumour-bearing rat. Endocrinology, 91, 1314-17, 1972.

Malarkey, W.B., Jacobs, L.S., Daughaday, W.H. Levodopa suppression of prolactin in non-puerperal galactorrhea. N. Engl. J. Med., 285, 1160-3, 1971.

Maletzky, B., Blachly, P.H. *The Use of Lithium in Psychiatry*. Chemical Rubber Co., 1971.

Malevski, Y., Yane, M.G., Sculthorpe, A., Sanger, V.L., Mickelsen, O. Hypothalamic and pituitary hormonal changes in rats injected with methylazoxy-methanol acetate. Fed. Proc. 31, 130-5, 1972.

Malven, P.V. Luteotrophic and luteolytic responses to prolactin in hypophysectomised rats. Endocrinology, 84, 1224-9, 1969.

Malven, P.V., Hansel, W., Sawyer, C.H. A mechanism antagonising the luteotrophic action of exogenous prolactin in rats. J. Reprod. Fertil., 13, 205-12, 1967.

Malven, P.V., Hoge, W.R. Effect of ergocornine on prolactin secretion by hypophysial homografts. Endocrinology, 88, 445-9, 1971.

Mandell, A.J., Spooner, C.E. Psychochemical research studies in man. Science, 162, 1442-53, 1968.

Manku, M.S. Responses of the rat mesenteric artery preparation to noradrenaline in the presence of prolactin. Unpublished, 1973.

Manku, M.S., Horrobin, D.F. An inhibitory action of prolactin on pregnant guinea pig myometrium. J. Int. Res. Comm., 1, 16, 1973a.

Manku, M.S., Horrobin, D.F. Effects of 2-bromo-α-ergokryptine on renal function in sheep. In preparation, 1973b.

Manku, M.S., Horrobin, D.F., Burstyn, P.G. Prolactin and ADH release. Lancet, 1, 1243, 1972.

Manku, M.S., Horrobin, D.F., Robertshaw, D. Actions of prolactin and aldosterone on renal function in normal and dehydrated sheep. Submitted for publication, 1973.

Manku, M.S., Mati, J.K.G., Horrobin, D.F. Action of prolactin on human myometrium. Unpublished, 1973.

Mannisto, P., Koivisto, V. Antidiabetic effects of lithium. Lancet, 2, 1031, 1972.

Manns, J.G., Boda, J.M. Effects of ovine growth hormone and prolactin on blood glucose, serum insulin, plasma non-esterified fatty acids and amino nitrogen in sheep. Endocrinology, 76, 1109-14, 1965.

Marsh, J.M., Telegdy, G., Savard, K. Effect of gonadotropins on steroidogenesis in rat ovaries at dioestrus. Nature (London), 212, 950-2, 1966.

Martinazzi, M., Baroni, C. The endocrine dependence of hemopoiesis. Research on pituitary dwarf mice. Haematologica, 47, 615-54, 1962.

Marzluff, W., McCarty, K.S., Turkington, R.W. Insulin-dependent synthesis of histones in relation to the mammary epithelial cell cycle. Biochim. Biophys. Acta, 190, 517-26, 1969.

Mason, N.R., Tinsley, F.C., Cochrane, R.L. Effect of prolactin and 5-bromo-2-thionyl-ethyl ketone thio-semicarbazone on ovarian progestin levels in the rat. Endocrinology, 85, 831-6, 1969.

Mati, J.K.G., Horrobin, D.F., Bramley, P.S. Induction of labour in sheep and humans by single injections of dexamethasone or of betamethasone into the amniotic fluid. Brit. Med. J. 2, 149-51, 1973.

Mauvais-Jarvis, P., De Lignieres, B. Hormone dependence of breast cancer. Nouv. Presse Med., 1, 1945-8, 1972.

Mears, E., Grant, E.C.G. Anovlar as an oral contraceptive. Brit. Med. J., 2, 75-9, 1962.

Medical Research Council Brain Metabolism Unit. Modified amine hypothesis for the aetiology of affective illness. Lancet, 2, 573-7, 1972.

Meers, P.D. Allergy and cancer. Lancet, i, 884, 1973.

Meier, A.H., Martin, D.D., MacGregor, R. Temporal synergism of corticosterone and prolactin controlling gonadal growth in sparrows. Science, 173, 1240-2, 1971.

Meier, A.H., Trobec, T.N., Joseph, M.M., John, T.M. Temporal synergism of prolactin and adrenal steroids in the regulation of fat stores. Proc. Soc. Exper. Biol. Med., 137, 408-15, 1971.

Meites, J. Maintenance of the mammary lobulo-alveolar system in rats after adreno-orchidectomy by prolactin and growth hormone. Endocrinology, 76, 1220-3, 1965.

Meites, J. Hypothalamic control of prolactin secretion. pp. 325-338 in *Lactogenic Hormones.* ed. G.E.W. Wolstenholme and J. Knight, Churchill Livingstone, 1972a.

Meites, J. Relation of prolactin to mammary tumourigenesis and growth in rats. *Prolactin and Carcinogenesis. 4th Tenovus Workshop.* ed. A.R. Boyns and K. Griffiths. Alpha Omega Alpha Publishing, Cardiff, 1972b.

Meites, J. Discussion pp. 176-7 in *Prolactin and Carcinogenesis. 4th Tenovus Workshop.* ed. A.R. Boyns and K. Griffiths, Alpha Omega Alpha Publishing, Cardiff, 1972c.

Meites, J. Relation of prolactin and estrogen to mammary tumorigenesis in the rat. J. Natl. Cancer Inst., 48, 1217-24, 1972d.

Meites, J., Cassell, E., Clark, J. Estrogen inhibition of mammary tumor growth in rats: counteraction by prolactin. Proc. Soc. Exp. Biol. Med., 137, 1225-7, 1971.

Meites, J., Clemens, J.A. Hypothalamic control of prolactin secretion. Vitam. Horm., 30, 165-221, 1972.

Meites, J., Hopkins, T.F., Talwalker, P.K., Induction of lactation in pregnant rabbits with prolactin, cortisol acetate or both. Endocrinology, 73, 261-4, 1963.

Meites, J., Kahn, R.H., Nicoll, C.S. Prolactin production by rat pituitary in vitro. Proc. Soc. Exp. Biol. Med., 108, 440-3, 1961.

Meites, J., Lu, K.H., Wuttke, W., Welsch, C.N., Nagasawa, H., Quadri, S.K. Recent studies on functions and control of prolactin secretion in rats. Rec. Prog. Horm. Res., 28, 471-516, 1972.

Meites, J., Nicoll, C.S. Adenohypophysis: prolactin. Ann. Rev. Physiol., 28, 57, 1966.

Meites, J., Sgouris, J.T. Effects of altering the balance between prolactin and ovarian hormones on initiation of lactation in rabbits. Endocrinology 55, 530-4, 1964.

Meites, J., Talwalker, P.K., Nicoll, C.S. Initiation of lactation in rats with hypothalamic or cerebral tissue. Proc. Soc. Exp. Biol. Med. 103, 298-300, 1960.

Melby, J.C., Dale, S.L., Wilson, T.E., Nicholas, A.S. Stimulation of aldosterone secretion by human placental lactogen. Clin. Res. 14, 283, 1966.

Mellerup, E.T., Plenge, P., Vendsborg, P., Rafaelsen, O.J., Kjeldsen, H., Agerbaek, H. Anti-diabetic effects of lithium. Lancet 2, 1367-8, 1972.

Mena, F., Beyer, C. Effect of high spinal section on established lactation in the rabbit. Amer. J. Physiol. 205, 313-6, 1963.

Mena, F., Grosvenor, C.E. Effect of number of pups upon suckling-induced fall in pituitary prolactin concentration and milk ejection in the rat. Endocrinology 82, 623-6, 1968.

Mena, F., Grosvenor, C.E. Effect of suckling and of exteroceptive stimulation upon prolactin release in the rat during late lactation. J. Endocr. 52, 11-22, 1972.

Mena, F., Maiweg, H., Grosvenor, C.E. Effect of ectopic pituitary glands upon prolactin concentration in the in situ pituitary of the lactating rat. Endocrinology 83, 1359-62, 1968.

Miall, W.E. Follow up study of arterial pressure in the population of a Welsh mining valley. Brit. Med. J. 2, 1204-10, 1959.

Milkovic, S., Garrison, M.M., Bates, R.W. Study of the hormonal control of body and organ size in rats with mammotropic tumors. Endocrinology 75, 670-91, 1964.

Minaguchi, H., Clemens, J.A., Meites, J. Changes in pituitary prolactin levels in rats from weaning to adulthood. Endocrinology 82, 555-8, 1968.

Minaguchi, H., Meites, J. Effects of suckling on hypothalamic LH-releasing factor and prolactin-inhibiting factor and on pituitary LH and prolactin. Endocrinology 80, 603-7, 1967a.

Minaguchi, H., Meites, J. Effects of a norethynodrel-mestranol combination (Enovid) on hypothalamic and pituitary hormones in rats. Endocrinology 81, 826-34, 1967b.

Minton, J.P., Dickey, R.P. Prolactin, FSH and LH in breast cancer: effect of levodopa and oophorectomy. Lancet, 1, 1069-70, 1972.

Mishkinsky, J., Kazhen, K., Sulman, F.G. Prolactin-releasing activity of the hypothalamus in post-partum rats. Endocrinology 82, 611-3, 1968.

Mishkinsky, J., Nir, I., Sulman, F.G. Internal feedback of prolactin in the rat. Neuroendocrinology 5, 48-52, 1970.

Mitnick, M., Reichlin, S. Thyrotropin-releasing hormone: biosynthesis by rat hypothalamic fragments in vitro. Science 172, 1241-3, 1971.

Mitsuda, Y. On the urinary excretion of pituitary prolactin. J. Jap. Obstet. Gynec. Soc. 17, 221-30, 1965.

Mittler, J.C., Meites, J. Effects of epinephrine and acetylcholine on hypothalamic content of prolactin-inhibiting factor. Proc. Soc. Exp. Biol. Med. 124, 310-1, 1967.

Mittra, B. Potassium, glucose and insulin in the treatment of myocardial infarction. Lancet 2, 607-9, 1965.

Mittra, B. Potassium, glucose and insulin in the treatment of heart block after myocardial infarction. Lancet 2, 1438-40, 1966.

Miyakawa, N. Luteolytic activity of prolactin in rats. Folia Endocr. Jap. 48, 265-7, 1972.

Mizuno, H., Talwalker, P.K., Meites, J. Influence of hormones on tumor growth and plasma prolactin levels in rats bearing a pituitary mammotropic tumor. Cancer Res. 24, 1433-6, 1964.

Moger, W.H., Geschwind, I.I. Plasma prolactin levels in fetal sheep. Experientia 27, 1479-80, 1971.

Moltz, H., Levin, R., Leon, M. Prolactin in the post partum rat: synthesis and release in the absence of suckling stimulation. Science **163**, 1083-4, 1969.

Moltz, H., Lubin, M., Leon, M., Numan, M. Hormonal induction of maternal behavior in the ovariectomized nulliparous rat. Physiol. Behav. **5**, 1373-7, 1970.

Moon, R.C., Young, S. Progestin secretion in 3-methylcholanthrene-treated rats. Int. J. Cancer **9**, 402-8, 1972.

Moore, R.O., Ball, E.G. Studies on the metabolism of adipose tissue: some in vitro effects of a prolactin preparation alone and in combination with insulin or adrenalin. Endocrinology **71**, 57-67, 1962.

Moses, A.M., Numan, P., Miller, M. Mechanism of chlorpropamide-induced antidiuresis in man: evidence for release of ADH and enhancement of peripheral action. Metabolism **22**, 59-66, 1973.

Muhlbock, O., Boot, L.M. The mode of action of ovarian hormones in the induction of mammary cancer in mice. Biochem. Pharm. **16**, 627-30, 1967.

Mulrow, P.J., Boyd, J.E. Hormonal effects on water and electrolyte metabolism excluding divalent cations and neurophyophysial hormones. pp 151-61 in *Clinical Disorders of Fluid and Electrolyte Metabolism*. ed. M.11. Maxwell & C.R. Kleeman, McGraw Hill, New York, 1972.

Mund, A., Simson, J., Rothfield, N. Effect of pregnancy on course of systemic lupus erythematosus. J. Am. Med. Ass. **183**, 917-20, 1963.

Murphy, D.L., Goodwin, F.K., Bunney, W.E. Aldosterone and sodium response to lithium administration. Lancet **2**, 458-61, 1969.

Murray, R.M.L., Mozaffarian, G., Pearson, O.H. Prolactin levels with L-dopa treatment in metastatic breast carcinoma. in *Prolactin and Carcinogenesis. 4th Tenovus Workshop*. ed. A.R. Boyns & K. Griffiths. Alpha Omega Alpha Publishing, Cardiff, 1972.

Musto, N., Hafiez, A.A., Bartke, A. Prolactin increases 17 β-hydroxysteroid dehydrogenase activity in the testis. Endocrinology **91**, 1106-8, 1972.

Nagasawa, H. Role of prolactin in experimental breast cancer. I. Clin. Endocr. (Tokyo) **19**, 625-9, 1971a.

Nagasawa, H. Role of prolactin in experimental breast cancer. II. Clin. Endocr. (Tokyo), **19**, 707-11, 1971b.

Nagasawa, H., Chen, C.L., Meites, J. Effects of estrogen implant in median eminence on serum and pituitary prolactin levels in the rat. Proc. Soc. Exp. Biol. Med. **132**, 859-61, 1969.

Nagasawa, H., Meites, J. Suppression by ergocornine and iproniazid of carcinogen-induced mammary tumors in rats: effects on serum and pituitary prolactin levels. Proc. Soc. Exp. Biol. Med. **135**, 469-72, 1970.

Nagasawa, H., Yanai, R. Reduction by pituitary isograft of inhibitory effect of large doses of estrogen on incidence of mammary tumors induced by carcinogen in ovariectomized rats. Int. J. Cancer **8**, 463-7, 1971.

Nagasawa, H., Yanai, R. Inhibitory effect of estrogen on mammary growth and its counteraction by pituitary isografts in mice. Endocr. Japon **19**, 107-10, 1972.

Nagasawa, H., Yanai, R. Promotion of pituitary prolactin release in rats by dibutyryl adenosine-3', 5'-monophosphate (cyclic AMP). J. Endocr. **55**, 215-6, 1972.

Nagasawa, H., Yanai, R., Iwahashi, H., Fujimoto, M., Kuretani, K. Difference in mammary gland susceptibility to prolactin between a high and a low mammary tumor strain of mice. Endocr. Japon **14**, 351-6, 1967.

Nagasawa, H., Yanai, R., Kuretani, K. Lack of effect of 7, 12-dimethylbenzanthracene on the prolactin secretory activity of the anterior pituitary in the rat. Gann **59**, 357-9, 1968.

Nagy, I., Kurcz, M., Kiss, C., Baranyai, P., Mosonyi, L., Halmy, L. The effect of suckling, stress and drugs on pituitary prolactin content in the rat. Acta Physiol. Acad. Sci. Hung. **38** 371-80, 1970.

Nandi, S., Bern, H.A. Relation between mammary gland responses to lactogenic hormone combinations and tumor susceptibility in various strains of mice. J. Nat. Cancer Inst., **24**, 907-24, 1960.

Nasr, H., Mozaffarian, G., Pensky, J., Pearson, O.H. Prolactin-secreting pituitary tumors in women. J. Clin. Endocr. **35**, 505-12, 1972.

Ndeti, C.S., Horrobin, D.F., Burstyn, P.G., Hopcraft, M.M. Salt to lower blood pressure. New Eng. J. Med. **286**, 782-3, 1972.

Neill, J.D. Effect of stress on serum prolactin and luteinizing hormone levels during the estrous cycle of the rat. Endocrinology **87**, 1192-7, 1970.

Neill, J.D. Comparison of plasma prolactin levels in the cannulated and decapitated rat. Endocrinology **90**, 568-72, 1972a.

Neill, J.D. Sexual differences in the hypothalamic regulation of prolactin secretion. Endocrinology **90**, 1154-9, 1972b.

Neill, J.D., Freeman, M.E., Tillson, S.A. Control of the proestrus surge of prolactin and luteinizing hormone secretion by estrogens in the rat. Endocrinology **89**, 1448-53, 1971.

Neill, J.D., Reichert, L.E. Development of radioimmunoassay for rat prolactin and evaluation of the NIAMD rat prolactin radioimmunoassay. Endocrinology **88**, 548-55, 1971.

Nejad, N.S., Chaikoff, I.L., Hill, R. Hormonal repair of defective lipogenesis from glucose in the liver of the hypophysectomised rat. Endocrinology **71**, 107-12, 1962.

Nelson, D.H., August, J.T. Abnormal response of oedematous patients to aldosterone or deoxycorticosterone. Lancet **2**, 883-5, 1959.

Newball, H., Byar, D. Unpublished, quoted by Farmsworth, 1972.

Niall, H.D. Revised primary structure for human growth hormone. Nature New Biol. **230**, 90-1, 1971.

Niall, H.D. The chemistry of human lactogenic hormones. in *Prolactin and Carcinogenesis. 4th Tenovus Workshop.* ed. A.R. Boyns & K. Griffiths, Alpha Omega Alpha, Cardiff, 1972.

Niall, H.D., Hogan, M.L., Sauer, R., Rosenblum, I.Y., Greenwood, F.C., Sequences of pituitary and placental lactogenic and growth hormones: evolution from a primordial peptide by gene duplication. Proc. Nat. Acad., Sci. USA **68**, 866-70, 1971.

Nicholson, P.M. Physiological variations in prolactin content of the mouse pituitary gland examined by disc electrophoresis and bioassay. J. Endocr. **47**, 403-9, 1970a.

Nicholson, P.M. A study of prolactin-like activity in individual human pituitary glands. J. Endocr. **48**, 639-47, 1970b.

Nicoll, C.S. Bioassay of prolactin. Analysis of the pigeon crop sac response to local prolactin injection by an objective and quantitative method. Endocrinology **80**, 641, 1967.

Nicoll, C.S. Bioassay of prolactin. Analysis of the pigeon crop sac response to systemic prolactin injection by an improved method of response quantification. Acta Endocrinol. (Kbh) **60**, 91, 1969.

Nicoll, C.S. Secretion of prolactin and growth hormone by adenohypophyses of rhesus monkeys in vitro. pp 257-68 in *Lactogenic Hormones.* ed. G.E.W. Wolstenholme & J. Knight, Churchill Livingstone, 1972.

Nicoll, C.S., Bern, H.A. On the actions of prolactin among the vertebrates: is there a common denominator? pp 299-317 in *Lactogenic Hormones.* ed. G.E.W. Wolstenholme & J. Knight, Churchill Livingstone, 1972.

Nicoll, C.S., Blair, S.M., Nichols, C.W., Russell, S.M., Taylor, M. Prolactin and growth hormone levels in serum from cavernous sinus of rhesus monkeys. J. Clin. Endocr. **34**, 1087-90, 1972.

Nicoll, C.S., Bryant, G.D. Physiological and immunological properties of prolactins. in *Prolactin and Carcinogenesis. 4th Tenovus Workshop.* ed. A.R. Boyns & K. Griffiths, Alpha Omega Alpha Publishing, Cardiff, 1972.

Nicoll, C.S., Meites, J. Estrogen stimulation of prolactin production by rat adenohypophysis in vitro. Endocrinology 70, 272-77, 1962a.

Nicoll, C.S., Meites, J. Failure of neurohypophysial hormones to influence prolactin secretion in vitro. Endocrinology 70, 927-9, 1962b.

Nicoll, C.S., Meites, J. Prolactin secretion in vitro: effects of thyroid hormones and insulin. Endocrinology 72, 544-51, 1963.

Nicoll, C.S., Meites, J. Prolactin secretion in vitro: effects of gonadal and adrenal cortical steroids. Proc. Soc. Exp. Biol. Med. 117, 579-83, 1964.

Nicoll, C.S., Parsons, J.A., Fiorindo, R.P. Estimation of prolactin and growth hormone levels by polyacrylamide disc electrophoresis. J. Endocr. 45, 183-96, 1969.

Nicoll, C.S., Parsons, J.A., Fiorindo, R.P., Nichols, C.W., Sakuma, M. Evidence of independent secretion of prolactin and growth hormone in vitro by adenohypophyses of rhesus monkeys. J. Clin. Endocr. 30, 512-9, 1970.

Nicoll, C.S., Talwalker, P.K., Meites, J. Initiation of lactation in rats by non-specific stresses. Amer. J. Physiol. 198, 1103-6, 1960.

Nicoll, C.S., Yaron, Z., Nutt, N., Daniels, E. Effects of ergotamine tartrate on prolactin and growth hormone secretion by rat adenohypophysis in vitro. Biol. Reprod. 5, 59-66, 1971.

Nikitovitch-Winer, M.B. Effect of hypophysial stalk transection on luteotropic hormone secretion in the rat. Endocrinology 77, 658-66, 1965.

Nikkari, T., Valavaara, M. Effects of androgens and prolactin on the rate of production and composition of sebum in hypophysectomised female rats. J. Endocr. 48, 373-8, 1970.

Niswender, G.D. The effect of ergocornine on reproduction in sheep. Biol. Reprod. 7, 138-9, 1972.

Noel, G.L., Suh, H.K., Frantz, A.G. Stimulation of prolactin release by stress in humans. Clin. Res. 19, 718, 1971.

Noel, G.L., Suh, H.K., Stone, J.G., Frantz, A.G. Human prolactin and growth hormone release during surgery and other conditions of stress. J. Clin. Endocr. 35, 840-51, 1972.

Nokin, J., Vekemans, M., L'Hermite, M., Robyn, C. Circadian periodicity of serum prolactin concentration in man. Brit. Med. J. 3, 561-2, 1972.

Obst, J.M., Seamark, R.F. Plasma oestrogen concentrations in ewes during parturition. J. Reprod. Fertil. 28, 161-2, 1972.

Oka, T., Topper, Y.J. Hormone-dependent accumulation of rough endoplasmic reticulum in mouse mammary epithelial cells in vitro. J. Biol. Chem. 246, 7701-7, 1971.

Oka, T., Topper, Y.J. Is prolactin mitogenic for mammary epithelium? Proc. Nat. Acad. Sci. USA 69, 1693-6, 1972.

Okamoto, R. Prolactin. Clin. Endocr. (Tokyo) 19, 788-91, 1971.

Oliver, M.F. Oral contraceptives and myocardial infarction. Brit. Med. J. 2, 210-3, 1970.

Orloff, M.J., Hutchin, P. Fluid and electrolyte response to trauma and surgery. pp 1063-88 in *Clinical Disorders of Fluid and Electrolyte Metabolism.* ed. M.H. Maxwell & C.R. Kleeman, McGraw Hill, New York, 1972.

Ormston, B.J., Garry, R., Cryer, R.J., Besser, G.M., Hall, R. Thyrotrophin-releasing hormone as a thyroid function test. Lancet 2, 10-14, 1971.

Ormston, B.J., Kilborn, J.R., Garry, R., Amos, J., Hall, R. Further observations on the effect of synthetic thyrotrophin-releasing hormone in man. Brit. Med. J. 2, 199-202, 1971.

Ota, K., Shinde, Y., Yokoyama, A. Relationship between oxytocin and prolactin secretion in maintenance of lactation in rats. Endocrinology **76**, 1-8, 1965.

Oxender, W.D. Serum growth hormone, LH and prolactin in the pregnant cow. J. Anim. Sci. **35**, 51-5, 1972a.

Oxender, W.D. Serum growth hormone, LH and prolactin in the bovine fetus and neonate. J. Anim. Sci. **35**, 56-61, 1972b.

Oxender, W.D., Convey, E.M., Hafs, H.D. Bovine fetal pituitary concentration and in vitro synthesis of prolactin, GH and LH. Proc. Soc. Exp. Biol. Med. **139**, 1017-21, 1972.

Papaioannou, A.N. Prolactin, levodopa and immune response in breast cancer. Lancet **2**, 226, 1972.

Pare, C.M.B., Yeung, D.P.H., Price, K., Stacey, R.S. 5-hydroxytryptamine, noradrenaline and dopamine in brainstem, hypothalamus and caudate nucleus of controls and of patients committing suicide by coal gas poisoning. Lancet **2**, 133, 1969.

Parsons, J.A. Calcium ion requirement for prolactin secretion by rat adenohypophysis in vitro. Amer. J. Physiol. **217**, 1599-603, 1969.

Parsons, J.A. Effects of cations on prolactin and growth hormone secretion by rat adenohypophyses in vitro. J. Physiol. (Lond.) **210**, 973-87, 1970.

Parsons, J.A., Nicoll, C.S. Mechanism of action of prolactin-inhibiting factor. Neuroendocrinology **8**, 213-27, 1971.

Pasteels, J.L. C.R. Acad. Sci. (Paris) **253**, 2140, 1961.

Pasteels, J.L. Recherches morphologiques et experimentales sur la secretion de prolactine. Arch. Biol. (Liege) **74**, 439, 1963.

Pasteels, J.L. Morphology of prolactin secretion. pp 241-55 in *Lactogenic Hormones*. ed. G.E.W. Wolstenholme & J. Knight, Churchill Livingstone, 1972a.

Pasteels, J.L. Tissue culture of human hypophyses: evidence of a specific prolactin in man. pp 269-77 in *Lactogenic Hormones*. ed. G.E.W. Wolstenholme and J. Knight, Churchill Livingstone, 1972b.

Pasteels, J.L., Brauman, H., Brauman, J. Comparative study of the secretion of somatotropic hormone by the human pituitary gland in vitro and of its lactogenic activity. C.R. Acad. Sci. (Paris) **256**, 2031-3, 1963.

Pasteels, J.L., Danguy, A., Frerotte, M., Ectors, F. Inhibition of prolactin secretion by ergocornine and 2-Br-α-ergokryptine: direct action on the pituitary in culture. Ann. d'Endocrinol. **32**, 188-92, 1971.

Pasteels, J.L., Ectors, F. Sensitivity of the anterior hypothalamus to progesterone and medroxyprogesterone. Ann. Endocr. (Paris) **29**, 663-78, 1968.

Pasteels, J.L., Ectors, F. The mode of action of ergocornine on the secretion of prolactin. Arch. Int. Pharmacodyn. **186**, 195-6, 1970.

Pasteels, J.L., Gausset, P., Danguy, A., Ectors, F. Immunofluorescent studies on prolactin and the pituitary. pp 128-136 in *Prolactin and Carcinogenesis. 4th Tenovus Workshop.* ed. A.R. Boyns & K. Griffiths, Alpha Omega Alpha Publishing, Cardiff, 1972.

Pasteels, J.L., Gauesset, P., Danguy, A., Ectors, F., Nicoll, C.S., Varavudhi, P. Morphology of the lactotropes and somatotropes of man and rhesus monkeys. J. Clin. Endocr. **34**, 959-67, 1972.

Pasteels, J.L., Robyn, C., Hubinont, P.O. An immune serum which neutralizes human prolactin. C.R. Acad. Sci. (Paris) **260**, 4381-4, 1965.

Patel, Y., Baker, G., Alford, F., Johns, M., Burger, H. Periodicity of serum prolactin concentration. Brit. Med. J. **4**, 110, 1972.

Peake, G.T., McKeel, D.W., Jarrett, L., Daughaday, W.H. Ultrastructural histologic and hormonal characterization of a prolactin-rich pituitary tumor. J. Clin. Endocr. **29**, 1383-93, 1969.

Pearce, M.L., Dayton, S. Incidence of cancer in men on a diet high in polyunsaturated fat. Lancet 1, 464-7, 1971.

Pearson, O.H., Llerena, O., Llerena, L., Molina, A., Butler, T. Prolactin-dependent rat mammary cancer: a model for man. Trans. Ass. Amer. Physicians 82, 225-38, 1969.

Pearson, O.H., Murray, R., Mozaffarian, G., Pensky, J. Prolactin and experimental breast cancer. in Prolactin and Carcinogenesis. 4th Tenovus Workshop. ed. A.R. Boyns & K. Griffiths, Alpha Omega Alpha, Cardiff, 1972.

Pearson, O.H., Ray, B.S., Results of hypophysectomy in the treatment of metastatic mammary carcinoma. Cancer 12, 85-92, 1959.

Pearson, O.H., West, C.D., Hollander, V.P., Treves, N. Evaluation of endocrine therapy for advanced breast cancer. J. Am. Med. Ass. 154, 234-9, 1954.

Pelletier, G., Lemay, A., Beraud, G., Labrie, F. Ultrastructural changes accompanying the stimulatory effect of N^6-monobutyryl adenosine $3'$, $5'$-monophosphate on the release of growth hormone, prolactin and adrenocorticotrophic hormone in rat anterior pituitary gland in vitro. Endocrinology 91, 1355-71, 1972.

Pendl, G. Cerebrovascular episodes in patients taking ovulation inhibitors. Munch. Med. Wschr. 115, 178-82, 1973.

Perera, G.A. Effect of continued desoxycorticosterone administration in hypertensive subjects. Proc. Soc. Exp. Biol. Med. 68, 48-50, 1948.

Peters, M.V. The effect of pregnancy on breast cancer. pp 65-81 in Prognostic Factors in Breast Cancer. ed. A.P.M. Forrest & P.B. Kunkler, Livingstone, 1968.

Peyre, A., Ravault, J.P., Laporte, P. Potentiating effect of prolactin on the response to testosterone of the sexual accessory glands in castrated rats. C.R. Soc. Biol. (Paris) 162, 1592-5, 1968.

Philbert, M. The cardiovascular manifestations of the premenstrual syndrome. Coeur Med. Intern. 1, 315-22, 1962.

Phillips, B.M. Oral contraceptive drugs and migraine. Brit. Med. J. 2, 99, 1968.

Picard, C. Why is normal pregnancy diabetogenic? Bull. Fed. Soc. Gynecol. Obstet. Lang. Fr. 20, 447-8, 1968.

Pimstone, B.L. LE cells after oral contraceptives. Lancet 1, 1153, 1968.

Pittinger, W.A., Talner, L., Ferris, T.F., Inappropriate secretion of antidiuretic hormone due to myxedema. New Eng. J. Med. 272, 362, 1965.

Pittman, J.A., Haigler, E.D., Hershman, J.M., Pittman, C.S. Hypothalamic hypothyroidism. New. Eng. J. Med. 285, 844-5, 1971.

Plotnikoff, N.P., Kastin, A.J., Anderson, M.S., Schally, A.V. DOPA-potentiation by a hypothalamic factor, MSH-releasing hormone (MIF). Life Sci. 10, 1279-84, 1971.

Plotnikoff, N.P., Prange, A.J., Breese, G.R. Anderson, M.S., Wilson, I.C. Science 178, 417, 1972.

Poirier, L.J., Sourkes, J.L., Bouvier, G., Boucher, R., Carabin, S. Striatal amines, experimental tremor and the effect of harmaline in the monkey. Brain 89, 37, 1966.

Polishuk, W.F., Kulesan, S. Effects of chlorpromazine on pituitary function. J. Clin. Endocr. 16, 292-3, 1956.

Poller, L., Thomson, J.M., Taniowo, A., Priest, C.M. Progesterone oral contraception and blood coagulation. Brit. Med. J. 1, 554-6, 1969.

Poplawski, A., Skorulska, M., Niewarowski, S. Increased platelet adhesiveness in hypertensive cardiovascular disease. J. Atheroscler. Res. 8, 721-3, 1968.

Potter, J.L., Duthie, J.J.R. Effects of environmental temperature upon capillary resistance in patients with rheumatoid arthritis and other individuals. Ann. Rheum. Dis. 20, 144-8, 1961.

Potter, J.L., Wigzell, F.W. Capillary resistance in rheumatoid arthritis. Ann. Rheum. Dis. 16, 357-64, 1957.

Poulson, E., Robson, J.M. The effect of amine oxidase inhibitors on pregnancy. J. Endocr. 27, 147-55, 1963.

Poulson, E., Robson, J.M. Effect of phenelzine and some related compounds on pregnancy and on sexual development. J. Endocr. 30, 205-15, 1964.

Prange, A.J., Wilson, I.C., Lara, P.P., Alltop, L.B., Breese, G.R. Effects of thyrotropin-releasing hormone in depression. Lancet 2, 999-1002, 1972.

Price, J.M., Thornton, M.J., Mueller, L.M. Tryptophan metabolism in women using steroid hormones for ovulation control. Amer. J. Clin. Nutr. 20, 452, 1967.

Quadri, S.K., Meites, J. LSD-induced decrease in serum prolactin in rats. Proc. Soc. Exp. Biol. Med. 137, 1242-3, 1971a.

Quadri, S.K., Meites, J. Regression of spontaneous mammary tumors in rats by ergot drugs. Proc. Soc. Exp. Biol. Med. 138, 999-1001, 1971.

Quinlan, J.T. Lactation following thoracotomy. Canad. J. Surg. 11, 60, 1968.

Rabii, J., Kragt, C.L. Plasma levels of prolactin, FSH and LH in the pseudo-pregnant rat. Proc. Soc. Exp. Biol. Med. 141, 359-62, 1972.

Rado, J.P., Szende, L., Borbely, L., Banos, C., Tako, J., Fischer, J. Different effects of frusemide administered during hypertonic saline infusions in healthy subjects and hypertensive patients. Clin. Sci. 39, 833-45, 1970.

Ragan, C. The syndrome of polydipsia and polyuria induced in normal animals by desoxycorticosterone acetate. Amer. J. Physiol. 131, 73, 1940.

Ramirez, V.D., McCann, S.M. Induction of prolactin secretion by implants of estrogen into the hypothalamo-hypophysial region of female rats. Endocrinology 75, 206-14, 1964.

Ramsay, T.A., Mendels, J., Stokes, J.W., Fitzgerald, R.G. Lithium carbonate and kidney function. A failure in renal concentrating ability. J. Am. Med. Ass. 219, 1446-9, 1972.

Ramsey, D.H., Bern, H.A. Stimulation by ovine prolactin of fluid transfer in everted sacs of rat small intestine. J. Endocr. 53, 453-9, 1972.

Rapoport, A., Husdan, H., Wilkins, G.E. A standardised test of renal concentrating ability in adults with some results in essential hypertension. Canad. Med. Ass. J. 101, 741-6, 1969.

Rassidakis, N.C., Kelepouris, M., Fox, S. Int. Ment. Hlth. Res. Newsletter 13, 1, 1971.

Rathgeb, I., Winkler, B., Steele, R., Altszuler, N. Effect of ovine prolactin administration on glucose metabolism and plasma insulin levels in the dog. Endocrinology 88, 718-22, 1971.

Ratner, A., Meites, J. Effects of hormone administration on milk production in underfed rats. Amer. J. Physiol. 204, 268-70, 1963.

Ratner, A., Meites, J. Depletion of prolactin-inhibiting activity of rat hypothalamus by estradiol or suckling stimulus. Endocrinology 75, 377-82, 1964.

Ratner, A., Talwalker, P.K., Meites, J. Effect of estrogen administration in vivo on prolactin release by rat pituitary in vitro. Proc. Soc. Exp. Biol. Med. 112, 12-15, 1963.

Ratner, A., Talwalker, P.K., Meites, J. Effect of reserpine on prolactin-inhibiting activity of rat hypothalamus. Endocrinology 77, 315-9, 1965.

Raud, H.R., Kiddy, C.A., Odell, W.D. The effects of stress upon the determination of serum prolactin by radioimmunoassay. Proc. Soc. Exp. Biol. Med. 136, 689-93, 1971.

Raud, H.R., Odell, W.D. Studies of the measurement of bovine and porcine prolactin in radioimmunoassay and by systemic pigeon crop sac bioassay. Endocrinology **88**, 991-1002, 1971.

Ravault, J.P., Peyre, A. Synergistic effect of the endogenous prolactin-nortestoerone combination on fructose and citric acid in the male accessory glands. J. Physiol. (Paris) Suppl. **1**, 6, 1969.

Rayyis, S.S., Horton, R. Effect of angiotensin II on adrenal and pituitary function in man. J. Clin. Endocr. **32**, 539-46, 1971.

Reddi, A.H. Role of prolactin in the growth and secretory activity of the prostate and other accessory glands of mammals. Gen. Comp. Endocr. Suppl. **2**, 81, 1969.

Rees, E.D., Higgins, C. Steroid influences on respiration, glycolysis and levels of pyridine nucleotide-linked dehydrogenases of experimental mammary cancers. Cancer Res. **20**, 963-71, 1960.

Reeves, B.D., Garvin, J.E., McElin, T.W. Premenstrual tension: symptoms and weight changes related to potassium therapy. Amer. J. Obstet. Gynec. **109**, 1036, 1971.

Reeves, J.J., Arimura, A. Serum prolactin and LH levels in the ewe during the estrous cycle. Fed. Proc. **29**, 440, 1970.

Reeves, J.J., Arimura, A., Schally, A.V. Serum levels of prolactin and luteinizing hormone in the ewe at various stages of the estrous cycle. Proc. Soc. Exp. Biol. Med. **134**, 938-42, 1970.

Refetoff, S., Block, M.B., Ehrlich, E.N., Friesen, H.G. Chiari-Frommel syndrome and primary adrenocortical insufficiency. New Eng. J. Med. **287**, 1326-8, 1972.

Reisfield, R.A., Tong, G.L., Riches, E.L., Brink, N.G., Steelman, S.L. Purification and characterization of sheep prolactin. J. Amer. Chem. Soc. **83**, 3717-9, 1961.

Relkin, R. Effects of variations in environmental lighting in pituitary and plasma prolactin levels in the rat. Neuroendocrinology **9**, 278-84, 1972.

Relkin, R., Adachi, M., Kahan, S.A. Effects of pinealectomy and constant light and darkness on prolactin levels in the pituitary and plasma and on pituitary ultrastructure of the rat. J. Endocr. **54**, 263-8, 1972.

Rennie, P., Davies, J., Friedrich, E. Failure of ovine prolactin to show luteotrophic or luteolytic effects in the rabbit. Endocrinology **75**, 622-6, 1964.

Rice, B.F., Hammerstein, J., Savard, K. Steroid hormone formation in the human ovary. II. Action of gonadotropins in vitro in the corpus luteum. J. Clin. Endocr. **24**, 606-15, 1964.

Richardson, B.P. Evidence for a physiological role of prolactin in osmoregulation in the rat. Proc. Brit. Pharmacol. Soc. Jan. 1973.

Riddle, O. Prolactin in vertebrate function and organization. J. Nat. Cancer Inst. **31**, 1039-110, 1963a.

Riddle, O. Prolactin or progesterone as the key to parental behavior: a review. Anim. Beghav. **11**, 419-32, 1963b.

Rimoin, D.L., Holzman, G.B., Merimee, T.J., Rabinowitz, D., Barnes, A.C., Tyson, J.E.A., McKusick, V.A. Lactation in the absence of human growth hormone. J. Clin. Endocr. **28**, 1183, 1968.

Rivera, E.M. Endocrine secretion in vitro: prolactin. In Vitro **5**, 28-39, 1970.

Rivera, E.M., Cummins, E.P. Hormonal induction of dehydrogenase enzymes in mammary gland in vitro. Gen. Comp. Endocr. **17**, 319-26, 1971.

Rivlin, S. Premenstrual varicose veins. Brit. Med. J. **2**, 618, 1955.

Robins, A.H. Melanocyte-stimulating hormone and Parkinsonism. Lancet **1**, 727, 1973.

Robinson, M. Salt in pregnancy, Lancet **1**, 178-81, 1958.

Robinson, R.W., Higano, N., Cohen, W.D., Long-term effects of high dosage estrogen therapy in men with coronary heart disease. J. Chron. Dis. 16, 155-61, 1963.

Robyn, C. Discussion on p150 in Boyns, Griffiths, 1972.

Rodbard, D., Rayford, P.L., Cooper, J.A., Ross, G.T. Statistical quality control of radioimmunoassays. J. Clin. Endocr. 28, 1412-8, 1968.

Roger, F.H. Secretion of prolactin induced by phenyl proprionate of 19-norandrostenolone in the castrated male rat. Ann. Endocr. (Paris) 31, 724-7, 1970.

Rosen, M., Mushin, W.W., Kilpatrick, G.S., Campbell, H., Davies, L.G.G., Harrison, E. Study of myocardial ischaemia in surgical patients. Brit. Med. J. 2, 1415-20, 1966.

Rosoff, B., Martin, C.R. Effect of gonadotrophins and of testosterone on organ weights and zinc-65 uptake in the male rat. Gen. Comp. Endocr. 10, 75-84, 1968.

Rothchild, I. The corpus luteum-pituitary relationship: the association between the cause of luteotrophic stimulation and the cause of follicular quiescence during lactation: the basis for a tentative theory of the corpus luteum-pituitary relationship in the rat. Endocrinology 67, 9-41, 1960.

Rovner, D.R., Conn, J.W., Knopf, R.F., Cohen, E.L., Hsueh, M.T.Y. Nature of renal escape from the sodium-retaining effect of aldosterone in primary aldosteronism and in normal subjects. J. Clin. Endocr. 25, 53-64, 1965.

Rowlands, I.W. The effect of oestrogens, prolactin and hypophysectomy on the corpora lutea and vagina of hysterectomized guinea pigs. J. Endocr. 24, 105-12, 1962.

Russell, G.F.M. Body weight and balance of water, sodium and potassium in depressed patients given electro-convulsive therapy. Clin. Sci. 19, 327-36, 1960.

Rybakowski, J., Sowinski, J. Free thyroxine index and absolute free thyroxine in affective disorders. Lancet 1, 889, 1973.

Sachar, E.J., Hellman, L., Roffwarg, H.P., Halpern, F.S., Fukushima, D.K., Gallagher, T.F. Disrupted 24 hour patterns of cortisol secretion in psychotic depression. Arch. Gen. Psychiat. 28, 19-24, 1973.

Sachson, R., Rosen, S.W., Cuatrecasas, P., Friesen, H. Prolactin stimulation by thyrotropin-releasing hormone in a patient with isolated thyrotropin deficiency. New Eng. J. Med. 287, 972-3, 1972.

Saito, M., Arimura, A., Sawano, S. Luteotrophic and luteolytic effects of prolactin in hypophysectomized rats. Endokrinologie 56, 129-39, 1970.

Salhanick, H.A., Holtrop, H.R. Gonadotropins in hirsutism. Clin. Obstet. Gynec. 7, 1092-108, 1964.

Salih, H., Flax, H., Brander, W., Hobbs, J.R. Prolactin dependence in human breast cancers. Lancet 2, 1103-5, 1972.

Salonen, I.S. Myocardial infarction caused by reserpine treatment. Sotilaslaak Aikak. 43, 95-7, 1968.

Sandler, M., Goodwin, B.L., Leask, B.G.S., Ruthven, C.R.J. Melanocyte – stimulating hormone and Parkinsonism: the role of hypothalamic releasing factors. Lancet 1, 612, 1973.

Sandstrom, B. Diabetes mellitus and menstruation. Nordisk Medicin 81, 727-8, 1969.

Sar. M., Meites, J. Changes in pituitary prolactin release and hypothalamic PIF content during the estrous cycle of rats. Proc. Soc. Exp. Biol. Med. 125, 1018-21, 1967.

Sar, M., Meites, J. Effects of progesterone, testosterone and cortisol on hypothalamic prolactin-inhibiting factor and pituitary prolactin content. Proc. Soc. Exp. Biol. Med. 127, 426-9, 1968.

Sar, M., Meites, J. Effects of suckling on pituitary release of prolactin, GH and TSH in post-partum lactating rats. Neuroendocrinology **4**, 25-31, 1969.

Sassin, J.F., Frantz, A.G., Weitzman, E.D., Kapen, S. Human prolactin: 24-hour pattern with increased release during sleep. Science **177**, 1205-7, 1972.

Saunders, G.A., Carey, R.J., Hewitt, G.C., Jones, W.A. Myocardial infarction in the elderly surgical patient. Geriatrics **26**, September, 122-8, 1971.

Savely. C., Modlinger-Odorfer, M., Szecsenyi-Nagy, L. Simultaneous occurence of a Chiari-Frommel syndrome and of hypothyroidism. Endokrinologie **48**, 129-41, 1965.

Sawyer, C.H., Haun, C.K., Hilliard, J., Radford, H.M., Kanematsu, S. Further evidence for the identity of hypothalamic areas controlling ovulation and lactation in the rabbit. Endocrinology **73**, 338-44, 1963.

Saxton, J.A., Kimball, G.C. Relation of nephrosis and other diseases of albino rats to age and to modifications of diet. Arch. Path. **32**, 951-65, 1941.

Sayar, B., Polvan, O. Epilepsy and bronchial asthma. Lancet **1**, 1038, 1968.

Schally, A.V., Arimura, A., Bowers, C.Y., Wakabayashi, I., Kastin, A., Redding, T.W., Mittler, J.C., Nair, R.M.G., Pizzolato, P., Segal, A.J. Purification of hypothalamic releasing hormones of human origin. J. Clin. Endocr. **31**, 291-300, 1970.

Schally, A.V., Kuroshima, A., Ishida, Y. The presence of prolactin-inhibiting factor in extracts of beef, sheep and pig hypothalami. Proc. Soc. Exp. Biol. Med. **118**, 350-2, 1965.

Schams, D. Prolactin levels in bovine blood influenced by milking, manipulation, genital stimulation and oxytocin administration with specific consideration of seasonal variations. Acta Endocr. (Kbh) **71**, 684-96, 1972.

Schams, D., Bohms, S., Karg, H. Studies on prolactin in cattle blood: release of prolactin after physiological stimuli and injection of oxytocin and oestrogens. Acta. Endocr. (Kbh) Suppl. **155**, 60, 1971.

Schams, D., Karg, H. Prolactin in cattle blood using a radioimmunological method of determination. Zentralb. Veterinaermed. **17**, 193-212, 1970.

Schams, D., Karg, H. The immediate response of the plasma prolactin level to oestrogen infusions in dairy cows. Acta Endocr. (Kbh) **69**, 47-52, 1972.

Schams, D., Reinhardt, V., Karg, H. Effects of 2-Br-α-ergokryptine on plasma prolactin level during parturition and onset of lactation in cows. Experientia **28**, 697-9, 1972

Schenkel-Hulliger, L., Krahenbuhl, C. Effects of gonadotrophins on progesterone secretion by hamster ovaries in vitro. Acta Endocr. (Kbh) Suppl. **155**, 57, 1971.

Schildkraut, J.J. The catecholamine hypothesis of affective disorders. Amer. J. Psychiat. **122**, 509-22, 1965.

Schleicher, E.M. LE cells after oral contraceptives. Lancet **1**, 821-2, 1968.

Schlough, J.S., Schuetz, A.W., Meyer, R.K. Induction of implantation in the hypophysectomized rat with gonadotrophins. Proc. Soc. Exp. Biol. Med. **120**, 458-63, 1965.

Schneider, H.P. Continual measurements of LH, FSH and prolactin in the plasma after the administration of gonadotrophin releasers and catecholamine precursors. Acta Endocr. (Kbh) Suppl. **152**, 3, 1971.

Schneider, H.P.G., McCann, S.M. Mono- and indolamines and control of LH secretion. Endocrinology **86**, 1127-32, 1970.

Schoonees, R., De Klerk, J.N., Murphy, G.P. The effect of prolactin on organ weights and zinc-65 uptake in male baboons. J. Surg. Oncol. **2**, 103-6, 1970.

Schottstaedt, W.W., Grace, W.J., Wolff, H.G. Life situations, behaviour, attitudes, emotions and renal regulation of fluid and electrolyte balance. J. Psychosom. Res. **1**. 287-91, 1956.

Schussler, G.C., Verso, M.A., Nemoto, T. Phosphaturia in hypercalcemic breast cancer patients. J. Clin. Endocr. **35**, 497-504, 1972.

Schwartz, W.B., Bennett, W., Curlop, S., Bartter, F.C. A syndrome of renal sodium loss and hyponatremia probably resulting from inappropriate secretion of antidiuretic hormone. Amer. J. Med. **23**, 529, 1957.

Schweppe, J.S., Jungmann, R.A., Lewin, I. Urine steroid excretion in post-menopausal cancer of the breast: response to corticotropin stimulation and dexamethasone suppression. Cancer **20**, 155-63, 1967.

Sealey, J.E., Laragh, J.H. Further studies of a natriuretic substance occurring in human urine and plasma. Circ. Res. **28-29**, Suppl. II, 32-43, 1971.

Seavey, B.K., Lewis, U.J. Bovine and ovine prolactins: a difference of two amino acids indicated by peptide maps. Biochem. Biophys. Res. Comm. **42**, 905-11, 1971.

Segaloff, A., Steelman, S.L. The human gonadotropins. Rec. Progr. Hormone Res. **15**, 127-34, 1959.

Segaloff, A., Steelman, S.L., Flores, A. Prolactin as factor in ventral prostate assay for luteinizing hormone. Endocrinology **59**, 233-40, 1956.

Serluca, F.P. Aspect of the alpha and beta cells of the pancreas after treatment with somatotropic hormone, prolactin and total placental extract. Ann. Ostet. Ginec. **84**, 486-507, 1962.

Shaar, C.J., Clemens, J.A. Inhibition of lactation and prolactin secretion in rats by ergot alkaloids. Endocrinology **90**, 285-8, 1972.

Shabanah, E.H. Treatment of premenstrual tension. Amer. J. Obstet. Gynec. **21**, 49-54, 1963.

Shani, J., Givani, Y., Sulman, F.G., Eshkol, A., Lunenfeld, B. Uptake of 121 I-labelled prolactin by rat mammary gland and pigeon crop mucoasa. J. Endocr. **52**, 397-8, 1972.

Shani, J., Givant, Y., Sulman, F.G., Eylath, U., Eckstein, B. Neuroendocrinology **8**, 307-16, 1971.

Shani, J., Zanbelman, L., Khazen, K., Sulman, F.G. Mammotropic and prolactin-like effects of rat and human placentae and amniotic fluid. J. Endocr. **46**, 15-20. 1970.

Shearman, R.P. Prolonged secondary amenorrhoea after oral contraceptive therapy. Lancet **2**, 64-6, 1971.

Shelesnyak, M.C. Ergotoxine inhibition of deciduomata formation and its reversal by progesterone. Amer. J. Physiol. **179**, 301-4, 1954.

Shelesnyak, M.C. Maintenance of gestation in ergotoxine-treated pregnant rats by exogenous prolactin. Acta Endocr. (Kbh) **27**, 99-109, 1958.

Sherman, L., Kim, S., Benjamin, F., Kolodny, H.D. Effect of chlorpromazine on serum growth hormone concentration in man. New Eng. J. Med. **284**, 72-4, 1971.

Sherwood, L.M. Similarities in the chemical structure of human placental lactogen and pituitary growth hormone. Proc. Nat. Acad. Sci. USA **58**, 2307-14, 1967.

Sherwood, L.M. Current concepts: human prolactin. New Eng. J. Med. **284**, 774-7, 1971.

Sherwood, L.M., Handwerger, S., McLaurin, W.D. The structure and function of human placental lactogen. pp 27-45 in *Lactogenic Hormones* ed. G.E.W. Wolstenholme & J. Knight. Churchill Livingstone, 1972.

Sherwood, L.M., Handwerger, S., McLaurin, W.D., Lanner, M. Amino acid sequence of human placental lactogen. Nature New Biol. **233**, 59-61, 1971.

Sherwood, L.M., Handwerger, S., McLaurin, W.D., Pang, E.C. in *Growth and Growth Hormone*, ed. A. Peale & E.E. Muller, Excerpta Medica, 1972.

Shield, H.H., Charme, L.S. Non-puerperal galactorrhea following hysterectomy. N.Y. State Med. J. **69**, 590-3, 1969.

Shiino, M., Williams, G., Rennels, E.G. Ultrastructural observation of pituitary release of prolactin in the rat by suckling stimulus. Endocrinology **90**, 176-87, 1972.

Short, R.V., McDonald, M.F., Rowson, L.E. Steroids in the ovarian venous blood of ewes before and after gonadotrophic stimulation. J. Endocr. **26**, 155-66, 1963.

Shuster, S., Burton, J.L., Thody, A.J., Plummer, N., Goolamali, S.K., Bates, D. Melanocyte stimulating hormones and Parkinsomism. Lancet **1**, 463-4, 1973.

Silberberg, M., Silberberg, R. Articular effects of somatotrophin and prolactin in male and female mice. Exp. Med. Surg. **20**, 165-73, 1962.

Siler, T.M., Morgesnstern, L.L., Greenwood, F.C. The release of prolactin and other peptide hormones from human anterior pituitary tissue cultures. pp 207-17, in *Lactogenic Hormones* ed. G.E.W. Wolstenholme & J. Knight, Churchill Livingstone, 1972.

Simkin, B., Arce, R. Prolactin activity in blood during the normal human menstrual cycle. Proc. Soc. Exp. Biol. Med. **113**, 485-8, 1963.

Simkin, B., Goodhart, D. Preliminary observations on prolactin activity in human blood. J. Clin. Endocr. **20**, 1095-1106, 1960.

Simpson, A.A., Schmidt, G.H. Effect of prolactin on nucleic acid metabolism during lactogenesis in the rabbit. J. Endocr. **51**, 265-70, 1971.

Simpson, F.O., Waal-Manning, H.J. Hypertension and depression: inter-related problems in therapy. J. Roy. Coll. Physicians Lond. **6**, 14-24, 1971.

Singh, D.V., Bern, H.A. Interaction between prolactin and thyroxine in mouse mammary gland lobulo-alveolar development in vitro. J. Endocr. **45**, 579-83, 1969.

Singh, D.V., Meites, K.J., Halmi, L., Kortright, K.H., Brennan, M.J. Effect of ergocornine on transplanted mammary tumor growth and pituitary prolactin level in BALB/c mice. J. Nat. Cancer. Inst. **48**, 1727-31, 1972.

Sinha, Y.N. Effect on thyroactive materials upon plasma corticoids, pituitary prolactin and mammary oxidative phosphorylation of lactating rats. J. Dairy Sci. **53**, 1077-82, 1970.

Sinha, Y.N., Lewis, U.J., Van der Laan, W.P. Effects of administering antisera to mouse growth hormone and prolactin on gain in litter weight and on mammary nucleic acid content of lactating C3H mice. J. Endocr. **55**, 31-40, 1972.

Sinha, D.K., Meites, J. Direct effects of a hypothalamic extract on hormone secretion by a pituitary mammo-somatotropic tumor. Endocrinology **80**, 131-4, 1967.

Sinha, Y.N., Sleby, F.W., Lewis, U.J., Vanderlaan, W.P. Studies of prolactin secretion in mice by a homologous radioimmunoassay. Endocrinology **91**, 1045-53, 1972.

Sinha, Y.N., Tucker, H.A. Pituitary prolactin content and mammary development after chronic administration of prolactin. Proc. Soc. Exp. Biol. Med. **128**, 84-8, 1968.

Sinha, Y.N., Tucker, H.A. Mammary development and pituitary prolactin level of heifers from birth through puberty and during the estrous cycle. J. Dairy Sci. **52**, 507-12, 1969.

Sinha, Y.N., Vanderlaan, W.P. Effects of gold thioglucose and bipiperydyl mustard on pituitary prolactin and growth hormone content of C3H mice. Proc. Soc. Exp. Biol. Med. **136**, 130-3, 1971.

Skutsch, G.M. Androgens and prolactin. Lancet **1**, 911, 1972a.

Skutsch, G.M. Prolactin and breast cancer. Lancet **2**, 1258, 1972b.

Sletton, I.W., Gershon, S. The premenstrual syndrome: a discussion of its pathophysiology and treatment with lithium ion. Compr. Psychiatry **7**, 197-202, 1966.

Soffer, L.J., Gabrilove, J.L. A simplified water loading test for the diagnosis of Addison's disease. Metabolism **1**, 504-10, 1952.

Soffer, L.J., Gabrilove, J.L., Jacobs, M.D. Further studies with the salt tolerance test in normal individuals and in patients with adrenal cortical hyperfunction. J. Clin. Invest. **28**, 1091-3, 1949.

Soffer, L.J., Lesnick, G., Sorkin, S.L., Sobotka, H.H., Jacobs, M. The utilization of intravenously injected salt in normals and in patients with Cushing's syndrome before and after administration of desoxycorticosterone acetate. J. Clin. Invest. **23**, 51-54, 1944.

Spaulding, S.W., Burrow, G.N., Bermudez, F., Himmelhoch, J.M. The inhibitory effect of lithium on thyroid hormone release in both euthyroid and thyrotoxic patients. J. Clin. Endocr. **35**, 905-11, 1972.

Spaulding, S.W., Burrow, G.N., Donabedian, R., Van Woert, M. L–DOPA suppression of thyrotropin-releasing hormone response in man. J. Clin. Endocr. **35**, 182-5, 1972.

Spies, H.G., Clegg, M.T. Pituitary as a possible site of prolactin feedback in autoregulation. Neuroendocrinology **8**, 205-12, 1971.

Spies, H.G., Forbes, Y.M., Clegg, M.T. The influence of coitus, suckling and prolactin injections on pregnancy in pelvic neurectomized rats. Proc. Soc. Exp. Biol. Med. **138**, 470-4, 1971.

Spies, H.G., Hilliard, J., Sawyer, C.H. Maintenance of corpora lutea and pregnancy in hypophysectomized rabbits. Endocrinology **83**, 354-67, 1968.

Spies, H.G., Niswender, G.D. Levels of prolactin, LH and FSH in the serum of intacts and pelvic-neurectomized rats. Endocrinology **88**, 937-43, 1971.

Stahelin, H., Burckhardt-Vischer, B., Fluckiger, E. Rat mammary cancer inhibition by a prolactin suppressor, 2-bromo- α -ergokryptine (CB 154). Experientia **27**, 915-6, 1971.

Stehlikova, J., Talas, M., Jezdinsky, J. Titration of luteotrophic hormone in the blood of women. Cesk. Gynek. **44**, 164-7, 1965.

Sterental, A., Dominquez, M., Weisman, C., Pearson, O.H. Pituitary role in the estrogen dependency of experimental mammary cancer. Cancer Res. **23**, 481-4, 1963.

Stitt, F.W., Clayton, D.G., Crawford, M.D., Morris, J.N. Clinical and biochemical indicators of cardiovascular disease among men living in hard and soft water areas. Lancet **1**, 122-6, 1973.

Stoll, B.A. Brain catecholamines and breast cancer: a hypothesis. Lancet **1**, 431, 1972.

Strauss, M.B., Earley, L.E. An enquiry into the role of "sodium-retaining" steroids in the homeostasis of body sodium in man. Trans. Ass. Amer. Physns. **72**, 200, 1959.

Strong, C., Dils, R., Forsyth, I.A. The effects of prolactin on fatty acid synthesis by rabbit mammary gland in vitro. J. Endocr. **51**, xxxii-iii, 1971.

Stupnicki, R., Stupnicka, E., Domanski, E. Effect of prolactin on the leukocytic picture of the peripheral blood in rats. Acta Physiol. Pol. **11**, 433-4, 1960.

Sud, S.C., Clemens, J.A., Meites, J. Suppression of prolactin release from adenohypophysis by prolactin: an in vitro study. Indian J. Exp. Biol. **9**, 260-1, 1971.

Sud, S.C., Meites, J. Induction of lactation in the guinea pig. J. Endocr. **51**, 221-2, 1971.

Sulman, F.G. *Hypothalamic Control of Lactation.* Heinmann, London, 1970.

Sulman, F.G., Winnik, H.Z. Hormonal depression due to treatment with chlorpromazine. Nature (Lond.) **178**, 365, 1956.

Sundsfjord, J.A., Aakvaag, A. Plasma angiotensin II and aldosterone excretion during the menstrual cycle. Acta Endocr. (Kbh) **64**, 452, 1970.

Superstine, E., Sulman, F.G. Endocrine effects of chlordiazepoxide, diazepam and guanethidine. Arch. Int. Pharmacodyn. **160**, 133-46, 1966.

Sutherland. H., Stewart, I. A critical analysis of the premenstrual syndrome. Lancet **1**, 1180, 1965.

Swanson, L.V. LH and prolactin in blood serum from estrus to ovulation in Holstein heifers. J. Anim. Sci. **33**, 1038-41, 1971.

Swearingen, K.C. Heterogeneous turnover of adenohypophysial prolactin. Endocrinology **89**, 1380-8, 1971.

Swearingen, K.C., Nicoll, C.S. Prolactin turnover in rat adenohypophyses in vivo: its evaluation as a method for estimating secretion rates. J. Endocr. **53**, 1-15, 1972.

Swingle, W.W., De Vanzo, J.P., Glenister, D., Osborne, M., Wagle, G. Role of gluco- and mineralocorticoids in salt and water metabolism of adrenalectomized dogs. Amer. J. Physiol. **199**, 412-6, 1090.

Takizawa, S., Furth, J.J., Furth, J. DNA synthesis in autonomous and hormone-responsive mammary tumours. Cancer Res. **30**, 206-210, 1970.

Talas, M. Luteotropic hormone levels in the blood of women with the Stein-Leventhal syndrome. Cesk. Gynek. **32**, 129, 1967.

Talas, M., Stehlikova, J., Jezdinsky, J. Pigeon crop weight responses to the application of extracts from the blood of women with Stein Leventhal syndrome, galactorrhoea and of those in the secretory phase of the menstrual cycle. Endokrinologie **52**, 387-94, 1968.

Talwalker, P.K., Meites, J., Mizuno, H. Mammary tumor induction by estrogen or anterior pituitary hormones in ovarietomized rate given 7, 12-dimethyl-1, 2-benzanthracene. Proc. Soc. Exp. Biol. Med. **116**, 531-4, 1964.

Talwalker, P.K., Ratner, A., Meites, J. In vitro inhibition of pituitary prolactin synthesis and release by hypothalamic extract. Amer. J. Physiol. **205**, 213-8, 1963.

Talwalker, P.K., Ratner, A., Meites, J. In vivo and in vitro prolactin secretion by transplanted rat mammotropic pituitary tumors. Cancer Res. **24**, 1723-6, 1964.

Tampan, R.K., Sundaram, K., Chanukattam, K. Fluid and electrolyte metabolism in pregnancy toxaemia. J. Obstet. Gynaec. India **7**, 14, 1956.

Tashjian, A.H., Barowsky, N.J., Jensen, D.K. Thyrotropin-releasing hormone: direct evidence for stimulation of prolactin production by pituitary cells in culture. Biochem. Biophys. Res. Comm. **43**, 516-23, 1971.

Tashjian, A.H., Bancroft, F.C., Levine, L. Production of both prolactin and growth hormone by clonal strains of rat pituitary tumor cells. Differential effects of hydrocortisone and tissue extracts. J.Cell. Biol. **47**, 61-70, 1970.

Taylor, W.H. Syndrome of inappropriate secretion of antidiuretic hormone. Lancet **1**, 970-1, 1971.

Terkel, J., Blake, C.A., Sawyer, C.H. Serum prolactin levels in lactating rats after suckling or exposure to ether. Endocrinology **91**, 49-53, 1972.

Thatcher, W.W., Tucker, H.A. Lactational performance of rats injected with oxytocin, cortisol-21-acetate, prolactin and growth hormone during prolonged lactation. Endocrinology **86**, 237-40, 1970.

Thatcher, W.W., Tucker, H.A. Adrenal function during prolonged lactation. Proc. Soc. Exp. Biol. Med. **134**, 915-8, 1970.

Thompson, H.E., Crean, G.P. Studies on the effect of hormone administration on body weight and on tibial epiphyseal cartilage width in intact, hypophysectomised and adrenalectomized rats. J. Endocr. **25**, 473-82, 1963.

Thompson, B.D., Edmonds, C.J. Comparison of effects of prolonged aldosterone administration on rat colon and renal electrolyte excretion. J. Endocr. **50**, 163-9, 1971.

Threlfall, W.R., Martin, C.E., Dale, H.E., Anderson, R.R., Krause, G.F. Pituitary prolactin and the oestrous cycle of sows. J. Reprod. Fertil. **31**, 201-4, 1972.

Tindal, J.S., Knaggs, G.S. Release of prolactin in the rabbit after electrical stimulation of the forebrain. J. Endocr. **48**, 32-3, 1970.

Tindal, J.S., Knaggs, G.S. Pathways in the forebrain of the rabbit concerned with the release of prolactin. J. Endocr. **52**, 253-63, 1972.

Tindal, J.S., Knaggs, G.S., Turvey, A. Central nervous control of prolactin secretion in the rabbit: effect of local oestrogen implants in the amygdaloid complex. J. Endocr. **37**, 279-87, 1967.

Tobon, H., Josimovich, J.B., Salazar, H. The ultrastructure of the mammary gland during prolactin-induced lactogenesis in the rabbit. Endocrinology **90**, 1569-77, 1972.

Topper, Y.J. Multiple hormone interactions in the development of mammary gland in vitro. Recent Progr. Hormone Res. **26**, 287-303, 1970.

Torghele, J.R. Premenstrual tension in psychotic women. Lancet **1**, 163-70, 1957.

Trautner, E.M., Pennycuik, P.P., Morr, R.J.H., Gershon, S., Shankly, K.H. The effects of prolonged sub-toxic lithium ingestion on pregnancy in rats. Aust. J. Exp. Biol. Med. Sci. **36**, 305-21, 1958.

Tucci, J.R., Lauler, D.P. Water, electrolyte and acid-base disorders in diseases of the adrenal cortex and thyroid gland. pp 923-70 in *Clinical Disorders of Fluid and Electrolyte Metabolism*, ed. M.H. Maxwell & C.R. Kleeman, McGraw Hill, New York, 1972.

Tupin, J.P., Schlagenhauf, G.K., Creson, D.L. Lithium effects on electrolyte excretion. Amer. J. Psychiat. **125**, 536, 1968.

Turkington, R.W. Inhibition of casein turnover by hydrocortisone during mammary gland differentiation in vitro. Biochem. Biophys. Acta **158**, 274-80, 1968a.

Turkington, R.W. Hormone-induced synthesis of DNA by mammary gland in vitro. Endocrinology **82**, 540-6, 1968b.

Turkington, R.W. Induction of milk protein synthesis by placental lactogen.and prolactin in vitro. Endocrinology **82**, 575-83, 1968c.

Turkington, R.W. Hormone-dependent differentiation of mammary gland in vitro. Curr. Top. Dev. Biol. **3**, 199-218, 1968d.

Turkington R.W. Homogeneous differentiation of mammary alveolar cells. Exp. Cell Res. **58**, 296-302, 1969a.

Turkington, R.W. Hormonal regulation of transfer ribonucleic acid and transfer ribonucleic acid-methylating enzymes during development of the mouse mammary gland. J. Biol. Chem. **244**, 5140-8, 1969b.

Turkington, R.W. Stimulation of RNA synthesis in isolated mammary cells by insulin and prolactin bound to Sepharose. Biochem. Biophys. Res. Comm. **41**, 1362-7, 1970a.

Turkington, R.W. Homogeneity of differentiated function in mammary carcinoma cell populations. Cancer Res. **30**, 1841-5, 1970b.

Turkington, R.W. Hormonal regulation of rapidly labelled ribonucleic acid in mammary cells in vitro. J. Biol. Chem. **245**, 6690-7, 1970c.

Turkington, R.W. Measurement of prolactin activity in human serum by the induction of specific milk proteins in mammary gland in vitro. J. Clin. Endocr. **33**, 210-16, 1971a.

Turkington, R.W. Ectopic production of prolactin. New Eng. J. Med. **285**, 1455-8, 1971b.

Turkington, R.W. Inhibition of prolactin secretion and successful therapy of the Forbes-Albright syndrome with L–DOPA. J. Lab. Clin. Med. **78**, 824-5, 1971c.

Turkington, R.W. Molecular biological aspects of prolactin. pp 111-27 in *Lactogenic hormones.* ed. G.E.W. Wolstenholme & J. Knight, Churchill Livingstone, 1972a.

Turkington, R.W. Measurement of prolactin activity in human serum by the induction of specific milk proteins in vitro: results in various clinical disorders. pp 169-84 in *Lactogenic Hormones.* ed. G.E.W. Wolstenholme & J. Knight Livingstone, 1972b.

Turkington, R.W. Discussion, pp 122-3 in Boyns, Griffiths, 1972c.

Turkington, R.W. Human prolactin: an ancient molecule provides new insights for clinical medicine. Amer. J. Med. **53**, 389-94, 1972d.

Turkington, R.W. Prolactin secretion in patients treated with various drugs: phenothiazines, tricyclic antidepressants, reserpine and methyldopa. Arch. Intern. Med. **130**, 349-54, 1972e.

Turkington, R.W. Serum prolactin levels in patients with gyecomastia. J. Clin, Endocr. **34**, 62-6, 1972f.

Turkington, R.W. Secretion of prolactin by patients with pituitary and hypothalamic tumors. J. Clin. Endocr. **34**, 159-64, 1972g.

Turkington, R.W. Phenothiazine stimulation test for prolactin reserve: the syndrome of isolated deficiency. J. Clin. Endocr. **34**, 247-9, 1972h.

Turkington, R.W. Inhibition of prolactin secretion and successful therapy of the Forbes-Albright syndrome with L-dopa. J. Clin. Endocr. **34**, 306-11, 1972i.

Turkington, R.W., Brew, D., Vanaman, T.C., Hill, R.L. The hormonal control of lactose synthetase in the developing mouse mammary gland. J. Biol. Chem. **243**, 3382-7, 1968.

Turkington, R.W., Frantz, W.L. The biochemical actions of prolactin. in *Prolactin and Carcinogenesis. 4th Tenovus Workshop.* ed. A.R. Boyns & K Griffiths, Alpha Omega Alpha Publishing, Cardiff, 1972.

Turkington, R.W., Hill, R.L. Lactose synthetase: progesterone inhibition of the introduction of α-lactalbumin. Science **163**, 1458-60, 1969.

Turkington, R.W., Juergens, W.G., Topper, Y.J. Hormone dependent synthesis of casein in vitro. Biochem. Biophys. Acta **111**, 573-6, 1965.

Turkington, R.W., MacIndoe, J. Hyperprolactinemia in sarcoidosis. Ann. Intern. Med. **76-**, 545-9, 1972.

Turkington, R.W., Ray, R., Costin, G. Discussion pp 107-11 in Boyns, Griffiths, 1972.

Turkington, R.W., Riddle, M. Hormone-dependent phosphorylation of nuclear proteins during mammary gland differentiation in vitro. J. Biol. Chem. **244**, 6040, -6, 1969.

Turkington, R.W., Riddle, M. Hormone-dependent formation of polysomes in mammary cells in vitro. J. Biol. Chem. **245**, 5145-52, 1970.

Turkington, R.W., Spielvogel, R.L. Methylation of deoxyribonucleic acid during hormonal stimulation of mammary cells in vitro. J. B iol. Chem. **246**, 3835-40, 1971.

Turkington, R.W., Underwood, L.E., Van Wyck, J. Elevated serum prolactin levels after pituitary stalk section in man. New Eng. J. Med. **285**, 707-10, 1971.

Turkington, R.W., Ward, O.T. Hormonal stimulation of RNA polymerase in mammary gland in vitro. Biochem. Biophys. Acta **174**, 291-301, 1969.

Tunrbull, J.G., Kent, G.C. Prolactin and the luteotropic complex in hamsters. Endocrinology **79**, 716-20, 1966.

Tyson, J.E., Austin, K.L., Forinhalt, J.W. Prolonged nutritional deprivation in pregnancy: change in human chorionic somatomammotropin and growth hormone secretion. Amer. J. Obstet. Gynec. **109**, 1080-2, 1971.

Tyson, J.E., Friesen, H.G., Anderson, M.S. Human lactational and ovarian response to endogenoi prolactin release. Science **177**, 897-900, 1972.

Tyson, J.E., Hwang, P., Guyda, H., Friesen, H.G. Studies of prolactin secretion in human pregnancy. Amer. J. Obstet. Gynec. **113**, 14-20, 1972.

Valverde, R.C., Chieffo, V., Reichlin, S. Prolactin-releasing factor in porcine and rat hypothalamic tissue. Endocrinology **91**, 982-93, 1972.

Van der Gugten, A.A. The effect of I-(morpholinomethyl)-4-phthalimido-piperidindione-2, 6-androstanolone propionate on the plasma prolactin concentration of oestrone-treated orchidectomized R-Amsterdam rats. Eur. J. Cancer **7**, 581-2, 1971.

Van der Gugten, A.A., Boot, L.M., Kwa, H.G. Effect of reserpine on plasma prolactin dependent on the presence of oestrogens. Acta Endocr. (Kbh) **65**, 309-15, 1970.

Vanderlaan, W.P. Direct effect of the anterior pituitary on the ventral prostate in rats. J. Clin. Invest. **32**, 609, 1953.

Van der Velde, C.D., Gordon, M. Manic-depressive illness, diabetes mellitus and lithium carbonate. Arch. Gen. Psychiat. **21**, 478-85, 1969.

Vanhaelst, L., Van Cauter, E., De Gaute, J.P., Golstein, J. Unpublished, quoted in L'Hermite et al. 1972

Van Maanen, J.H., Smelik, P.G. Induction of pseudopregnancy in rats following local depletion of monoamines in the median eminence of the hypothalamus. Neuroendocrinology **3**, 177-86, 1968.

Van Woert, M.H., Palmer, S.H. Inhibition of growth of mouse melanoma by chlorpromazine. Cancer Res. 29, 1952-5, 1969.

Van Wyck, J.J., Grumbach, M.M. Syndrome of precocious menstruation and galactorrhea in juvenile hypothyroidism: an example of hormonal overlap in pituitary feedback. J. Pediat. **57**, 416-35, 1960.

Varavudhi, P., Lobel, B.L., Shelesnyak, M.C. Studies on the mechanism of nidation. XXIII. Effect of ergocornine in pregnant rats during experimentally induced delayed nidation. J. Endocr. **34**, 425-30, 1966.

Varga, L., Lutterbeck, P.M., Pryor, J.S., Wenner, R., Erb, H. Suppression of puerperal lactation with an ergot alkaloid: a double blind study. Brit. Med. J. **2**, 743-4, 1972.

Verheyden, C. Action of the adrenal cortex on prolactin secretion. Ann. Endocr. (Paris) **25**, 356-60, 1964.

Vesin, P. Water, electrolyte and acid-base disorders in liver disease. pp 873-95, in *Clinical Disorders of Fluid and Electrolyte Metabolism,* ed. M.H. Maxwell & C.R. Kleeman, McGraw Hill, New York, 1972.

Vessey, M.P., Doll, R. Investigation of relation between use of oral contraceptives and thrombo-embolic disease: a further report. Brit. Med. J. **2**, 651-7, 1969.

Veterans Administration Cooperative Urological Research Group. Threatment and survival of patients with cancer of the prostate. Surg. Gynec. Obstet. **124**, 1011-7, 1967.

Vilar, O., Alvarez, B., Davidson, O., Mancini, R.E. Incorporation by the kidney of fluorescent pituitary hormones. J. Histochem. Cytochem. **12**, 621-7, 1964.

Vodian, M.A., Distribution of prolactin and growth hormone in rat and guinea pig adenohypophyses. Life Sci. **9**,. 443-9, 1970.

Volpe, R., Killinger, D., Bird, C., Clark, A.F., Friesen, H.G. Idiopathic galactorrhea and mild hypogonadism in a young adult male. J. Clin. Endocr. **35**, 684-92, 1972.

Voogt, J.L., Chen, C.L., Meites, J. Serum and pituitary prolactin levels before, during and after puberty in female rats. Amer. J. Physiol. **218**, 396-9, 1970.

Voogt, J.L., Clemens, J.A., Meites, J. Stimulation of pituitary FSH release in immature female rats by prolactin implant in median eminence. Neuroendocrinology **4**, 157-63, 1969.

Voogt, J.L., Meites, J. Effects of an implant of prolactin in median eminence of pseudopregnant rats on serum and pituitary LH, FSH and prolactin. Endocrinology **88**, 286-92, 1971.

Voogt, J.L., Sar, M., Meites, J. Influence of cycling, pregnancy, labor and suckling on corticosterone and ACTH levels. Amer. J. Physiol. **216**, 655-8, 1969.

Voors, A.W. Does lithium depletion cause atherosclerotic heart disease? Lancet **2**, 1337-9, 1969.

Voors, A.W. Lithium in the drinking water and atherosclerotic heart death: epidemiologic argument for protective effect. Amer. J. Epidem. **92**, 164-71, 1970.

Wakabayashi, I., Arimura, A., Schally, A.V. Effect of pentobarbital and ether stress on serum prolactin in rats. Proc. Soc. Exp. Biol. Med. **137**, 1189-93, 1971.

Wakabayashi, I., Arimura, A., Schally, A.V. Different effect of potassium and calcium ion on the release of growth hormone and prolactin from isolated rat pituitaries in vitro. Endokrinologie **59**, 69-76, 1972.

Wallis, M. Structural relationships among growth hormones and prolactins. Biochem. J. **125**, 54-6P, 1971.

Walsh, P.C., Gittes, R.F. Inhibition by antiandrogens of the prostatic growth stimulated by adrenal androgens and pituitary prolactin in castrate rats. Surg. Forum **20**, 518-9, 1969.

Wang, D.Y., Hallowes, R.C., Bealing, J., Strong, C., Dils, R. Effect of growth hormone and prolactin on fatty acid synthesis in mouse mammary gland explants in organ culture. J. Endocr. **51**, xxx-i, 1971.

Wang, D.Y., Hallowes, R.C., Bealing, J., Strong, C.R., Dils, R. The effect of prolactin and growth hormone on fatty acid synthesis by pregnant mouse mammary gland in organ culture. J. Endocr. **53**, 311-21, 1972.

Wang, D.Y., Hallowes. R.C., Smith, R.H., Amor, V., Lewis, D.J. A biochemical comparison of the lactogenic effect of prolactin and growth hormone on mouse mammary gland in organ culture. J. Endocr. **52**, 349-58, 1972.

Watanabe, A.M., Parks, L.C., Kopin, I.J., Weise, V.K. Modification of the cardiovascular effects of L-DOPA by decarboxylase inhibitors. J. Clin. Invest. **50**, 1322-8, 1971.

Watson, J.T., Krulich, L., McCann, S.M. Effect of crude rat hypothalamic extract on serum gonadotropin and prolactin levels in normal and orchidectomozed male rats. Endocrinology **89**, 1412-8, 1971.

Waxler, E.B., Kimbiris, D., Van den Broeck, H., Segal, B.L., Likoff, W. Myocardial infarction and oral contraceptive agents. Amer. J. Cardiol. **28**, 96-101, 1971.

Weil-Malherbe, H., Szara, S.I. *The Biochemistry of Functional and Experimental Psychoses.* Charles C. Thomas, Springfield, 1971,

Weir, R.J., Briggs, E., Browning, J., Mack, A., Naismith, L., Taylor, L., Wilson, E. Blood pressure in women after one year of oral contraception. Lancet 1, 467-70, 1971.

Weir, R.J., Brown, J.J., Fraser, R., Kraszewski, A., Lever, A.F., McIlwaine, G.M., Morton, J.J., Robertson, J.I.S., Tree, M. Plasma renin, renin substrate, angiotensin II, and aldosterone in hypertensive disease of pregnancy. Lancet 1, 291-5, 1973.

Weiss, S. Myocardial infarction a..u oral contraceptives. New Eng. J. Med. 286, 436-7, 1972.

Weissman, P.N., Shenkman, L., Gregerman, R.I. Chlorpropamide hyponatremia: drug-induced inappropriate antidiuretic hormone activity. New Eng. J. Med. 284, 65-71, 1971.

Welsch, C.W., Clemens, J.A., Meites, J. Effects of multiple pituitary homo-grafts or progesterone on 7, 12-dimethylbenz(a)anthracene-induced mammary tumors in rats. J. Nat. Cancer Inst. 41, 465-71, 1968.

Welsch, C.W., Clemens, J.A., Meites, J. Effects of hypothalamic and amygdaloid lesions on development and growth of carcinogen-induced mammary tumors in the female rat. Cancer Res. 29, 1541-9, 1969.

Welsch, C.W., Jenkins, T.W., Meites, J. Increased incidence of mammary tumors in the female rat grafted with multiple pituitaries. Cancer Res. 30,, 1024-9, 1970.

Welsch, C.W., Meites, J. Effects of a norethynodrel-mestranol combination (Enovid) on development and growth of carcinogen-induced mammary tumors in female rats. Cancer 23, 601-7, 1969.

Welsch, C.W., Meites, J. Effects of reserpine on development of 7, 12-dimethylbenzanthracene-induced mammary tumors in female rats. Experientia 26, 1133-4, 1970.

Welsch, C.W., Negro-Vilar, A., Meites, J. Effects of pituitary homografts on host pituitary prolactin and hypothalamic PIF levels. Neuroendocrinology 3, 238-45, 1968.

Welsch, C.W., Rivera, E.M. Differential effects of estrogen and prolactin on DNA synthesis in organ cultures of DMBA-induced rat mammary carcinoma. Proc. Soc. Exp. Biol. Med. 139, 623-6, 1972.

Welsch, C.W., Squiers, M.D., Cassell, E., Chen, C.L., Meites, J. Median eminence lesions and serum prolactin: influence of overiectomy and ergocornine. Amer. J. Physiol. 221, 1714-7 1971.

Wenner, R., Varga, L. Prolactinhemmung mittels Ergocryptin. Acta Endocr. (Kbh) Suppl. 159, 40, 1972.

Weston, R.E. Pathogenesis and treatment of edema with special reference to use of diuretics. pp 163-214 in Clinical Disorders of Fluid and Electrolyte Metabolism. ed. M.H. Maxwell & C.R. Kleeman, McGraw Hill, New York, 1972.

White, A. The chemistry and physiology of adenohypophyseal luteotropin (prolactin). Vitam. Horm. 7, 253, 1949.

Whitfield, J.F., Perris, A.D., Youdale, T. The calcium-mediated promotion of mitotic activity in rat thymocyte populations by growth hormone, neuro-hormones, parathyroid hormone and prolactin. J. Cell Physiol. 73, 203-11, 1969.

Williams, G.H., Lauler, D.P. Water, electrolyte and acid-base disorders in congestive heart failure and hypertension. pp 835-72 in Clinical Disorders of Fluid and Electrolyte Metabolis ed. M.H. Maxwell & C.R. Kleeman, McGraw Hill, New York, 1972.

Williams, W.F., Weisshaar, A.G., Lauterbach, G.E. Lactogenic hormone effects on plasma nonesterified fatty acids and blood glucose concentrations. J Dairy Sci 49, 106-7, 1966.

Wilson, R.G., Singhal, V.K., Percy-Robb, I., Forrest, A.P.M., Cole, E.N., Boyns, A.R., Griffiths, K. Response of plasma prolactin and growth hormone to insulin hypoglycaemia. Lancet 2, 1283-5, 1972.

Winegrad, A.I., Shaw, W.N., Lukens, F.D., Stadie, W.C. Effects of prolactin in vitro on fatty acid synthesis in rat : adipose tissue. J. Biol. Chem. 234, 3111-4, 1959.

Winkler, B., Rathgeb, I., Steele, R., Altszuler, N. Effect of ovine prolactin administration on free fatty acid metabolism in the normal dog. Endocrinology **88**, 1349-52, 1971.

Winnik, H., Tennenbaum, L. Appearance of galactorrhea during treatment with Largactil. Presse Med. **63**, 1092, 1955.

Winston, F. Oral contraceptives and depression. Lancet **1**, 1209, 1969.

Witorsch, R.J., Kitay, J.I. Pituitary hormones affecting adrenal 5 α -reductase activity: ACTH, growth hormone and prolactin. Endocrinology **91**, 764-9, 1972.

Woods, J.W. Oral contraceptives and hypertension. Lancet **2**, 653-4, 1967.

Wright, H.P. Changes in the adhesiveness of blood platelets following parturition and surgical operations. J. Path. Bact. **54**, 461, 1942.

Wurtman, R.J., Axelrod, J., Chu, E.W. Melatonin synthesis in the pineal gland: control by light. Science **142**, 1071-3, 1963.

Wuttke, W., Cassell, E., Meites, J. Effects of ergocornine on serum prolactin and LH and on hypothalamic content of PIF and LRF. Endocrinology **88**, 737-41, 1971.

Wuttke, W., Gelato, M., Meites, J. Metabolism of pentobarbital actions on prolactin release. Endocrinology **89**, 1191-4, 1971.

Wuttke, W., Meites, J. Effects of ether and pentobarbital on serum prolactin and LH levels in proestrous rats. Proc. Soc. Exp. Biol. Med. **135**, 648-52, 1970.

Wuttke, W., Meites, J. Luteolytic role of prolactin during the estrous cycle of the rat. Proc. Soc. Exp. Biol. Med. **137**, 988-91, 1971.

Wuttke, W., Meites, J. Induction of pseudopregnancy in the rat with no rise in serum prolactin. Endocrinology **90**, 438-43, 1972.

Yamamoto, K., Taylor, L.M., Cole, F.E. Synthesis and release of GH and prolactin from the rat anterior pituitary in vitro as functions of age and sex. Endocrinology **87**, 21-6, 1970.

Yamini, G., Chard, T., Blake, M.E. Some biological effects of antisera to human placental lactogen in rodents. J. Endocr. **55**, xxx, 1972.

Yanai, R., Nagasawa, H. Effects of ergocornine and 2-Br-α -ergokryptin (CB 154) on the formation of mammary hyperplastic alveolar nodules and pituitary prolactin levels in mice. Experientia **26**, 649-50, 1970a.

Yanai, R., Nagasawa, H. Suppression of mammary hyperplastic nodule formation and pituitary prolactin secretion in mice induced by ergocornine or 2-Br-α -ergokryptine. J. Nat. Cancer Inst. **45**, 1105-12, 1970b.

Yanai, R., Nagasawa, H. Inhibition by ergocornine and 2-Br-α -ergokryptine of spontaneous mammary tumor appearance in mice. Experientia **27**, 934-5, 1971.

Yanai, R., Nagasawa, H. Inhibition of mammary tumorigenesis by ergot alkaloids and promotion of mammary tumorigenesis by pituitary isografts in adreno-ovariectomized mice. J. Nat. Cancer.Inst. **48**, 715-9, 1972.

Yokoro, K., Furth, J., Haran-Ghera, N. Induction of mammotropic pituitary tumors by X-rays in rats and mice: the role of mammotropes in development of mammary tumors. Cancer Res. **21**, 178-86, 1961.

Yokoyama, A., Prolactin surge on the afternoon of proestrus in the rat and its blockade by phenobarbitone. Experientia **27**, 578-9, 1971.

Yokoyama, A., Tomogane, H., Ota, K. Effects of ovariectomy and of oestrogen administration on the decrease in pituitary prolactin content which occurs on the afternoon of proestrus in the rat. Experientia **27**, 1221-2, 1971.

Yokoyama, A., Tomogane, H., Ota, K. Ergocornine blockade of the surge of prolactin at proestrus failed to block ovulation in cycling rats. Proc. Soc. Exp. Biol. Med. **140**, 169-71, 1972.

Yoshida, K. The effects of reserpine on reproductive function in female rats. Endocr. Japon **11**, 216-36, 1964.

Yoshinaga, K., Grieves, S.A., Short, R.V. Steriodogenic effects of luteinizing hormone and prolactin on the rat ovary in vivo. J. Endocr. **38**, 423-30, 1967.

Yoshinaga, K., Moudgal, N.R., Greep, R.O. Progestin secretion by the ovary in lactating rats: effect of LH antiserum, LH and prolactin. Endocrinology **88**, 1126-30, 1971.

Zarrow, M.X., Brown-Grant, K. Inhibition of ovulation in the gonadotrophin-treated immature rat by chlorpromazine. J. Endocr. **30**, 87-95, 1964.

Zarrow, M.X., Clark, J.H. Gonadotropin regulation of ovarian cholesterol levels in the rat. Endocrinology **84**, 340-6, 1969.

Zarrow, M.X., Farooq, A., Denenberg, V.H., Sawin, P.B., Ross, S. Maternal behaviour in the rabbit: endocrine control of maternal nest building. J. Reprod. Fertil. **6**, 375-83, 1963.

Zarrow, M.X., Grota, L.J., Denenberg, V.H. Maternal behaviour in the rat: survival of newborn fostered young after hormonal treatment of the foster mother. Anat. Rec. **157**, 13-7, 1967.

Zarrow, M.X., Sawin, P.B., Ross, S., Denenberg, V.H., Crary, D., Wilson, E.D., Farooq, A. Maternal behaviour in the rabbit: evidence for an endocrine basis of maternal nest building and additional data on maternal nest building in the Dutch belted race. J. Reprod. Fertil. **2**, 152, 1961.

Zolman, J., Convey, E.M. Bovine pituitary LH and prolactin release during superfusion in vitro. Proc. Soc. Exp. Biol. Med. **140**, 194-8, 1972.

INDEX

Prolactin as such is not listed in the index since all the entries refer to it in one way or another